# Gallbladder Disease

*Guest Editor*

CYNTHIA W. KO, MD, MS

# GASTROENTEROLOGY CLINICS OF NORTH AMERICA

www.gastro.theclinics.com

June 2010 • Volume 39 • Number 2

SAUNDERS an imprint of ELSEVIER, Inc.

**W.B. SAUNDERS COMPANY**

*A Division of Elsevier Inc.*

Elsevier Inc. ● 1600 John F. Kennedy Blvd., Suite 1800 ● Philadelphia, Pennsylvania 19103-2899

http://www.theclinics.com

GASTROENTEROLOGY CLINICS OF NORTH AMERICA Volume 39, Number 2
June 2010 ISSN 0889-8553, ISBN-13: 978-1-4377-1911-6

Editor: Kerry Holland
Developmental Editor: Theresa Collier

*Gastroenterology Clinics of North America* (ISSN 0889-8553) is published quarterly by Elsevier Inc., 360 Park Avenue South, New York, NY 10010-1710. Months of issue are March, June, September, and December. Business and Editorial Offices: 1600 John F. Kennedy Blvd., Suite 1800, Philadelphia, PA 19103-2899. Customer Service Office: 6277 Sea Harbor Drive, Orlando, FL 32887-4800. Periodicals postage paid at New York, NY and additional mailing offices. Subscription prices are $264.00 per year (US individuals), $135.00 per year (US students), $416.00 per year (US institutions), $290.00 per year (Canadian individuals), $507.00 per year (Canadian institutions), $366.00 per year (international individuals), $186.00 per year (international students), and $507.00 per year (international institutions). Foreign air speed delivery is included in all *Clinics* subscription prices. All prices are subject to change without notice. **POSTMASTER**: Send address changes to *Gastroenterology Clinics of North America*, Elsevier Health Sciences Division, Subscription Customer Service, 3251 Riverport Lane, Maryland Heights, MO 63043. Telephone: 1-800-654-2452 (U.S. and Canada); 314-447-8871 (outside U.S. and Canada). Fax: 314-447-8029. E-mail: journalscustomerservice-usa@elsevier.com (for print support); journalsonlinesupport-usa@elsevier.com (for online support).

*Reprints.* For copies of 100 or more, of articles in this publication, please contact the Commercial Reprints Department, Elsevier Inc., 360 Part Avenue South, New York, New York 10010-1710. Tel. (212) 633-3813, Fax: (212) 462-1935, E-mail: reprints@elsevier.com.

*Gastroenterology Clinics of North America* is also published in Italian by Il Pensiero Scientifico Editore, Rome, Italy; and in Portuguese by Interlivros Edicoes Ltda., Rua Commandante Coelho 1085, 21250 Cordovil, Rio de Janeiro, Brazil.

*Gastroenterology Clinics of North America* is covered in *MEDLINE/PubMed (Index Medicus), Excerpta Medica, Current Contents/Clinical Medicine, Science Citation Index, ISI/BIOMED,* and *BIOSIS.*

Printed and bound by CPI Group (UK) Ltd, Croydon, CR0 4YY
Transferred to Digital Print 2011

# Contributors

## GUEST EDITOR

**CYNTHIA W. KO, MD, MS**
Associate Professor, Department of Medicine, Division of Gastroenterology, University of Washington, Seattle, Washington

## AUTHORS

**NEZAM H. AFDHAL, MD**
Associate Professor of Medicine, Liver Center and Gastroenterology Division, Department of Medicine, Beth Israel Deaconess Medical Center, Harvard Medical School, Boston, Massachusetts

**PHILIP S. BARIE, MD, MBA, FIDSA, FCCM, FACS**
Professor of Surgery and Public Health, Division of Critical Care and Trauma, Department of Surgery; Division of Medical Ethics, Department of Public Health, Anne and Max A. Cohen Surgical Intensive Care Unit, New York-Presbyterian Hospital, Weill Cornell Medical College, New York, New York

**JONATHAN W. BERLIN, MD**
Department of Radiology, NorthShore University Health System; Associate Professor of Radiology, University of Chicago Pritzker School of Medicine, Evanston, Illinois

**LEONILDE BONFRATE, MD**
Research Fellow, Clinica Medica "A. Murri" Department of Internal and Public Medicine, University Medical School, Policlinico, Bari, Italy

**JASON D. CONWAY, MD, MPH**
Assistant Professor of Medicine, Section on Gastroenterology, Wake Forest University School of Medicine, Winston-Salem, North Carolina

**BRIAN R. DAVIDSON, FRCS**
Professor of HPB and Liver Transplantation Surgery, Department of Surgery, Royal Free Campus, UCL Medical School, Royal Free Hospital, London, United Kingdom

**JOHN K. DIBAISE, MD**
Professor of Medicine, Division of Gastroenterology and Hepatology, Mayo Clinic, Scottsdale, Arizona

**AGOSTINO DI CIAULA, MD**
Internist, Division of Internal Medicine, Hospital of Bisceglie, Bari, Italy

**SOUMITRA R. EACHEMPATI, MD, FACS**
Associate Professor of Surgery and Public Health, Division of Critical Care and Trauma, Department of Surgery; Division of Medical Ethics, Department of Public Health, Anne and Max A. Cohen Surgical Intensive Care Unit, New York-Presbyterian Hospital, Weill Cornell Medical College, New York, New York

**GUY D. ESLICK, PhD, MMedSc(Clin Epi), MMedStat**
Discipline of Surgery, The University of Sydney, Sydney Medical School, Nepean, Penrith, and School of Public Health, New South Wales, Australia; Department of Nutrition, Harvard School of Public Health, Boston, Massachusetts

**WILLIAM C. GALLAHAN, MD**
Fellow, Section on Gastroenterology, Wake Forest University Health Sciences, Winston-Salem, North Carolina

**RICHARD M. GORE, MD**
Department of Radiology, Chief of Gastrointestinal Radiology, NorthShore University Health System; Professor of Radiology, University of Chicago Pritzker School of Medicine, Evanston, Illinois

**KURINCHI S. GURUSAMY, MRCS**
Clinical Research Fellow, Department of Surgery, Royal Free Campus, UCL Medical School, Royal Free Hospital, London, United Kingdom

**STEPHANIE L. HANSEL, MD, MS**
Assistant Professor of Medicine, Division of Gastroenterology and Hepatology, Mayo Clinic, Rochester, Minnesota

**WILLIAM R. JARNAGIN, MD**
Hepatopancreatobiliary Service, Department of Surgery, Memorial Sloan-Kettering Cancer Center, New York, New York

**SHIVA JAYARAMAN, MD, MESc**
Hepatopancreatobiliary Service, Department of Surgery, Memorial Sloan-Kettering Cancer Center, New York, New York

**GLEN A. LEHMAN, MD**
Professor of Medicine and Radiology, Division of Gastroenterology/Hepatology, Department of Medicine, Indiana University Hospital, Indianapolis, Indiana

**UDAY K. MEHTA, MD**
Department of Radiology, NorthShore University Health System; Assistant Professor of Radiology, University of Chicago Pritzker School of Medicine, Evanston, Illinois

**ROBERT P. MYERS, MD, MSc, FRCPC**
Associate Professor of Medicine, Division of Gastroenterology, Department of Medicine, Faculty of Medicine, University of Calgary, Calgary, Alberta, Canada

**GERALDINE M. NEWMARK, MD**
Department of Radiology, Chief of Body Imaging, NorthShore University Health System; Associate Professor of Radiology, University of Chicago Pritzker School of Medicine, Evanston, Illinois

**PIERO PORTINCASA, MD, PhD**
Associate Professor of Medicine, Clinica Medica "A. Murri" Department of Internal and Public Medicine, University Medical School, Policlinico, Bari, Italy

**DARBY E. ROBINSON O'NEILL, MD**
Senior Fellow, Division of Gastroenterology, University of Washington Medical Center, Seattle, Washington

**MICHAEL D. SAUNDERS, MD**
Clinical Associate Professor, Director of Digestive Disease Center, Division of Gastroenterology, University of Washington Medical Center, Seattle, Washington

**ELDON A. SHAFFER, MD, FRCPC**
Professor of Medicine, Division of Gastroenterology, Department of Medicine, Faculty of Medicine, University of Calgary, Calgary, Alberta, Canada

**LAURA M. STINTON, MD, MSc**
Gastroenterology Fellow, Division of Gastroenterology, Department of Medicine, Faculty of Medicine, University of Calgary, Calgary, Alberta, Canada

**KIRAN H. THAKRAR, MD**
Department of Radiology, NorthShore University Health System; Assistant Professor, University of Chicago Pritzker School of Medicine, Evanston, Illinois

**KAREL JOHANNES VAN ERPECUM, MD, PhD**
Department of Gastroenterology and Hepatology, University Medical Center Utrecht, Utrecht, The Netherlands

**NIELS GERARD VENNEMAN, MD, PhD**
Department of Gastroenterology and Hepatology, University Medical Center Utrecht, Utrecht, The Netherlands

**DAVID Q.H. WANG, MD, PhD**
Assistant Professor of Medicine, Liver Center and Gastroenterology Division, Department of Medicine, Beth Israel Deaconess Medical Center, Harvard Medical School and Harvard Digestive Diseases Center, Boston, Massachusetts

**HELEN H. WANG, MS**
Research Associate, Liver Center and Gastroenterology Division, Department of Medicine, Beth Israel Deaconess Medical Center, Harvard Medical School, Boston, Massachusetts

**KYO-SANG YOO, MD**
ERCP Research fellow, Division of Gastroenterology/Hepatology, Department of Medicine, Indiana University Hospital, Indianapolis, Indiana

# Contents

identification of many candidate *LITH* genes. Because there is exceptionally close homology between mouse and human genomes, the orthologous human *LITH* genes can be identified from the mouse study. The discovery of *LITH* genes and more fundamental knowledge concerning the genetic determinants and molecular mechanisms underlying the formation of cholesterol gallstones in humans will pave the way for critical diagnostic and prelithogenic preventive measures for this exceptionally prevalent digestive disease.

Bile duct stone management has greatly changed in the past 2 decades. Open surgical techniques have mostly been replaced by transoral endoscopic techniques. Routine common bile duct stones can be managed by standard biliary endoscopic sphincterotomy and extraction. Various advanced transoral techniques can also manage most difficult ductal stones. In skilled centers, laparoscopic ductal stone management has assumed a back-up role.

Currently there is no evidence for prophylactic cholecystectomy to prevent gallstone formation (grade B). Cholecystectomy cannot be recommended for any group of patients having asymptomatic gallstones except in those undergoing major upper abdominal surgery for other pathologies (grade B). Laparoscopic cholecystectomy is the preferred treatment for all patient groups with symptomatic gallstones (grade B). Patients with gallstones along with common bile duct stones treated by endoscopic sphincterotomy should undergo cholecystectomy (grade A). Laparoscopic cholecystectomy with laparoscopic common bile duct exploration or with intraoperative endoscopic sphincterotomy is the preferred treatment for obstructive jaundice caused by common bile duct stones, when the expertise and infrastructure are available (grade B).

Gallstone disease is a frequent condition throughout the world and, cholesterol stones are the most frequent form in Western countries. The standard treatment of symptomatic gallstone subjects is laparoscopic cholecystectomy. The selection of patients amenable for nonsurgical, medical therapy is of key importance; a careful analysis should consider the natural history of the disease and the overall costs of therapy. Only patients with mild symptoms and small, uncalcified cholesterol gallstones in a functioning gallbladder with a patent cystic duct are considered for oral litholysis by hydrophilic ursodeoxycholic acid, in the hope of achieving cholesterol desaturation of bile and progressive stone dissolution. Recent studies have raised the possibility that cholesterol-lowering agents that inhibit hepatic cholesterol synthesis (statins) or intestinal cholesterol absorption (ezetimibe), or drugs acting on specific nuclear receptors involved in cholesterol and bile acid homeostasis, may offer, alone or in combination, additional medical therapeutic tools for treating cholesterol gallstones. Recent perspectives on medical treatment of cholesterol gallstone disease are discussed in this article.

The treatment of gallbladder disease has been revolutionized by improvements in laparoscopic surgery as well as endoscopic and radiologic interventional techniques. Therapeutic success is dependent on accurate radiologic assessment of gallbladder pathology. This article describes recent technical advances in ultrasonography, multidetector computed tomography, magnetic resonance imaging, positron emission tomography, and scintigraphy, which have significantly improved the accuracy of noninvasive imaging of benign and malignant gallbladder disease. The imaging findings of common gallbladder disorders are presented, and the role of each of the imaging modalities is placed in perspective for optimizing patient management.

In recent years, endoscopic ultrasonography (EUS) has emerged as an important tool for the diagnosis and management of pancreaticobiliary disease. The close proximity of the echoendoscope to the biliary system allows detailed imaging of the gallbladder and adjacent structures. EUS is useful for the detection of occult cholelithiasis and biliary sludge and in the evaluation of suspected choledocholithiasis. It can be used to classify and predict neoplasia in polypoid lesions of the gallbladder and also to diagnose and stage gallbladder carcinoma. This article reviews the use of EUS in these diseases of the gallbladder.

Gallbladder cancer is the most common biliary tract cancer. The highest incidence rates occur in Chile, which also has the highest mortality rates. This lethal gastrointestinal cancer has a predilection among adult women and older subjects of both sexes, and also among populations throughout central and Eastern Europe and certain racial groups, such as Native American Indians. Unfortunately, prospects are poor for preventing this form of cancer.

**THE CLINICS ARE NOW AVAILABLE ONLINE!**

Access your subscription at:
**www.theclinics.com**

## FORTHCOMING ISSUES

**September 2010**
Pharmacologic Therapies for
Gastrointestinal Disease
Richard Hunt, MD, Guest Editor

**December 2010**
Advances in Chemotherapy
Karl Kreutzer, MD, Guest Editor

## RECENT ISSUES

**March 2010**
Gastroenterologic Issues in the Obese Patient
David A. Johnson, MD,
Guest Editor

**December 2009**
Endoscopy in Inflammatory
Bowel Disease
Maria Regueiro, MD, and
Arthur M. Barrie III, MD, PhD,
Guest Editors

**September 2009**
Gastroenterology in the Elderly
Nicholas J. Talley, MD, PhD, and
Eric G. Tangalos, MD, Guest Editors

### ISSUES OF RELATED INTEREST

Ultrasound Clinics July 2007 (Vol. 2, No. 3)
Abdominal Ultrasound
M. Spicer, Guest Editor

## THE CLINICS ARE NOW AVAILABLE ONLINE!

Access your subscription at:
www.theclinics.com

# Preface
# Gallbladder Disease

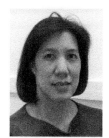

Cynthia W. Ko, MD, MS
*Guest Editor*

Gallbladder diseases, particularly gallstone-related syndromes, are common clinical problems facing practicing gastroenterologists and surgeons. Our understanding of the pathogenesis of gallbladder disease, including gallstones, acalculous cholecystitis, gallbladder dysmotility, and gallbladder cancer, continues to advance at a rapid pace. Furthermore, our ability to diagnose and treat gallbladder diseases is rapidly evolving.

In this issue, recognized experts discuss recent advances in the epidemiology; pathogenesis; and endoscopic, surgical, and medical therapies for gallstones. Additional articles address evolving methods to image the gallbladder, including computed tomography, magnetic resonance imaging, and endoscopic ultrasound. Finally, articles address other important but less well-understood gallbladder diseases, covering the epidemiology, diagnosis, and management of gallbladder cancer and polyps, acalculous cholecystitis, and dysmotility.

I hope the articles in this issue provide a balanced, state-of-the-art review of current knowledge and issues in management of gallbladder diseases and stimulate further research and investigation into their pathogenesis and treatment.

I am grateful for the enthusiasm and fine contributions of each of the authors. I also extend my sincere gratitude to Kerry Holland and her editorial staff at Elsevier for their assistance.

Cynthia W. Ko, MD, MS
Department of Medicine
Division of Gastroenterology
University of Washington
Seattle, WA, USA

E-mail address:
cwko@u.washington.edu

doi:10.1016/j.gtc.2010.02.013
**gastro.theclinics.com**

# Epidemiology of Gallstones

Laura M. Stinton, MD, MSc, Robert P. Myers, MD, MSc, FRCPC,
Eldon A. Shaffer, MD, FRCPC*

KEYWORDS

• Gallstones • Gallbladder disease • Biliary stones
• Epidemiology • Cholesterol • Cholecystectomy

Gallstone disease is a major health problem that is escalating. To identify risk factors in a given population, epidemiologic studies must first define the frequency of disease. Such information should not only direct public health initiatives but also reveal causal relationships; biologic plausibility reaffirms correlations and this then drives research to advance health care.

The prevalence of gallstones (ie, the number of individuals harboring gallstones at a certain point in time) is best determined by studies in well-defined patient populations that use ultrasonography, a noninvasive and safe method.[1] Ultrasonography eliminates the bias of autopsy, which implies death, and of clinical diagnosis, which requires biliary symptoms, yet only 20% ever experience symptoms.[2] The frequency of cholecystectomy, another potential measure of disease burden, has only a limited relationship to the prevalence of gallstone disease in a population, limited by the perceived threshold for surgery (largely doctor driven) and patient access to care.[3] Less well studied is its incidence, the risk of developing gallstones within a certain period of time or per person-years.

## BURDEN OF GALLSTONE DISEASE

Gallstones are an ancient entity, having occurred more than 3500 years ago according to autopsies performed on Egyptian and Chinese mummies. Gallbladder disease today is a common problem: 20 to 25 million Americans harbor gallstones, representing 10% to 15% of the adult population.[1] It constitutes a major health burden, with direct plus indirect costs of approximately $6.2 billion annually in the United States.[4] This burden has increased more than 20% since the 1980s and accounts for an estimated 1.8 million ambulatory care visits. Gallstone disease is now a leading cause of hospital admissions for gastrointestinal problems,[5] yielding 622,000 discharges (according to the most responsible diagnosis) each year in the United States.[4] This

Division of Gastroenterology (TRW Building, Room 6D29), Department of Medicine, Faculty of Medicine, University of Calgary, 3280 Hospital Drive NW, Calgary, Alberta, T2N 4N1, Canada
* Corresponding author.
E-mail address: shaffer@ucalgary.ca

Gastroenterol Clin N Am 39 (2010) 157–169
doi:10.1016/j.gtc.2010.02.003
0889-8553/10/$ – see front matter © 2010 Elsevier Inc. All rights reserved.

hospital burden is actually an underestimate; most admissions occur for laparoscopic cholecystectomy, commonly done without an overnight stay and thus not included in hospitalization statistics. Gallstone disease has a low mortality rate of 0.6%, but considering the burden of the disease, there were still an estimated 1092 gallstone-related deaths in 2004. Case fatality rates have steadily diminished from more than 5000 deaths in 1950, falling more than 50% between 1979 and 2004. This decline represents the greatest decrease for any digestive disease.[4]

Although most gallstones are clinically silent, 20% of people harboring stones experience true biliary symptoms at some time; 1% to 2% of patients each year experience complications and require surgical removal of the gallbladder.[6] Yet the number of operations for cholelithiasis has increased since 1950 in developed countries.[7] During the mid-twentieth century, the frequency of gallbladder surgeries was 6 times higher in the United States than in Western Europe. Gallstone disease in Europe, however, is similar to that in the United States, with a median prevalence in large population surveys ranging from 5.9% to 21.9%.[8] The reason for this discrepancy does not lie in the prevalence of cholelithiasis but most likely represent differences in surgical practice.[9] The introduction of laparoscopic cholecystectomy in 1989 further increased the cholecystectomy rate in the United States and the United Kingdom[7,10] From 1990 to 1993, there was a 28% escalation in the numbers of cholecystectomies performed.[11] A likely explanation for this increase is that laparoscopy is less invasive, providing a lower surgical risk and better patient acceptance compared with conventional (open) surgery, therefore leading to more surgeries in patients previously thought too high a risk or in those with minimal symptoms. Although there is undoubtedly an element of overuse, cholecystectomy is now the most common elective abdominal surgery performed in the United States, with more than 750,000 operations annually.

## ETHNICITY AND GALLSTONE DISEASE

The highest prevalence of gallstone disease has been described in North American Indians: 64.1% of women and 29.5% of men have gallstones **(Table 1)**.[1,12] This apparent epidemic reaches a high of 73% in Pima Indian women over age 30.[13] Similar high occurrences have been reported among the aboriginal populations of South America.[14] In the native Mapuche of Chile, gallstone disease afflicts 49.4% of women and 12.6% of men, exceeding 60% in women in their 50s. Mexican Americans are also at an increased risk when compared with white Americans.[15] As elsewhere in the Americas, this risk is directly related to the degree of Amerindian admixture. White Americans have a prevalence of 16.6% in women and 8.6% in men.[15,16] In Northern Europe, prevalence is somewhat higher at 20%, whereas lower rates are evident in Italy at 11%.[8,17] Intermediate prevalence rates occur in Asian populations and black Americans (13.9% of women; 5.3% of men).[16] The lowest frequencies occur in sub-Saharan black Africans (<5%)[18]; the entity is virtually nonexistent in the Masai and the Bantu.[19]

Ethnicity is a major determinant of the type of stones that form, why they develop, and where they reside in the biliary system **(Table 2)**. In developed countries, the majority (>85%) consist predominantly of cholesterol, whereas the remainder constitutes black pigment (calcium bilirubinate). Cholesterol and black pigment stones form within the gallbladder. Cholesterol gallstone formation begins with the liver producing bile supersaturated with cholesterol, which precipitates as microcrystals in the gallbladder. Here, excessive mucin and impaired gallbladder motility retain these crystals that then aggregate and grow into macroscopic stones. Black pigment stones also

**Table 1**
**Prevalence of gallstones worldwide**

| Population | Examples | Prevalence (%) Male | Prevalence (%) Female | Study |
|---|---|---|---|---|
| **High Prevalence** | | | | |
| North American Indians | | 29.5 | 64.1 | Everhart et al. Hepatology 2002;35(6):1507–12. |
| | Pima Indians | | 73 | Sampliner et al. N Engl J Med 1970;283(25):1358–64. |
| **South American Indians** | | | | |
| | Chile—Mapuche Indians | 12.6 | 49.4 | Miquel et al. Gastroenterology 1998;115(4):937–46. |
| Mexican Americans | | 8.9 | 26.7 | Everhart et al. Gastroenterology 1999;117(3):632–9. |
| White Americans | | 8.6 | 16.6 | Everhart et al. Gastroenterology 1999;117(3):632–9. |
| **Europe** | | | | |
| | Stockholm, Sweden | 4–15 | 11–25 | Muhrbeck et al. Scand J Gastroenterol 1995;30(11):1125–8. |
| | Sirmione, Italy | 6.7 | 14.4 | Barbara et al. Hepatology 1987;7(5):913–7. |
| **Intermediate Prevalence** | | | | |
| **Asia** | | | | |
| | Chandigarh, India | 6.2 | 21.6 | Singh et al. J Gastroenterol Hepatol 2001;16(5):560–3. |
| | Taipei, Taiwan | 10.7 | 11.5 | Chen CY et al. Age Ageing 1998;27(4):437–41. |
| Black Americans | United States | 5.3 | 13.9 | Everhart et al. Gastroenterology 1999;117(3):632–9. |
| **Low Prevalence** | | | | |
| Black Africans | Sudan | 5.6 | 5.1 | Bagi Abdel et al. Gastroenterology 1991;100:A307. 2009. |

develop in the gallbladder but consist primarily of bilirubin polymers (calcium bilirubinate). These are associated with advanced age, cirrhosis, cystic fibrosis, and increased red blood cell destruction (chronic hemolytic states, such as sickle cell anemia; ineffective erythropoesis).

Bile duct stones can originate in the gallbladder or develop primarily in the biliary system. In Western societies, 10% to 15% of patients with gallstones have concomitant stones found in the common bile duct, having secondarily migrated there from the gallbladder. Risk factors for such biliary stones coexisting with (and originating from) stones in the gallbladder are increasing age, Asian descent, chronic bile duct inflammation, and possibly hypothyroidism. These common bile duct stones are

**Table 2**
**Types of stones: characteristics and clinical associations**

| | Cholesterol Gallstones | Black Pigment Stones | Brown Pigment Stones |
|---|---|---|---|
| Composition | 50%–100% cholesterol | Calcium bilirubinate polymer | Unconjugated bilirubin, calcium soaps (palmitate, stearate) cholesterol and mucin |
| Color | Yellow-brown | Black | Brown |
| Consistency | Crystalline | Hard | Soft, greasy |
| Location | Gallbladder ± common duct (approximately 10%) | Gallbladder ± common duct | Bile ducts |
| Radiodensity | Lucent (85%) | Opaque (>50%) | Lucent (100%) |
| Clinical Associations | Metabolic: family history (genetic traits), obesity, female gender, aging (excessive cholesterol secretion) | Increased red cell destruction (hemolysis), cirrhosis, cystic fibrosis, Crohn disease, advanced age (excessive bilirubin excretion) | Infection, inflammation, infestation (stasis, strictures) |

usually composed of cholesterol. Choledocholithiasis can also develop de novo in the bile ducts associated with biliary strictures and the attendant stasis and inflammation/infection in the form of brown pigment stones.

The situation differs in East Asia where brown pigment stones predominate and originate in the bile ducts. Such brown pigment stones consist of calcium bilirubinate, fatty acids, cholesterol, and mucin (glycoproteins primarily from bacterial biofilms). They form in the common bile duct (choledocholithiasis) or the intrahepatic bile ducts (hepatolithiasis). Bacterial infection, biliary parasites (*Clonorchis sinensis, Opisthorchis* species, and *Fasciola hepatica*) and stasis (from partial biliary obstruction) are key factors in the development of these primary bile duct stones. Brown pigment stones are the predominant type in Asia and can cause Oriental cholangiohepatitis: biliary obstruction with recurrent cholangitis, dilatation, and stricturing of the biliary tree. In hepatolithiasis, stones are present in the intrahepatic bile ducts, regardless of any coexistent stones residing elsewhere in the biliary system (ie, the extrahepatic ducts or the gallbladder). These intrahepatic brown pigment stones have higher cholesterol content and less bilirubin than when arising in extrahepatic sites, presumably due to a different basis for their formation. The frequency of hepatolithiasis, as a proportion of all biliary tract stones, varies from a high of 20% in China and Taiwan to 2% to 3% in Japan, Singapore, and Hong Kong.[20] There has been, however, a recent shift from pigment to cholesterol stones in developing Asian countries. This has been attributed to consumption of a more Westernized diet and a decreased rate of chronic biliary infections.[1]

## RISK FACTORS FOR GALLSTONE FORMATION

Gallstone formation is multifactorial, including constitutional and environmental factors. Some factors, such as diet, activity, rapid weight loss, and obesity, are modifiable, whereas others (eg, age, female gender, genetics, and ethnicity) cannot change.

Several case-control studies, which compare those with gallstones versus those without, have identified important associations for harboring gallstones (**Table 3**).[1]

### Age

Gallstone disease is rare in neonates and young children. Once thought only related to pigment stones developing in the setting of hemolysis, cholesterol stones are becoming increasingly more common in children.[21,22] Risk factors for gallstone disease in children include female gender, obesity, and Mexican American origin. The frequency of gallstones increases with age, rising noticeably after age 40 to become 4 to 10 times more likely in older individuals.[1] Although age correlates positively with increased cholesterol secretion and saturation, the stone type found in advanced age tends to be pigment. Although gallstones are inclined to be clinically silent, symptoms and severe complications increase with age, leading to cholecystectomy in more than 40% of those above age 40 in a report from Germany.[23] High prevalence rates of gallstones can occur in such older women (70 to 79 years old): 57% have a history of cholecystectomy or current sonographic evidence for gallstones.

### Gender and Female Sex Hormones

Female gender is one of the most powerful influences on gallstone disease, with women almost twice as likely as men to form stones.[1] This is especially true for women in their fertile years, with the gap narrowing into the postmenopausal period when men catch up. Women are also more likely to undergo cholecystectomy. The basis for this finding seems related to the female sex hormones, because parity, oral contraceptive use, and estrogen replacement therapy are risk factors for gallstone disease.[24] During pregnancy, biliary sludge can appear in 5% to 30% of women; gallstones develop in 2% to 5%.[25] In the puerperium, sludge disappears in two-thirds whereas small gallstones (<1 cm) resolve in one-third. Additional risk factors include obesity (prepregnancy weight), reduced levels of high-density lipoprotein (HDL) cholesterol, parity, and insulin resistance (the metabolic syndrome). Female sex hormones adversely influence hepatic bile secretion and gallbladder function. Estrogens increase cholesterol secretion and diminish bile salt secretion. Progestins act by reducing bile salt secretion and impairing gallbladder emptying leading to stasis.

### Obesity

Obesity connotes excess body fat, an entity that cannot be directly measured. Hence, it is best defined as a body mass index (BMI), which is used to express weight adjusted for height, as kilograms divided by height in meters squared ($kg/m^2$). The normal range

| Table 3 | |
|---|---|
| **Risk factors for gallstone disease** | |
| **Modifiable** | **Nonmodifiable** |
| Diet | Familial/genetic |
| Female sex hormone use | Ethnicity |
| Obesity/metabolic syndrome | Female gender |
| Rapid weight loss | |
| Low physical activity | |
| Underlying disease: cirrhosis, Crohn disease | |
| Drugs | |
| TPN | |

of BMI is 20 to 25. Overweight is a BMI of 25 to 30. Obesity (>30) may be further divided into severe (>35–39) or extreme (morbid) when BMI is greater than 35 and accompanied by comorbid conditions, such as diabetes or cardiovascular disease, or when the BMI is greater than 40. Overweight for children and adolescents is a BMI for age at or above the 95th percentile of a specified reference population of 30 or greater.[26] The prevalence of obesity has risen drastically over the past several decades, acquiring the status of an epidemic not only in developed counties, such as the United States, but also in developing nations, such as China. Obesity is a major, well-established risk factor for gallstone disease, particularly abdominal/centripetal obesity (eg, as measured by waist-to-hip ratio). The risk is especially high in women and rises linearly with increasing obesity.[27] Women with extreme obesity have a 7-fold elevation in the development of gallstones compared with nonobese controls; their annual incidence of developing gallstones is 2%. Obesity earlier in life (late teens) carries the greatest risk, whereas slimness protects against cholelithiasis.[1,27] Obesity is associated with increased cholesterol synthesis and secretion into bile.

### Dyslipidemia, Diabetes Mellitus, and the Metabolic Syndrome

Given that cholesterol gallstone disease is a metabolic problem, it should correlate with lipid abnormalities, diabetes mellitus, and adiposity. Although most gallstones in the Western world consist of cholesterol, there is no definite association with hypercholesterolemia.[1] Rather, a low HDL cholesterol carries an increased risk of developing stones, as does hypertriglyceridemia.

The association between diabetes mellitus and gallstones is confounded by age, obesity, and a family history of gallstones.[1] The link between diabetes, obesity, and gallstones most likely comes through the metabolic syndrome. The metabolic syndrome characterizes a specific body phenotype (abdominal obesity), insulin resistance (type 2 diabetes mellitus), and dyslipidemia (hypertriglyceridemia), all risks for cardiovascular disease. Insulin resistance predisposes to cholesterol gallstone disease,[28,29] suggesting that hepatic insulin resistance must somehow affect cholesterol and bile salt metabolism.

### Rapid Weight Loss

At least 25% of morbidly obese individuals have evidence of gallstone disease even before undergoing weight reduction surgery.[30] Low calorie diets and rapid weight loss (particularly after bariatric surgery), ironically, are then associated with the development of gallstones in 30% to 71% of these obese individuals losing weight.[1,31,32] Weight loss exceeding 1.5 kg/week after bariatric surgery particularly increases the risk for stone formation.[33] Furthermore, stones are most likely to become apparent during the first 6 weeks after surgery when weight loss is most profound.[34] Such gallstones are usually clinically silent; sludge in the gallbladder and small stones (microlithiasis) often disappear. Following bariatric surgery, only 7% to 16% develop symptoms, best predicted by a weight loss exceeding 25% of their preoperative body weight.[30] Strategies for ameliorating this complication have ranged from routine prophylactic cholecystectomy, through regular ultrasound surveillance to detect even asymptomatic stones, to low-dose ursodeoxycholic acid for preventing stone formation.[30,35,36] Even less extreme weight fluctuations create a risk for stone formation, as is a history of dieting.[37]

### Diet

Although nutrition, intuitively, should represent a key factor contributing to gallstone formation, findings are often conflicting and difficult to examine.[38] Other than energy intake as calories leading to obesity, the importance of dietary content is unclear. Diets high in cholesterol, fatty acids, carbohydrates, or legumes seem to increase the risk of cholelithiasis. In contrast, unsaturated fats, coffee, fiber, ascorbic acid (vitamin C), calcium, and moderate consumption of alcohol reduce the risk.[1] The shift to a more Western diet, high in refined carbohydrates and fat (triglycerides) and low in fiber, best explains the profound increase in cholesterol gallstones in American Indians (unmasking their presumed genetic burden) and in post–World War II European countries; this also may underline the shift from pigment to cholesterol stones in Asian countries. Genetic variations, especially in those genes controlling cholesterol metabolism, presumably underscore why some respond to dietary change by developing cholesterol gallstones.[39]

### Total Parental Nutrition

Total parental nutrition (TPN) is a well-known risk factor for developing microlithiasis (biliary sludge) and gallstone disease, along with acalculous cholecystitis in critically ill patients.[40] In an intensive care setting, biliary sludge appears after 5 to 10 days of fasting. After 4 weeks of TPN, half of those on TPN develop gallbladder sludge; after 6 weeks all show evidence of sludge. Most are asymptomatic. Fortunately, sludge resolves within 4 weeks of discontinuing TPN and resuming an oral intake, a pattern similar to sludge appearing during pregnancy and rapid weight loss: sludge disappearing after the inciting event resolves.[41] A possible explanation for this relates to loss of the enteric stimulation of the gallbladder in the absence of eating, leading to gallbladder stasis.[40] Additionally, ileal disorders, such as Crohn disease or ileal resection, in which TPN is frequently required, can affect the enterohepatic cycling of bile acids and thus augment bilirubin absorption and excessive pigment secretion.[42]

### Lifestyle Factors and Socioeconomic Status

It is controversial if an association between gallbladder disease and socioeconomic status exists.[1] Any inverse relation likely reflects socioeconomic status as an indirect marker for other risk factors, such as obesity and dietary issues. Physical activity helps prevent cholelithiasis, independent of its role in weight loss.[43] Reduced activity heightens the risk. The role of smoking in cholelithiasis is unclear.

### Family History and Genetics

Familial and epidemiologic studies demonstrate that genetic susceptibility is important in the formation of gallstones.[44] Occurrence within families can be a product of genetic and shared environmental factors. Familial studies reveal an increased frequency in family clusters (about 5 times more common in families of affected persons) and relatives of gallstone patients, but more convincingly in monozygotic (12%) as opposed to dizygotic twins (6%).[45] Genetic effects account for 25%, shared environmental effects for 13%, while unique environmental effects for 62% of the phenotypic variance.[46] The extraordinary susceptibility of American Indians might relate to thrifty genes that conferred a survival advantage when Paleo-Indians migrated across the land bridge from Asia to the Americas during the last great ice age (50,000–10,000 years ago). This might also explain their proclivity to acquire the metabolic syndrome and its sequelae.[1]

The search for gene variants has implicated polymorphisms of apolipoprotein E4 being associated with biliary cholesterol supersaturation and cholesterol stones[47]; other studies, however, failed to find such a correlation.[48] The frequency of reputed lithogenic genetic variants may coincide with the gallstone prevalence in certain populations[44] but none has reached common recognition in population studies.

The search for single gene mutation, lithogenic alleles associated with cholesterol gallstones has focused on the adenosine triphosphate–binding cassette (ABC) transporters located in the hepatocyte canalicular membrane. Specific mutations have been identified for cholesterol gallstone formation in animal models and seem to be a susceptibility factor for human gallstone formation. The ABCB4 gene mutation (impairing lecithin secretion) represents a risk factor causing the low phospholipid-associated cholelithiasis (LPAC) syndrome: symptomatic and recurring cholelithiasis in young patients (<40 years).[49] This monogenetic defect however is an uncommon cause of cholelithiasis in young adults, evident in less than 2% of cases.[50] More promising is the genome analysis that identified ABCG8 19H and ABCB4 variants (for cholesterol secretion) as susceptibility factors for human gallstones.[51,52] This confers odds ratios of 2 to 3 and 7 for heterozygous and homozygous carriers, respectively, but accounts for only 11% of their total gallstone risk. Further, a genome-wide search has uncovered 2 susceptibility loci, at least for symptomatic gallbladder disease, located on chromosome 1p of Mexican Americans.[53] Cholelithiasis seems to be a polygenetic disorder.

## Underlying Chronic Diseases

### Liver disease
Cirrhosis is a well-established risk factor for gallstones particularly in the more advanced stages.[54,55] The overall prevalence is much higher than the general population at 25% to 30%.[56] Increasing Child-Pugh score and obesity are more likely associated with gallstones. Most stones in cirrhosis are of the black pigment type.[57] The biologic mechanism likely relates to altered pigment secretion, abnormal gallbladder motility, or increased estrogen levels.[1] The threat of these stones becoming symptomatic seems higher in women, those more advanced in age, and patients with viral hepatitis compared with alcohol-related cirrhosis.[58] Gallstone disease is also associated with hepatitis C virus (even when not yet cirrhotic)[59] and nonalcoholic fatty liver disease, the connection being the metabolic syndrome and obesity.[60]

### Crohn disease
Crohn disease, when associated with extensive ileal disease or loss, conveys a 2 to 3 fold increased risk of developing gallstones.[61] Although once believed due to bile acid malabsorption and depletion leading to cholesterol gallstones, recent studies have found an increased frequency of pigment stones. Unabsorbed bile acids that escape into the colon function as a biologic detergent to solubilize bilirubin and thus increase its absorption and enterohepatic cycling. The resultant increased pigment in bile then promotes stone formation.[62]

### Cystic fibrosis
The gallstone prevalence in cystic fibrosis is increased: 10% to 30% versus less than 5% in age-matched controls.[62] Like ileal Crohn disease, cystic fibrosis is associated with bile acid malabsorption; in this instance, the bile salts bind to undigested dietary nutrients. Such bile salt depletion could lead to cholesterol stone formation or the escape of bile salts into the colon might enhance bilirubin absorption, resulting in pigment stones.

### Other diseases
In the irritable bowel syndrome (IBS), cholecystectomy is a more common operation because of diagnostic confusion leading to inappropriate surgery[63] or because the IBS symptoms are a consequence of the surgery.

Spinal cord injury is associated with a 3-fold increase in gallstones, presumably related to gallbladder stasis (ie, forming sludge) and intestinal hypomotility (by augmenting secondary bile acids, such as deoxycholic acid, that then adversely influence bile).[64]

## Drugs

### Octreotide

More than 50% of patients receiving octreotide (eg, acromegalic and cancer patients) or those with a somatostatinoma develop cholelithiasis; the majority are asymptomatic.[65] Somatostatin abrogates the postprandial release of cholecystokinin, presumably leading to gallbladder stasis.

### Ceftriaxone

The third-generation cephalosporin antibiotic, ceftriaxone, is secreted unmetabolized into bile reaching high concentrations and producing biliary sludge.[66] Usually, patients remain asymptomatic; sludge resolves once the medication is discontinued.

### Statins

Drugs that inhibit hydroxymethylglutaryl–coenzyme A (HMG-coA) reductase not only diminish cholesterol synthesis in the liver but also decrease its secretion into bile, seeming to prevent cholesterol gallstone disease.[67]

## THE FUTURE

The true frequency of gallstone disease at any point in time (ie, prevalence) has advanced with the use of ultrasonographic surveys as opposed to clinical and necropsy studies. These studies have better defined important risk factors and ethnic differences. Cholelithiasis is rampant in American Indians and Hispanics, fostering the concept of a genetic basis for the racial differences. There is also an increased heritability in those who develop cholelithiasis early in life. The complicated pathogenesis of gallstone formation renders identification of genes causing stones difficult. Well-defined monogenic forms of gallstone disease affecting the ABC transporters are rare, or if more common, such as the *ABCG8 19H* gene variant (responsible for hepatic cholesterol secretion), exhibit an attributable risk that only reaches 11%. Future epidemiologic studies should, therefore, clarify genetic susceptibility factors and their frequency, leading to new means for risk assessment, prevention, and treatment. Identifying gene variants for the gallstone phenotype would then require action: better defining the role of diagnostic imaging (ultrasonography to detect stone development), strategies for prevention (like ursodeoxycholic acid for LPAC syndrome), and the value of modifying environmental factors.

The implications of changing environmental risk factors predict an increase in the numbers of individuals with gallstones. An aging population plus the rising epidemic of obesity and the metabolic syndrome are certain to aggravate the frequency and complications of gallstone disease. Identifying risk factors that can be altered (ie, extreme obesity, rapid weight loss, sedentary lifestyle, and key dietary factors) will provide an opportunity for the prevention of cholelithiasis.

## REFERENCES

1. Shaffer EA. Gallstone disease: epidemiology of gallbladder stone disease. Best Pract Res Clin Gastroenterol 2006;20(6):981–96.

2. Gracie WA, Ransohoff DF. The natural history of silent gallstones: the innocent gallstone is not a myth. N Engl J Med 1982;307(13):798–800.

3. Pedersen G, Hoem D, Andren-Sandberg A. Influence of laparoscopic cholecystectomy on the prevalence of operations for gallstones in Norway. Eur J Surg 2002;168(8–9):464–9.

4. Everhart JE, Ruhl CE. Burden of digestive diseases in the United States part I: overall and upper gastrointestinal diseases. Gastroenterology 2009;136(2): 376–86.

5. Shaheen NJ, Hansen RA, Morgan DR, et al. The burden of gastrointestinal and liver diseases, 2006. Am J Gastroenterol 2006;101(9):2128–38.

6. Ransohoff DF, Gracie WA, Wolfenson LB, et al. Prophylactic cholecystectomy or expectant management for silent gallstones. A decision analysis to assess survival. Ann Intern Med 1983;99(2):199–204.

7. Legorreta AP, Silber JH, Costantino GN, et al. Increased cholecystectomy rate after the introduction of laparoscopic cholecystectomy. JAMA 1993;270(12): 1429–32.

8. Aerts R, Penninckx F. The burden of gallstone disease in Europe. Aliment Pharmacol Ther 2003;18(Suppl):349–53.

9. Plant JC, Percy I, Bates T, et al. Incidence of gallbladder disease in Canada, England, and France. Lancet 1973;2(7823):249–51.

10. Kang JY, Ellis C, Majeed A, et al. Gallstones—an increasing problem: a study of hospital admissions in England between 1989/1990 and 1999/2000. Aliment Pharmacol Ther 2003;17(4):561–9.

11. Nenner RP, Imperato PJ, Rosenberg C, et al. Increased cholecystectomy rates among Medicare patients after the introduction of laparoscopic cholecystectomy. J Community Health 1994;19(6):409–15.

12. Everhart JE, Yeh F, Lee ET, et al. Prevalence of gallbladder disease in American Indian populations: findings from the Strong Heart Study. Hepatology 2002;35(6): 1507–12.

13. Sampliner RE, Bennett PH, Comess LJ, et al. Gallbladder disease in pima indians. Demonstration of high prevalence and early onset by cholecystography. N Engl J Med 1970;283(25):1358–64.

14. Miquel JF, Covarrubias C, Villaroel L, et al. Genetic epidemiology of cholesterol cholelithiasis among Chilean Hispanics, Amerindians, and Maoris. Gastroenterology 1998;115(4):937–46.

15. Everhart JE. Gallstones and ethnicity in the Americas. J Assoc Acad Minor Phys 2001;12(3):137–43.

16. Everhart JE, Khare M, Hill M, et al. Prevalence and ethnic differences in gallbladder disease in the United States. Gastroenterology 1999;117(3):632–9.

17. Barbara L, Sama C, Morselli Labate AM, et al. A population study on the prevalence of gallstone disease: the Sirmione Study. Hepatology 1987;7(5): 913–7.

18. Bagi Abdel M. Prevalence of gallbladder disease in Sudan: first sonographic field study in adult population [abstract]. Arabi M ARB editor. Gastroenterology 1991; 100:A307. 2009.

19. Biss K, Ho KJ, Mikkelson B, et al. Some unique biologic characteristics of the Masai of East Africa. N Engl J Med 1971;284(13):694–9.

20. Shoda J, Tanaka N, Osuga T. Hepatolithiasis—epidemiology and pathogenesis update. Front Biosci 2003;8:e398–409.

21. Palasciano G, Portincasa P, Vinciguerra V, et al. Gallstone prevalence and gallbladder volume in children and adolescents: an epidemiological

ultrasonographic survey and relationship to body mass index. Am J Gastroenterol 1989;84(11):1378–82.

22. Kaechele V, Wabitsch M, Thiere D, et al. Prevalence of gallbladder stone disease in obese children and adolescents: influence of the degree of obesity, sex, and pubertal development. J Pediatr Gastroenterol Nutr 2006;42(1):66–70.

23. Volzke H, Baumeister SE, Alte D, et al. Independent risk factors for gallstone formation in a region with high cholelithiasis prevalence. Digestion 2005;71(2):97–105.

24. Cirillo DJ, Wallace RB, Rodabough RJ, et al. Effect of estrogen therapy on gallbladder disease. JAMA 2005;293(3):330–9.

25. Maringhini A, Ciambra M, Baccelliere P, et al. Biliary sludge and gallstones in pregnancy: incidence, risk factors, and natural history. Ann Intern Med 1993; 119(2):116–20.

26. Ogden CL, Yanovski SZ, Carroll MD, et al. The epidemiology of obesity. Gastroenterology 2007;132(6):2087–102.

27. Maclure KM, Hayes KC, Colditz GA, et al. Weight, diet, and the risk of symptomatic gallstones in middle-aged women. N Engl J Med 1989;321(9):563–9.

28. Ruhl CE, Everhart JE. Association of diabetes, serum insulin, and C-peptide with gallbladder disease. Hepatology 2000;31(2):299–303.

29. Nervi F, Miquel JF, Alvarez M, et al. Gallbladder disease is associated with insulin resistance in a high risk Hispanic population. J Hepatol 2006;45(2): 299–305.

30. Li VK, Pulido N, Fajnwaks P, et al. Predictors of gallstone formation after bariatric surgery: a multivariate analysis of risk factors comparing gastric bypass, gastric banding, and sleeve gastrectomy. Surg Endosc 2009;23(7):1640–4.

31. Everhart JE. Contributions of obesity and weight loss to gallstone disease. Ann Intern Med 1993;119(10):1029–35.

32. Broomfield PH, Chopra R, Sheinbaum RC, et al. Effects of ursodeoxycholic acid and aspirin on the formation of lithogenic bile and gallstones during loss of weight. N Engl J Med 1988;319(24):1567–72.

33. Weinsier RL, Wilson LJ, Lee J. Medically safe rate of weight loss for the treatment of obesity: a guideline based on risk of gallstone formation. Am J Med 1995; 98(2):115–7.

34. Al-Jiffry BO, Shaffer EA, Saccone GT, et al. Changes in gallbladder motility and gallstone formation following laparoscopic gastric banding for morbid obestity. Can J Gastroenterol 2003;17(3):169–74.

35. Wudel LJ Jr, Wright JK, Debelak JP, et al. Prevention of gallstone formation in morbidly obese patients undergoing rapid weight loss: results of a randomized controlled pilot study. J Surg Res 2002;102(1):50–6.

36. Miller K, Hell E, Lang B, et al. Gallstone formation prophylaxis after gastric restrictive procedures for weight loss: a randomized double-blind placebo-controlled trial. Ann Surg 2003;238(5):697–702.

37. Syngal S, Coakley EH, Willett WC, et al. Long-term weight patterns and risk for cholecystectomy in women. Ann Intern Med 1999;130(6):471–7.

38. Mendez-Sanchez N, Zamora-Valdes D, Chavez-Tapia NC, et al. Role of diet in cholesterol gallstone formation. Clin Chim Acta 2007;376(1–2):1–8.

39. Rudkowska I, Jones PJ. Polymorphisms in ABCG5/G8 transporters linked to hypercholesterolemia and gallstone disease. Nutr Rev 2008;66(6):343–8.

40. Angelico M, Della GP. Review article: hepatobiliary complications associated with total parenteral nutrition. Aliment Pharmacol Ther 2000;14(Suppl):254–7.

41. Shaffer EA. Gallbladder sludge: what is its clinical significance? Curr Gastroenterol Rep 2001;3(2):166–73.

42. Lambou-Gianoukos S, Heller SJ. Lithogenesis and bile metabolism. Surg Clin North Am 2008;88(6):1175–94, vii.
43. Leitzmann MF, Rimm EB, Willett WC, et al. Recreational physical activity and the risk of cholecystectomy in women. N Engl J Med 1999;341(11):777–84.
44. Lammert F, Miquel JF. Gallstone disease: from genes to evidence-based therapy. J Hepatol 2008;48(Suppl 1):S124–35.
45. Sarin SK, Negi VS, Dewan R, et al. High familial prevalence of gallstones in the first-degree relatives of gallstone patients. Hepatology 1995;22(1):138–41.
46. Katsika D, Grjibovski A, Einarsson C, et al. Genetic and environmental influences on symptomatic gallstone disease: a Swedish study of 43,141 twin pairs. Hepatology 2005;41(5):1138–43.
47. Bertomeu A, Ros E, Zambon D, et al. Apolipoprotein E polymorphism and gallstones. Gastroenterology 1996;111(6):1603–10.
48. Mella JG, Schirin-Sokhan R, Rigotti A, et al. Genetic evidence that apolipoprotein E4 is not a relevant susceptibility factor for cholelithiasis in two high-risk populations. J Lipid Res 2007;48(6):1378–85.
49. Rosmorduc O, Hermelin B, Boelle PY, et al. ABCB4 gene mutation-associated cholelithiasis in adults. Gastroenterology 2003;125(2):452–9.
50. Nakken KE, Labori KJ, Rodningen OK, et al. ABCB4 sequence variations in young adults with cholesterol gallstone disease. Liver Int 2009;29(5):743–7.
51. Buch S, Schafmayer C, Volzke H, et al. A genome-wide association scan identifies the hepatic cholesterol transporter ABCG8 as a susceptibility factor for human gallstone disease. Nat Genet 2007;39(8):995–9.
52. Grunhage F, Acalovschi M, Tirziu S, et al. Increased gallstone risk in humans conferred by common variant of hepatic ATP-binding cassette transporter for cholesterol. Hepatology 2007;46(3):793–801.
53. Puppala S, Dodd GD, Fowler S, et al. A genomewide search finds major susceptibility loci for gallbladder disease on chromosome 1 in Mexican Americans. Am J Hum Genet 2006;78(3):377–92.
54. Acalovschi M, Badea R, Dumitrascu D, et al. Prevalence of gallstones in liver cirrhosis: a sonographic survey. Am J Gastroenterol 1988;83(9):954–6.
55. Conte D, Barisani D, Mandelli C, et al. Cholelithiasis in cirrhosis: analysis of 500 cases. Am J Gastroenterol 1991;86(11):1629–32.
56. Conte D, Fraquelli M, Fornari F, et al. Close relation between cirrhosis and gallstones: cross-sectional and longitudinal survey. Arch Intern Med 1999;159(1):49–52.
57. Alvaro D, Angelico M, Gandin C, et al. Physico-chemical factors predisposing to pigment gallstone formation in liver cirrhosis. J Hepatol 1990;10(2):228–34.
58. Acalovschi M, Blendea D, Feier C, et al. Risk factors for symptomatic gallstones in patients with liver cirrhosis: a case-control study. Am J Gastroenterol 2003; 98(8):1856–60.
59. Acalovschi M, Buzas C, Radu C, et al. Hepatitis C virus infection is a risk factor for gallstone disease: a prospective hospital-based study of patients with chronic viral C hepatitis. J Viral Hepat 2009;16(12):860–6.
60. Loria P, Lonardo A, Lombardini S, et al. Gallstone disease in non-alcoholic fatty liver: prevalence and associated factors. J Gastroenterol Hepatol 2005;20(8):1176–84.
61. Whorwell PJ, Hawkins R, Dewbury K, et al. Ultrasound survey of gallstones and other hepatobiliary disorders in patients with Crohn's disease. Dig Dis Sci 1984;29(10):930–3.
62. Vitek L, Carey MC. Enterohepatic cycling of bilirubin as a cause of 'black' pigment gallstones in adult life. Eur J Clin Invest 2003;33(9):799–810.

63. Kennedy TM, Jones RH. Epidemiology of cholecystectomy and irritable bowel syndrome in a UK population. Br J Surg 2000;87(12):1658–63.
64. Xia CS, Han YQ, Yang XY, et al. Spinal cord injury and cholelithiasis. Hepatobiliary Pancreat Dis Int 2004;3(4):595–8.
65. Trendle MC, Moertel CG, Kvols LK. Incidence and morbidity of cholelithiasis in patients receiving chronic octreotide for metastatic carcinoid and malignant islet cell tumors. Cancer 1997;79(4):830–4.
66. Bickford CL, Spencer AP. Biliary sludge and hyperbilirubinemia associated with ceftriaxone in an adult: case report and review of the literature. Pharmacotherapy 2005;25(10):1389–95.
67. Tsai CJ, Leitzmann MF, Willett WC, et al. Statin use and the risk of cholecystectomy in women. Gastroenterology 2009;136(5):1593–600.

# Pathogenesis of Gallstones

Niels Gerard Venneman, MD, PhD,
Karel Johannes van Erpecum, MD, PhD*

**KEYWORDS**

- Bilirubin • Bile salt • Cholesterol • Crystallization
- FXR • Gallbladder • Motility

Gallstone disease is very common in the Western world with an estimated prevalence of 10% to 15% in white adults, leading to significant morbidity, mortality, and considerable health care costs. In the Western world, approximately 70% of gallstone carriers exhibit cholesterol gallbladder stones (cholesterol content >50%), and 30% exhibit black pigment gallbladder stones. In East Asia, there is a high prevalence of brown pigment stones residing in the bile ducts, and causing potentially devastating cholangitis. Nevertheless, also in these countries, prevalence of cholesterol gallstones increases, supposedly caused by the introduction of Western diet. Because of increased prevalence of overweight or a higher proportion of elderly subjects in the population, the prevalence of gallstone disease may further increase in the near future. This article focuses on the pathogenesis of cholesterol gallstones. Cholesterol crystal nucleation is considered the earliest step in cholesterol gallstone formation. Various conditions affecting the crystallization process are discussed, such as biliary cholesterol supersaturation, excess pronucleating proteins, or shortage of nucleation-inhibiting proteins, and factors related to the gallbladder, such as hypomotility. Pigment gallstone pathogenesis is briefly discussed.

## PHYSICAL-CHEMICAL ASPECTS OF BILIARY CHOLESTEROL SOLUBILIZATION AND CHOLESTEROL CRYSTALLIZATION

Although solubility of cholesterol in aqueous solutions is extremely limited, in gallbladder bile a relatively large amount (approximately $20 \times 10^{-3}$ M) of the sterol can be kept in solution. This significant increase in solubility is explained by incorporation of cholesterol in mixed micelles, together with bile salts and phospholipids (mainly phosphatidylcholine). Supersaturation occurs when either too much cholesterol or not enough solubilizing bile salt and phosphatidylcholine molecules are secreted to allow complete micellar solubilization of all cholesterol. Excessive cholesterol may

Department of Gastroenterology and Hepatology, University Medical Center Utrecht, HP. F.02.618, PO Box 85500, 3508 GA Utrecht, The Netherlands
* Corresponding author.
*E-mail address:* k.j.vanerpecum@umcutrecht.nl

Gastroenterol Clin N Am 39 (2010) 171–183
doi:10.1016/j.gtc.2010.02.010
0889-8553/10/$ – see front matter © 2010 Elsevier Inc. All rights reserved.

be kept in vesicles (ie, spherical bilayers of cholesterol and phospholipids, without bile salts) or in cholesterol crystals. Cholesterol crystal nucleation is thought to occur in general from vesicles supersaturated with cholesterol (ie, vesicular cholesterol/phospholipid ratio >1).[1] First, small unilamellar supersaturated vesicles aggregate or fuse into larger multilamellar vesicles ("liquid crystals"), with subsequent phase-separation of cholesterol crystals.[2] Pivotal information on the process of cholesterol crystal nucleation, the earliest step in cholesterol gallstone formation,[3] has been obtained from in vitro studies in model bile systems. Wang and Carey[4] found that cholesterol crystallization pathways and sequences in human gallbladder biles are identical to model biles matched for all relevant physical-chemical conditions, underlining the relevance of the model bile data. Based on these model bile data, the equilibrium bile salt–phospholipid–cholesterol ternary phase diagram was constructed, which allows one to predict behavior of mixtures of the three biliary lipids when present in various proportions.[5] As shown in **Fig. 1**, the phase diagram contains a bottom one-phase zone (only micelles);

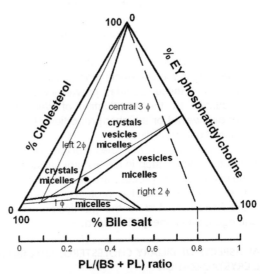

**Fig. 1.** Equilibrium bile salt–phospholipid–cholesterol phase diagram. The components are expressed in mol percent. Depicted are a one-phase (micellar) zone at the bottom; a left two-phase zone (containing micelles and crystals); a central three-phase zone (containing micelles, vesicles and crystals); and a right two-phase zone (containing micelles and vesicles). Phospholipid/(bile salt + phospholipid) ratios are given at the bottom axis, and going from left to right indicates increased relative amounts of phospholipids compared with bile salts, with increased vesicular cholesterol solubilization. Any line connecting the bottom axis with the top of the triangle (100% cholesterol) represents identical phospholipid/(bile salt + phospholipid) ratio, with increased relative amounts of cholesterol when moving from bottom to top. For example, in the Figure, all biles plotting on the coarse interrupted line exhibit identical phospholipid/(bile salt + phospholipid) ratio of 0.8. In the Figure, fine lines indicate zones in case of diluted bile, hydrophilic bile salts or saturated phospholipid acyl chains. Thick lines indicate zones in case of concentrated bile, hydrophobic bile salts, or unsaturated phospholipid acyl chains. Under the latter circumstances, cholesterol crystallization is promoted by an expansion of the crystal-containing zones to the right. The bile sample initially plotting in the right two-phase zone (indicated by the dot) now plots in the central three-phase zone (cholesterol crystal-containing zone), despite identical relative lipid composition.

a left two-phase (micelles and cholesterol crystals containing) zone; a central three-phase (micelles, vesicles, and cholesterol crystals containing) zone; and a right two-phase (micelles and vesicles containing) zone. Going from baseline to top in the phase diagram the relative percentage of cholesterol increases, with progressive tendency of cholesterol crystallization as a result. Second, a shift from left to right in the phase diagram increases relative amounts of phospholipids compared with bile salts, allowing more solubilization of cholesterol in vesicles, lower vesicular cholesterol/phospholipid ratios, and less cholesterol crystallization as a result. If gallstones are present in supersaturated bile, competition may occur between the gallstone surface (gallstone growth) and the surrounding bile for available cholesterol molecules.[6] Three factors strongly affect the ternary equilibrium bile salt–phospholipid–cholesterol ternary phase diagram, with potential consequences for in vivo cholesterol crystallization: (1) increased bile concentration, (2) increased bile salt hydrophobicity, and (3) phospholipids containing unsaturated acyl chains all strongly promote cholesterol crystallization. Corresponding effects on the ternary equilibrium bile salt–phospholipid–cholesterol ternary phase diagram are in all three cases an increase of the bottom one-phase (micellar) zone, an expansion of the cholesterol crystal–containing zones to the right, and a decrease of the vesicles-containing zones (see **Fig. 1**).[5,7]

## BILE CONCENTRATION

Water is a major component of bile. Significant net water absorption occurs during bile transfer through the bile ducts and during prolonged storage in the gallbladder. As a result, bile water content decreases from 97% weight in the bile ducts to 90% weight in the gallbladder. This threefold to fourfold concentration of bile enhances cholesterol crystallization and gallstone formation considerably.[8,9] During the process of bile formation, detergent bile salt monomers first induce formation of nascent cholesterol-phospholipid vesicles in the bile canalicular space. These vesicles are stable because they are relatively cholesterol-poor (cholesterol/phospholipid ratio <1), and cholesterol crystallization does not occur. During bile concentration in the bile ducts and gallbladder, mixed cholesterol–phospholipid–bile salt micelles are increasingly formed, because bile salt concentrations now progressively exceed critical micellar concentrations required for micelle formation. Cholesterol and phospholipid transfer then occurs from vesicles to these mixed micelles. Because solubilizing capacity of micelles for phospholipids is much higher than for cholesterol, however, there is preferential phospholipid transfer. Although fewer vesicles remain, they are now cholesterol supersaturated (ie, cholesterol/phospholipid ratio >1) and may nucleate cholesterol crystals. This sequence explains why gallstones are generally formed in the gallbladder rather than in the bile ducts.

## BILE SALT HYDROPHOBICITY

More hydrophobic bile salts strongly promote cholesterol crystallization, by affecting the ternary phase diagram in a similar way as bile concentration (increased micellar cholesterol solubilization, shift of crystal-containing zones to the right, cholesterol supersaturated vesicles, promotion of cholesterol crystallization[5]). In the animal kingdom, human bile exhibits the most hydrophobic bile salt composition, with strong propensity to gallstone formation. Nevertheless, there is considerable variation in hydrophobicity of human bile salt composition (especially amounts of deoxycholate). In gallbladder bile of cholesterol gallstone patients, increased amounts of the hydrophobic bile salt deoxycholate are associated with fast crystallization.[10] The primary bile salts cholate and chenodeoxycholate are synthesized from cholesterol in the liver, and secondary bile salts (mainly deoxycholate) are formed from primary bile salts in the intestine by bacterial 7α-dehydroxylase activity. Interestingly, gallstone patients exhibit larger amounts of bacteria and more 7α-dehydroxylase activity in cecal aspirates in conjunction with higher colonic pH values and prolonged small and large bowel transit times, all favoring solubilization and absorbtion of deoxycholate into the enterohepatic circulation.[11] Because of the presence of *Lith* genes, male C57L inbred mice are highly susceptible to cholesterol gallstone formation during lithogenic diet, provided that a hydrophobic biliary bile salt composition (quite hydrophilic at baseline) is obtained by dietary measures (15% fat, 1% cholesterol, 0.5% cholic acid), supporting a role for bile salt composition in gallstone formation.[12] Modulating biliary bile salt composition may have therapeutic consequences. In selected patients with cholesterol gallstones, treatment with the hydrophilic bile salt ursodeoxycholate may dissolve their stones. Under these circumstances, 30% to 60% of the total bile salt pool consists of ursodeoxycholate, with the result that cholesterol crystallization is inhibited.

## BILIARY PHOSPHOLIPID COMPOSITION

In in vitro studies with model biles, phospholipid class and phospholipid acyl chain composition exert profound effects on cholesterol crystallization. Similar to increased bile concentration and increased bile salt hydrophobicity, phospholipids with more unsaturated acyl chains affect the ternary equilibrium bile salt–phospholipid–cholesterol ternary phase diagram by increasing the bottom one-phase (micellar) zone, expanding the cholesterol crystal–containing zones to the right and decreasing the vesicles-containing zones, with the result that cholesterol supersaturated vesicles and cholesterol crystallization occur (see **Fig. 1**).[7] The underlying physical-chemical explanation for these findings is that phospholipids with saturated acyl chains by their "*trans*" configuration fit easily in the vesicular cholesterol-phospholipid bilayer, which is not the case for phospholipids with *cis*-unsaturated acyl chains with a bend in the molecule (leading to preferential micellar containment). Human biliary phospholipid composition is tightly regulated, however, and almost exclusively composed of phosphatidylcholine with unsaturated acyl chains (mainly 16:0 acyl chains on *sn*-1 position, 18:2 > 18:1 > 20:4 acyl chains on *sn*-2 position), contributing to human vulnerability for gallstone formation.[13] Although modification of biliary phospholipids toward a more saturated acyl chain composition is in theory attractive, dietary modifications to accomplish this have not been successful.

## BILIARY NUCLEATION PROMOTING AND INHIBITING PROTEINS

During the last decades, numerous biliary proteins have been suggested to enhance or inhibit cholesterol crystallization in gallbladder bile, based on their in vitro or ex vivo effects. Immunoglobulins M and G,[14,15] haptoglobin,[16] $\alpha_1$-acid glycoprotein,[17,18] aminopeptidase-N,[19] $\alpha_1$-antichymotrypsin, and mucin[20] are regarded as pronucleating proteins. By contrast, human apolipoprotein A-I[21] and IgA[22] have been postulated to exert antinucleating activity. Cholesterol crystallization often occurs much faster in bile of patients with (especially multiple) cholesterol stones than in bile of patients with pigment stones or subjects without stones, or in model biles, even in case of comparable relative lipid composition. Excess biliary pronucleating compared with crystallization-inhibiting proteins could contribute to this phenomenon. Nevertheless, in more recent years, a growing number of publications have marshaled experimental evidence arguing against a role of most of these biliary proteins in cholesterol gallstone formation. In a recent study on a large number of gallstone patients, cholesterol saturation was an independent predictor of speed of crystallization, which was not the case for biliary protein, immunoglobulins, $\alpha_1$-acid glycoprotein, or aminopeptidase-N content.[23] Also, Wang and coworkers[24] showed that after the extraction of biliary lipids from human bile and their reconstitution in buffer solution, the resulting model system displayed the same speed and pattern of crystallization as the original bile sample. Of note, whereas subsequent addition of purified concanavalin A–binding glycoprotein fraction did not affect speed of cholesterol crystallization, the nucleation process was markedly enhanced by adding purified mucin. Furthermore, in the inbred mouse model, most pronucleating proteins in bile (again with the exception of mucin) were found to decrease during the earliest stages of gallstone formation, arguing against an appreciable role of these biliary proteins in gallstone pathogenesis.[25] Mucin remains one of the few candidate proteins with a potential role in human gallstone formation. Marked hypersecretion of mucin occurs in the earliest stages of human and experimental gallstone formation.[12,20] Several MUC genes are expressed in human gallbladder mucosa, including MUC1, MUC2, MUC3, MUC4, MUC5AC, MUC5B, and MUC6. Upregulation of these MUC genes could lead to the observed increased gallbladder mucin concentrations. Mucin may increase bile viscosity leading to the formation of a gel matrix that can entrap cholesterol crystals in the gallbladder.[26] Mucin may also enhance cholesterol crystallization by offering low-affinity binding sites for cholesterol. Indeed, *Lith* genes have been identified that control mucin accumulation, cholesterol crystallization, and gallstone formation in the mouse model.[27,28] Also, decreasing biliary mucin content with aspirin decreases risk of gallstones in the prairie dog model[29] and risk of gallstone recurrence after nonsurgical treatment in humans.[30] Ursodeoxycholic acid also decreases biliary mucin contents.[31]

## GALLBLADDER AND INTESTINAL MOTILITY

Meal ingestion induces considerable gallbladder emptying (up to 70%–80% of fasting gallbladder volumes) by releasing the hormone cholecystokinin from the upper intestine. Impaired gallbladder emptying may prolong residence of bile in the gallbladder, allowing more time for nucleation of cholesterol crystals from supersaturated bile. Furthermore, in case of adequate emptying, cholesterol crystals that have nucleated may be ejected to the duodenum, whereas in case of impaired gallbladder emptying, these crystals may aggregate into macroscopic gallstones. Several studies have shown that gallstone patients may be divided into a group with severely impaired or even absent postprandial emptying ("bad contractors") and a group with good postprandial gallbladder emptying ("good contractors"). Patients with good postprandial contraction often have increased fasting and residual gallbladder volumes compared with normal controls.[32] Prospective studies also indicate that impaired postprandial gallbladder motility is an independent risk factor for gallstone recurrence after successful treatment with extracorporeal shockwave lithotripsy.[33] It is less well appreciated that significant periodic gallbladder emptying also occurs during the fasting state (20%–30% emptying in the fasting state vs 70%–80% emptying after a meal) at 1- to 2-hour intervals, associated with the cycle of the intestinal migrating motor complex and with a rise of plasma motilin levels.[34] It has been found that gallstone patients show a pattern of less frequent migrating motor complex cycles, with absent interdigestive gallbladder emptying and altered motilin release compared with controls.[35] A similarly prolonged migrating motor complex cycle has been found in the ground squirrel model of gallstone formation.[36] The fasting state (ie, the night) seems to be the most vulnerable period for gallstone formation. During this period, biliary cholesterol saturation is highest, because of relatively low bile salt secretion and relatively high cholesterol secretion. There is also a progressive concentration of gallbladder bile during this period, which is partially counteracted by periodic interdigestive gallbladder contraction in association with antral phase 3 of the migrating motor complex of the intestine.

There is increasing insight into pathogenesis of impaired gallbladder motility. Significant absorbtion of cholesterol seems to occur from supersaturated bile in the gallbladder.[37,38] Excess cholesterol is then incorporated within the sarcolemmal plasma membrane of the gallbladder smooth muscle cell, with decreased membrane fluidity, impaired contractility, and impaired relaxation as a result.[39] In addition, the gallbladder wall is exposed to detergent bile salts, unesterified cholesterol, and bacteria.[40,41] As a result, a proinflammatory Th1 immune response may occur, which contributes to hypomotility. Although impaired motility could be in many cases secondary to biliary cholesterol supersaturation, it may still facilitate the process of gallstone formation. Gallbladder motility is often impaired in high-risk situations for gallstone formation, such as pregnancy, obesity, diabetes mellitus, gastric surgery, treatment with the somatostatin analogue octreotide, very low calorie dieting, and total parenteral nutrition.

## PATHOPHYSIOLOGY OF CHOLESTEROL GALLSTONE FORMATION

It is not surprising, that in a polygenetic disorder as cholesterol gallstone disease, several underlying mechanisms may be involved in its pathogenesis. Nevertheless, the common theme remains excess biliary cholesterol compared with solubilizing bile salts or phospholipids. In Chilean patients (especially of Amerindian descent), increased bile salt and cholesterol synthesis have been reported.[42] The defect was supposed to be secondary to increased intestinal loss of bile salts, and preceded gallstone formation. Interestingly, decreased expression of ileal bile salt transport proteins apical sodium-dependent bile acid transporter, cytosolic ileal lipid binding protein, and basolateral organic solute transporter α and β were recently described in female nonobese patients as a possible explanation of these findings.[43,44] It has also been reported that high dietary cholesterol increases biliary cholesterol secretion and decreases bile acid synthesis and pool in cholesterol gallstone subjects but not in controls.[45] These findings point to the importance of intestinal cholesterol absorbtion in gallstone pathogenesis. Interestingly, increased expression of the intestinal cholesterol uptake protein NPC1L1 (Niemann-Pick C1–like protein 1) was recently reported in gallstone patients.[46] Also, inhibiting cholesterol absorbtion with etezimibe prevents gallstone formation in the mouse model and decreases biliary cholesterol saturation in gallstone patients with slower crystallization as a result.[47] Nevertheless, current evidence points to hepatic hypersecretion of cholesterol as the primary defect in most Western patients with cholesterol gallstones.[48] In vivo, biliary lipid composition is determined to a large extent at the level of the hepatocyte canalicular membrane. The process of nascent bile formation is maintained by an elaborate network of adenosine triphosphate–binding cassette (ABC) transporters in the hepatocyte canalicular membrane that regulate biliary secretion of cholesterol, bile salts, and phospholipids (**Fig. 2**). The *ABCG5/G8* genes encode protein half-transporters that heterodimerize to form the functional transporter localized in the canalicular membrane of hepatocytes and facilitating cholesterol secretion into bile.[49] Recently, in genome-wide association studies, the ABCG8 19H allele was found to be associated with gallstone formation.[50,51] ABCG5/G8 is also present in the intestine, and decreases net cholesterol absorbtion by transfer of cholesterol molecules taken up by the intestinal cell back to the lumen.[52] ABCG5/G8 polymorphisms associated with increased gallstone risk

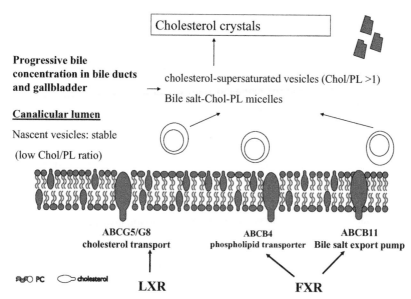

**Fig. 2.** Nascent bile formation at the hepatocytic canalicular membrane. ABCG5-G8 transports cholesterol into bile, and is regulated by nuclear receptor LXR. ABCB11 and ABCB4 transport bile salts and phosphatidylcholine into bile, and are regulated by nuclear receptor FXR. Excess hepatic cholesterol secretion or insufficient bile salt–phosphatidylcholine secretion lead to biliary cholesterol supersaturation. Subsequently, cholesterol supersaturated vesicles may form, which is promoted by bile concentration, hydrophobic bile composition, or unsaturated phospholipid acyl chains. Nucleation of cholesterol crystals may occur from aggregated or fused supersaturated vesicles.

could also affect intestinal cholesterol absorption. The bile salt export pump (current nomenclature ABCB11) pumps bile salts over the membrane into bile.[53] Severe mutations in ABCB11 lead to progressive intrahepatic cholestasis in the first decade of life that rapidly leads to liver failure (PFIC2), whereas less severe mutations may lead to benign recurrent cholestasis (BRIC2) and intermittent intractable pruritus. A considerable number of patients with BRIC2 exhibit associated gallstones, supposedly caused by insufficient amounts of biliary bile salts.[54] The human MDR3 (multidrug resistance 3) P-glycoprotein (current nomenclature ABCB4) functions as a "floppase," translocating phosphatidylcholine molecules from the inner to the outer leaflet of the canalicular membrane, enabling their secretion into bile.[55] Recently, a subset of gallstone patients has been identified with intrahepatic and bile duct stones at young age (<40 years) and high risk of recurrent biliary symptoms after cholecystectomy. The underlying pathogenetic mechanism of this so-called "low phospholipid-associated cholelithiasis" is thought to be relative biliary phospholipid deficiency caused by a missense mutation in the MDR3 gene.[56]

## NUCLEAR RECEPTORS AND CHOLESTEROL GALLSTONE FORMATION

In their turn, the lipid transport proteins in the hepatocytic canalicular membrane are regulated by nuclear receptors (see **Fig. 2**). Farnesoid X receptor ([FXR] NR1H4) is a member of the nuclear receptor superfamily[57] and functions as a bile salt receptor that regulates transcription of numerous genes involved in maintaining cholesterol and bile salt homeostasis.[58] The primary bile salt chenodeoxycholic acid is the highest affinity endogenous ligand characterized for FXR in the enterohepatic system.[59] In the liver, the activation of FXR by endogenous bile salts inhibits through intermediate small heterodimer partner the transcription of the gene encoding cholesterol 7α-hydroxylase, the rate-limiting enzyme in the major synthetic pathway of bile salts.[60] The FXR–small heterodimer partner signaling pathway is an important molecular basis for the feedback repression of bile salt synthesis. FXR has also been shown to regulate expression of ABCB11 and ABCB4, affecting amounts of solibilizing bile salts and phospholipids in bile. As expected, FXR "knockout" mice are highly susceptible to gallstone formation on a lithogenic diet, because of low relative amounts of biliary bile salts and phospholipids. Also, gallstone formation can be prevented in wild-type mice by the synthetic FXR agonist GW4064, because increased amounts of solubilizing bile salts and phospholipids prevent cholesterol supersaturation.[61] Data on role of FXR in human cholesterol gallstone formation are limited. FXR is also expressed in the ileal cell, and regulates activity of transport proteins involved in bile salt reabsorption into the enterohepatic circulation: apical sodium-dependent bile acid transporter, cytosolic ileal lipid binding protein, and basolateral organic solute transporter α and β. Decreased expression of these ileal transport proteins occurs in female nonobese gallstone patients, with an associated decreased expression of FXR.[43,44] Data on gene polymorphisms for FXR have revealed controversial results. In a Mexican population, the most common haplotype NR1H4_1 was associated with gallstone prevalence. In contrast, NR1H4_1 displayed no association with gallstone prevalence in a German population, whereas in a Chilean population a trend toward a protective effect of NR1H4_1 was observed.[62]

Another subfamily of nuclear receptors, liver X receptor (LXR), regulates expression of ABCG5/G8 cholesterol transport protein. In the murine model, activation of LXR increases risk of gallstone formation.[63] In a limited number of human gallstone patients, hepatic mRNA levels of ABCG5, ABCG8, and LXRα were increased by 51%, 59%, and 102%, respectively, and significantly correlated with cholesterol saturation index.[64] Further research is needed on the role of nuclear receptors in gallstone pathogenesis and the therapeutic feasibility of nuclear receptor agonists.

## PATHOGENESIS OF PIGMENT GALLSTONES

In the Western world, approximately 30% of gallstone carriers exhibit black pigment gallbladder stones (<20% cholesterol content). Whereas black gallbladder pigment stones are extremely rare below age 50 years, there is a progressive relative contribution of this stone type at older age.[65] In East Asia, there is a relatively high prevalence of brown pigment stones residing in the bile ducts, and causing potentially devastating cholangitis.

### Black Pigment Stones

Black pigment stones are formed in sterile bile in the gallbladder. In contrast to cholesterol gallstones, impaired gallbladder motility does not contribute to pathogenesis. Black pigment stones are primarily composed of calcium bilirubinate. Other important components are calcium carbonate and calcium phosphate in polymer-like complexes with mucin glycoproteins. Normally most bilirubin, the breakdown product of hemoglobin, is conjugated in the liver to bilirubin monoglucuronide and subsequently to water-soluble bilirubin diglucuronide. Unconjugated bilirubin is poorly soluble in water. In case of hemolysis, biliary excretion of bilirubin may increase 10-fold with increased risk of calcium bilirubinate precipitation. This phenomenon explains the high prevalence of black pigment stones in chronic hemolytic disorders, such as sickle cell anemia, hereditary spherocytosis, and Gilbert syndrome. Concomitant presence of Gilbert syndrome is associated with increased gallstone prevalence in sickle cell disease.[66] Evidence from experimental animal models indicates that enterohepatic cycling of bilirubin may contribute to high frequency of pigment stones in patients with ileal Crohn disease, especially in case of ileal resection. The proposed mechanism is that increased amounts of bile salts reach the cecum and solubilize unconjugated bilirubin, allowing their reabsorbtion with subsequent hyperbilirubinobilia.[67–69] A similar mechanism could contribute to increased incidence of pigment stones in patients with cystic fibrosis.[70] Interestingly, prevalence of Gilbert syndrome is increased in patients with cystic fibrosis and gallstones, suggesting that hemolysis could also contribute to pigment stone formation in this patient category.[71] Last, insufficient acidification of bile in the gallbladder and reduced buffering capacity of mucin gel also promote biliary calcium supersaturation and pigment stone formation.[72]

### Brown Pigment Stones

In contrast to black pigment stones, their brown pigment counterparts are formed in the bile ducts.[73] They are primarily composed of calcium salts of unconjugated bilirubin and varying amounts of cholesterol and protein. Brown pigment stones are associated with chronic bacterial infection of the bile ducts by *Escherichia coli*, *Bacteroides* spp, and *Clostridium* spp, and parasites *Opisthorchis veverrini*, *Clonorchis sinensis*, and *Ascaris lumbricoides*. Bacteria in the bile ducts produce β-glucoronidase, phospholipase A, and bile acid hydrolase leading to increased amounts of unconjugated bilirubin, palmitic and stearic acids, and unconjugated bile acids, which can complex with calcium, resulting in stone formation. Parasites in the bile ducts may stimulate stone formation by the calcified overcoat of the parasitis egg, which may serve as a nidus and enhance precipitation of calcium bilirubinate.

## REFERENCES

1. Somjen GJ, Gilat T. Contribution of vesicular and micellar carriers to cholesterol transport in human bile. J Lipid Res 1985;26:699–704.
2. Halpern Z, Dudley MA, Kibe A, et al. Rapid vesicle formation and aggregation in abnormal human biles: a time-lapse video-enhanced contrast microscopy study. Gastroenterology 1986;90:875–85.
3. Holan KR, Holzbach RT, Hermann RE, et al. Nucleation time: a key factor in the pathogenesis of cholesterol gallstone disease. Gastroenterology 1979;77: 611–7.
4. Wang DQH, Carey MC. Characterization of crystallization pathways during cholesterol precipitation from human gallbladder bile: identical pathways to corresponding model biles with three predominating sequences. J Lipid Res 1996; 37:2539–49.
5. Wang DQH, Carey MC. Complete mapping of crystallization pathways during cholesterol precipitation from model bile: influence of physical-chemical variables of pathophysiologic significance and identification of a stable liquid-crystalline state in cold, dilute and hydrophilic bile salt-containing systems. J Lipid Res 1996;37:606–30.
6. Venneman NG, van Kammen M, Renooij W, et al. Effects of hydrophobic and hydrophilic bile salts on gallstone growth and dissolution in model biles. Biochim Biophys Acta 2005;1686(3):209–19.

7. van Erpecum KJ, Carey MC. Influence of bile salts on molecular interactions between sphingomyelin and cholesterol: relevance to bile formation and stability. Biochim Biophys Acta 1997;1345:269–82.

8. van Erpecum KJ, vanBerge-Henegouwen GP, Stoelwinder B, et al. Bile concentration is a key factor for nucleation of cholesterol crystals and cholesterol saturation index in gallbladder bile of gallstone patients. Hepatology 1990;11:1–6.

9. van Erpecum KJ. Biliary lipids, water and cholesterol gallstones. Biol Cell 2005; 97(11):815–22.

10. Hussaini SH, Pereira SP, Murphy GM, et al. Deoxycholic acid influences cholesterol solubilization and microcrystal nucleation time in gallbladder bile. Hepatology 1995;22:1735–44.

11. Thomas LA, Veysey MJ, Bathgate T, et al. Mechanism for the transit-induced increase in colonic deoxycholic acid formation in cholesterol cholelithiasis. Gastroenterology 2000;119(3):806–15.

12. Wang DQH, Paigen B, Carey MC. Phenotypic characterization of Lith genes that determine susceptibility to cholesterol cholelithiasis in inbred mice: physical-chemistry of gallbladder bile. J Lipid Res 1997;38:1395–411.

13. Hay DW, Calahane MJ, Timofeyeva N, et al. Molecular species of lecithins in human gallbladder bile. J Lipid Res 1993;34:759–68.

14. Harvey PRC, Upadhya GA, Strasberg SM. Immunoglobulins as nucleating proteins in the gallbladder bile of patients with cholesterol gallstones. J Biol Chem 1991;266:13996–4003.

15. Abei M, Schwarzendrube J, Nuutinen H, et al. Cholesterol crystallization-promoters in human bile: comparative potencies of immunoglobulins, α1-acid glycoprotein, phospholipase C, and aminopeptidase N. J Lipid Res 1993;34:1141–8.

16. Yamashita G, Ginanni Corradini S, Secknus R, et al. Biliary haptoglobin, a potent promoter of cholesterol crystallization at physiological concentrations. J Lipid Res 1995;36:1325–33.

17. Abei M, Nuutinen H, Kawczak P, et al. Identification of human biliary α1-acid glycoprotein as a cholesterol crystallization promotor. Gastroenterology 1994; 106:231–8.

18. Nuutinen H, Corradini SG, Jüngst D, et al. Correlation between biliary α1-acid glycoprotein concentration and cholesterol crystal nucleation time in gallstone disease. Dig Dis Sci 1995;40:1174–8.

19. Offner GW, Gong D, Afdahl NH. Identification of a 130-kilodalton human biliary concanavalin A binding protein as aminopeptidase N. Gastroenterology 1994; 106:755–62.

20. Lee SM, LaMont JT, Carey MC. Role of gallbladder mucus hypersecretion in the evolution of cholesterol gallstones. Studies in the prairie dog. J Clin Invest 1981; 67:1712–23.

21. Kibe A, Holzbach RT, LaRusso NF, et al. Inhibition of cholesterol crystal formation by apolipoproteins in supersaturated model bile. Science 1984;255:514–6.

22. Busch N, Lammert F, Matern S. Biliary secretory immunoglobulin A is a major constituent of the new group of cholesterol crystal-binding proteins. Gastroenterology 1998;115:129–38.

23. Miquel JF, Nunez L, Amigo L, et al. Cholesterol saturation, not proteins or cholecystitis, is critical for crystal formation in human gallbladder bile. Gastroenterology 1998;114:1016–23.

24. Wang DQH, Cohen DE, Lammert F, et al. No pathophysiologic relationship of soluble biliary proteins to cholesterol crystallization in human bile. J Lipid Res 1999;40:415–25.

25. van Erpecum KJ, Wang DQ-H, Lammert F, et al. Phenotypic characterization of Lith genes that determine susceptibility to cholesterol cholelithiasis in inbred mice: soluble pronucleating proteins in gallbladder and hepatic biles. J Hepatol 2001;35:444–51.

26. Smith BF. Gallbladder mucin as a pronucleating agent for cholesterol monohydrate crystals in bile. Hepatology 1990;12:183S–6S.

27. Lammert F, Carey MC, Paigen B. Chromosomal organization of candidate genes involved in cholesterol gallstone formation: a murine gallstone map. Gastroenterology 2001;120:221–38.

28. Lammert F, Wang DQ, Wittenburg H, et al. Lith genes control mucin accumulation, cholesterol crystallization, and gallstone formation in A/J and AKR/J inbred mice. Hepatology 2002;36(5):1145–54.

29. Lee SP, Carey MC, LaMont JT. Aspirin prevention of cholesterol gallstone formation in prairie dogs. Science 1981;211:1429–31.

30. Hood K, Gleeson D, Ruppin DC, et al. Prevention of gallstone recurrence by non-steroidal anti- inflammatory drugs. Lancet 1988;2:1223–5.

31. van Erpecum KJ, Portincasa P, Eckhardt E, et al. Ursodeoxycholic acid reduces protein levels and nucleation-promoting activity in human gallbladder bile. Gastroenterology 1996;110:1225–37.

32. van Erpecum KJ, vanBerge-Henegouwen GP, Stolk MFJ, et al. Fasting gallbladder volume, postprandial emptying and cholecystokinin release in gallstone patients and normal subjects. J Hepatol 1992;14:194–202.

33. Pauletzki J, Althaus R, Holl J, et al. Gallbladder emptying and gallstone formation: a prospective study on gallstone recurrence. Gastroenterology 1996;111:765–71.

34. Stolk MFJ, van Erpecum KJ, Smout AJ, et al. Motor cycles with phase III in antrum are associated with high motilin levels and prolonged gallbladder emptying. Am J Physiol 1993;264:G596–600.

35. Stolk MF, van Erpecum KJ, Peeters TL, et al. Interdigestive gallbladder emptying, antroduodenal motility, and motilin release patterns are altered in cholesterol gallstone patients. Dig Dis Sci 2001;46(6):1328–34.

36. Xu Q-W, Scott RB, Tan DTM, et al. Altered migrating myoelectrical complex (MMC) in an animal model of cholesterol gallstone disease [abstract]. Gastroenterology 1997;112:A1417.

37. Corradini SG, Elisei W, Giovannelli L, et al. Impaired human gallbladder lipid absorption in cholesterol gallstone disease and its effect on cholesterol solubility in bile. Gastroenterology 2000;118(5):912–20.

38. Corradini SG, Ripani C, Della Guardia P, et al. The human gallbladder increases cholesterol solubility in bile by differential lipid absorption: a study using a new in vitro model of isolated intra-arterially perfused gallbladder. Hepatology 1998;28:314–22.

39. Yu P, Chen Q, Biancani P, et al. Excess membrane cholesterol impairs gallbladder muscle contraction. Gastroenterology 1995;108:A442.

40. van Erpecum KJ, Wang DQ, Moschetta A, et al. Gallbladder histopathology during murine gallstone formation: relation to motility and concentrating function. J Lipid Res 2006;47(1):32–41.

41. Maurer KJ, Carey MC, Fox JG. Roles of infection, inflammation, and the immune system in cholesterol gallstone formation. Gastroenterology 2009;136(2):425–40.

42. Galman C, Miquel JF, Perez RM, et al. Bile acid synthesis is increased in Chilean Hispanics with gallstones and in gallstone high-risk Mapuche Indians. Gastroenterology 2004;126(3):741–8.

43. Bergheim I, Harsch S, Mueller O, et al. Apical sodium bile acid transporter and ileal lipid binding protein in gallstone carriers. J Lipid Res 2006;47(1): 42–50.

44. Renner O, Harsch S, Strohmeyer A, et al. Reduced ileal expression of OSTalpha-OSTbeta in non-obese gallstone disease. J Lipid Res 2008;49(9):2045–54.

45. Kern F Jr. Effects of dietary cholesterol on cholesterol and bile acids homeostasis in patients with cholesterol gallstones. J Clin Invest 1994;93:1186–94.

46. Jiang ZY, Jiang CY, Wang L, et al. Increased NPC1L1 and ACAT2 expression in the jejunal mucosa from Chinese gallstone patients. Biochem Biophys Res Commun 2009;379(1):49–54.

47. Wang HH, Portincasa P, Mendez-Sanchez N, et al. Effect of ezetimibe on the prevention and dissolution of cholesterol gallstones. Gastroenterology 2008; 134(7):2101–10.

48. Wang DQ, Cohen DE, Carey MC. Biliary lipids and cholesterol gallstone disease. J Lipid Res 2009;50(Suppl):S406–11.

49. Yu L, Hammer RE, Li-Hawkins J, et al. Disruption of Abcg5 and Abcg8 in mice reveals their crucial role in biliary cholesterol secretion. Proc Natl Acad Sci U S A 2002;99(25):16237–42.

50. Buch S, Schafmayer C, Volzke H, et al. A genome-wide association scan identifies the hepatic cholesterol transporter ABCG8 as a susceptibility factor for human gallstone disease. Nat Genet 2007;39(8):995–9.

51. Grunhage F, Acalovschi M, Tirziu S, et al. Increased gallstone risk in humans conferred by common variant of hepatic ATP-binding cassette transporter for cholesterol. Hepatology 2007;46(3):793–801.

52. Berge KE, Tian H, Graf GA, et al. Accumulation of dietary cholesterol in sitosterolemia caused by mutations in adjacent ABC transporters. Science 2000; 290(5497):1771–5.

53. Gerloff T, Stieger B, Hagenbuch B, et al. The sister of P-glycoprotein represents the canalicular bile salt export pump of mammalian liver. J Biol Chem 1998;273: 10046–50.

54. van Mil SW, van der Woerd WL, van der BG, et al. Benign recurrent intrahepatic cholestasis type 2 is caused by mutations in ABCB11. Gastroenterology 2004; 127(2):379–84.

55. Smit JJM, Schinkel AH, Oude Elferink RPJ, et al. Homozygous disruption of the murine mdr2 P-glycoprotein gene leads to a complete absence of phospholipid from bile and to liver disease. Cell 1993;75:451–62.

56. Rosmorduc O, Hermelin B, Boelle PY, et al. ABCB4 gene mutation-associated cholelithiasis in adults. Gastroenterology 2003;125(2):452–9.

57. Mangelsdorf DJ, Thummel C, Beato M, et al. The nuclear receptor superfamily: the second decade. Cell 1995;83(6):835–9.

58. Lu TT, Repa JJ, Mangelsdorf DJ. Orphan nuclear receptors as eLiXiRs and FiXeRs of sterol metabolism. J Biol Chem 2001;276(41):37735–8.

59. Makishima M, Okamoto AY, Repa JJ, et al. Identification of a nuclear receptor for bile acids. Science 1999;284(5418):1362–5.

60. Lu TT, Makishima M, Repa JJ, et al. Molecular basis for feedback regulation of bile acid synthesis by nuclear receptors. Mol Cell 2000;6(3):507–15.

61. Moschetta A, Bookout AL, Mangelsdorf DJ. Prevention of cholesterol gallstone disease by FXR agonists in a mouse model. Nat Med 2004;10(12):1352–8.

62. Kovacs P, Kress R, Rocha J, et al. Variation of the gene encoding the nuclear bile salt receptor FXR and gallstone susceptibility in mice and humans. J Hepatol 2008;48(1):116–24.

63. Uppal H, Zhai Y, Gangopadhyay A, et al. Activation of liver X receptor sensitizes mice to gallbladder cholesterol crystallization. Hepatology 2008;47(4): 1331–42.

64. Jiang ZY, Parini P, Eggertsen G, et al. Increased expression of LXR alpha, ABCG5, ABCG8, and SR-BI in the liver from normolipidemic, nonobese Chinese gallstone patients. J Lipid Res 2008;49(2):464–72.

65. van Erpecum KJ, vanBerge-Henegouwen GP, Stoelwinder B, et al. Cholesterol and pigment gallstone disease: comparison of the reliability of three bile tests for differentiation between the two stone types. Scand J Gastroenterol 1988;23: 948–54.

66. Haverfield EV, McKenzie CA, Forrester T, et al. UGT1A1 variation and gallstone formation in sickle cell disease. Blood 2005;105(3):968–72.

67. Brink MA, Mendez-Sanchez N, Carey MC. Bilirubin cycles enterohepatically after ileal resection in the rat. Gastroenterology 1996;110(6):1945–57.

68. Mendez-Sanchez N, Brink MA, Paigen B, et al. Ursodeoxycholic acid and cholesterol induce enterohepatic cycling of bilirubin in rodents. Gastroenterology 1998; 115(3):722–32.

69. Brink MA, Slors JF, Keulemans YC, et al. Enterohepatic cycling of bilirubin: a putative mechanism for pigment gallstone formation in ileal Crohn's disease. Gastroenterology 1999;116(6):1420–7.

70. Freudenberg F, Broderick AL, Yu BB, et al. Pathophysiological basis of liver disease in cystic fibrosis employing a DeltaF508 mouse model. Am J Physiol Gastrointest Liver Physiol 2008;294(6):G1411–20.

71. Wasmuth HE, Keppeler H, Herrmann U, et al. Coinheritance of Gilbert syndrome-associated UGT1A1 mutation increases gallstone risk in cystic fibrosis. Hepatology 2006;43(4):738–41.

72. Gleeson D, Hood KA, Murphy GM, et al. Calcium and carbonate ion concentrations in gallbladder and hepatic bile. Gastroenterology 1992;102:1707–16.

73. Lambou-Gianoukos S, Heller SJ. Lithogenesis and bile metabolism. Surg Clin North Am 2008;88(6):1175–94, vii.

# *Lith* Genes and Genetic Analysis of Cholesterol Gallstone Formation

Helen H. Wang, MS[a], Piero Portincasa, MD, PhD[b],
Nezam H. Afdhal, MD[c], David Q.H. Wang, MD, PhD[d],*

**KEYWORDS**

- Bile • Cholesterol • Lipid transporter • Liquid crystal
- *Lith* gene • Micelle • Mucin • Nucleation

Cholesterol cholelithiasis is one of the most prevalent digestive diseases, resulting in a considerable financial and social burden worldwide. In the United States, at least 20 million Americans (12% of adults) are affected.[1,2] Each year, approximately 1 million new cases are discovered, and more than 700,000 cholecystectomies are performed, making this one of the most common elective abdominal operations.[1] Although many gallstones are silent, approximately one-third eventually cause symptoms and complications. In addition, the unavoidable complications result in 3000 deaths (0.12% of all deaths) annually. In the year 2000, more than 750,000 outpatient clinic visits and more than 250,000 hospitalizations were the result of gallstone-induced gastrointestinal symptoms.[3] As a result, there was a median inpatient charge of $11,584, and medical expenses for the treatment of gallstones exceeded $6 billion.[1] Because the prevalence of gallstones is increasing because of the worldwide obesity epidemic with

This work was supported in part by research grants DK54012 and DK73917 (DQ-HW) from the National Institutes of Health (US Public Health Service), and FIRB 2003 RBAU01RANB002 (PP) from the Italian Ministry of University and Research. PP was a recipient of the short-term mobility grant 2005 from the Italian National Research Council (CNR).

[a] Liver Center and Gastroenterology Division, Department of Medicine, Beth Israel Deaconess Medical Center, Harvard Medical School, 330 Brookline Avenue, DA 601, Boston, MA 02215, USA

[b] Department of Internal Medicine and Public Medicine, Clinica Medica "A. Murri," University of Bari Medical School, Policlinico Hospital, Piazza Giulio Cesare 11, 70124 Bari, Italy

[c] Liver Center and Gastroenterology Division, Department of Medicine, Beth Israel Deaconess Medical Center, Harvard Medical School, 110 Francis Street, Suite 8E, Boston, MA 02215, USA

[d] Liver Center and Gastroenterology Division, Department of Medicine, Beth Israel Deaconess Medical Center, Harvard Medical School and Harvard Digestive Diseases Center, 330 Brookline Avenue, DA 601, Boston, MA 02215, USA

* Corresponding author.

*E-mail address:* dqwang@caregroup.harvard.edu

associated insulin resistance, a key feature of the metabolic syndrome, it is imperative to find potential ways to prevent the formation of gallstones.[4,5]

During the past 50 years, it has been established that the primary pathophysiologic defect in most cholelithogenic humans is hepatic hypersecretion of biliary cholesterol, which may be accompanied by normal, high, or (less commonly) low secretion rates of biliary bile salts or phospholipids, inducing unphysiological cholesterol supersaturation of gallbladder bile.[2] Recent studies on humans and mouse models have shown that interactions of 5 defects (**Fig. 1**) result in nucleation and crystallization of cholesterol monohydrate crystals in bile and eventually gallstone formation.[6] These are (1) genetic factors and *Lith* genes; (2) unphysiological supersaturation with cholesterol due to hepatic hypersecretion of biliary lipids; (3) accelerated phase transitions of cholesterol; (4) dysfunctional gallbladder motility accompanied by immune-mediated gallbladder inflammation, as well as hypersecretion of mucins and accumulation of

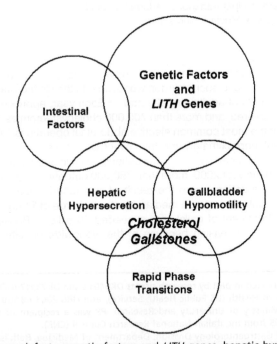

**Fig. 1.** Five primary defects: genetic factors and *LITH* genes, hepatic hypersecretion, gallbladder hypomotility, rapid phase transitions, and intestinal factors. The hypothesis is that hepatic cholesterol hypersecretion into bile is the primary defect and is the outcome in part of a complex genetic predisposition. The downstream effects include gallbladder hypomotility and rapid phase transitions. A major result of gallbladder hypomotility is alteration in the kinetics of the enterohepatic circulation of bile salts (intestinal factors), resulting in increased cholesterol absorption and reduced bile salt absorption that lead to abnormal enterohepatic circulation of bile salts and diminished biliary bile salt pool size. Gallbladder hypomotility facilitates nucleation and allows the gallbladder to retain cholesterol monohydrate crystals. Although a large number of candidate *Lith* genes have been identified in mouse models, the identification of human *LITH* genes in humans and their contributions to gallstones require further investigation. (*From* Wang DQ-H, Afdhal NH. Gallstone disease. In: Feldman M, Friedman LS, Brandt LJ, editors. Sleisenger and Fordtran's gastrointestinal and liver disease. 9th edition. Philadelphia: Elsevier; 2010; with permission.)

mucin gel in the gallbladder lumen; and (5) increased amounts of cholesterol from the intestinal source due to high efficiency of cholesterol absorption or slow intestinal motility which aids hydrophobe absorption and augments second bile salt synthesis by the anaerobic microflora. Growth of solid platelike cholesterol monohydrate crystals to form gallstones is a consequence of persistent hepatic hypersecretion of biliary cholesterol together with gallbladder mucin hypersecretion and gel formation and with incomplete evacuation by the gallbladder as a result of its impaired motility function.

Epidemiologic investigations, clinical observations, and family and twin studies in humans, as well as gallstone prevalence investigations in inbred mouse models, have clearly shown that a complex genetic basis could play a key role in determining individual predisposition to develop cholesterol gallstones in response to environmental factors.[7] A powerful genetic technique, quantitative trait locus (QTL) analysis has been successfully used to identify, localize, and analyze the lithogenic effects of pathophysiologically relevant gallstone (*Lith*) genes in inbred strains of mice.[8] These genetic analyses of cholesterol gallstones in mice have provided many novel insights into the complex pathophysiological mechanisms that are involved in the formation of cholesterol gallstones in humans. On the basis of these studies, a new view has been proposed that hepatic hypersecretion of biliary cholesterol could be induced by multiple *Lith* genes in mice and humans, as well as insulin resistance as part of the metabolic syndrome, all interacting with cholelithogenic environmental factors to cause the phenotype. This review summarizes recent progress in searching for *Lith* genes by a strategy of the combined genomic and phenotypic studies in inbred strains of mice, which has been proven to be a powerful approach to understand the complex pathophysiology of this common disease, as well as in elucidating the genetic mechanisms of cholesterol gallstone disease in humans.

## QTL STUDY AND *LITH* GENES IN MICE

In 1964, Tepperman and colleagues[9] first established a mouse model of cholesterol gallstones by feeding a special lithogenic diet containing 1% cholesterol and 0.5% cholic acid. Later, Fujihira and colleagues[10] found that at 8 weeks on the lithogenic diet, gallstone prevalence rates varied from 0% to 100% in 7 strains of mice. Alexander and Portman[11] further observed that feeding the lithogenic diet for a longer time, from 8 weeks to 12 weeks, strain differences in gallstone formation still existed in mice. Khanuja and colleagues[8] also found a striking strain difference in gallstone prevalence rates in 9 strains of inbred mice. By using a mouse backcross strategy and QTL analysis, they observed that differences in gallstone susceptibility between gallstone-susceptible C57L/J and resistant AKR/J strains were determined by at least 2 *Lith* genes, with *Lith1* (for lithogenic gene 1) and *Lith2* mapping on mouse chromosomes 2 and 19, respectively.[8] These studies show that the mouse is an excellent model for gallstone studies and also permits the investigation of genetics of cholesterol cholelithiasis.

On the basis of these mouse studies, it has been proposed that cholesterol gallstone formation is most likely to result from complex interactions of environmental factors and the effects of multiple, but as yet unknown, genes.[7,12,13] Thus, methods for studying genetics of gallstones, a complex genetic trait, could differ from those that are used to discover genes for simple Mendelian defects. To study quantitative polygenic traits, conventional genetic mapping methods are inadequate because they are designed for single-gene traits. As a result, genetic analysis of affected sibling pairs or families is hampered by multiple modes of inheritance of the trait, genetic heterogeneity, and large variations in environmental conditions. It has been proposed[7] that the strategy for identifying the genetic defects underlying the metabolic abnormalities in cholesterol gallstones in inbred strains of mice includes the following steps: (1) QTL analysis in inbred mice with different gallstone prevalence is performed to identify the chromosomal regions that contain *Lith* genes; (2) all candidate genes in regions that have putative lithogenic effects, and that are colocated with the chromosomal regions of the QTLs, are determined; and (3) the candidate genes are individually evaluated by studying their lithogenic actions in knockout, transgenic, or congenic mice, and, accordingly, their cholelithogenic mechanisms are identified at a molecular level.

The QTL technique provides a useful and powerful method that can be used to identify, locate, and analyze the lithogenic effects of candidate genes in several chromosomal regions.[8,14–16] An additional advantage of the QTL technique is that it can be used to discover new genes, whereas knockout and transgenic mice usually provide information only on known genes. The QTL method is used to investigate linkages of the candidate genes to polymorphic genetic markers on the mouse genome. The polymorphic genetic markers are short, variable DNA sequences (ie, microsatellite markers) or even single nucleotides that differ among inbred strains of mice.[17–19] During the past decades, a systematic mapping of murine genes relevant to the phenotypes of common diseases became possible with the construction of a dense genetic map that consists of thousands of microsatellite markers with known chromosomal localizations.[20,21] The goal of QTL analysis is to identify the genes underlying these polygenic traits and to gain a better understanding of their lithogenic actions on gallstone formation.

The first QTL analysis of cholesterol gallstones was successfully performed between inbred strains of C57L/J and AKR/J mice.[8,22] The results from this study showed that (1) gallstone susceptibility in the C57L/J strain is determined by at least 2 unlinked genes; (2) 2 major genes, designated *Lith1* and *Lith2*, are mapped on mouse chromosomes 2 and 19, respectively; and (3) gallstone formation is determined by a dominant trait. Additional QTLs in other strains of inbred mice with different susceptibility to gallstones have been investigated, and so far, 25 *Lith* genes have been identified, which are distributed from chromosomes 1 to X, designated *Lith1* to *Lith25*.[7,12,13,23,24]

Compared with AKR/J mice,[25,26] C57L/J mice of both genders displayed biliary cholesterol hypersecretion, early cholesterol supersaturation, accumulation of mucin gel, large gallbladder size, rapid cholesterol crystallization, and early onset and high gallstone prevalence rate.[22,25,27] On the lithogenic diet, C57L/J mice failed to down-regulate activities of hepatic 3-hydroxy-3-methylglutaryl coenzyme A (HMG-CoA) reductase controlling cholesterol biosynthesis, and cholesterol 7$\alpha$-hydroxylase and sterol 27-hydroxylase, regulatory enzymes in 2 bile salt synthesis pathways, became profoundly suppressed.[26] The biliary secretion study found that there is absolute and relative biliary cholesterol hypersecretion leading to increased cholesterol saturation index in the face of upregulated bile salt and phospholipid secretion rates in C57L/J mice. C57L/J mice displayed significantly greater absorption of cholesterol from the small intestine, more rapid plasma clearance of chylomicrons and chylomicron remnants, higher activities of lipoprotein lipase and hepatic lipase, greater hepatic uptake of chylomicron remnants, and faster secretion of chylomicron remnant cholesterol from plasma into bile.[28] This finding shows that cholesterol absorbed from the intestine provides an important source for biliary hypersecretion. These data provide important clues for further exploring the roles of *Lith* genes in pathogenesis of cholesterol cholelithiasis, and for investigating the phenotypes of individual *Lith* genes.

To confirm whether *Lith1* and *Lith2* could induce gallstones, congenic strains that carry the C57L/J alleles only in the *Lith1* or the *Lith2* regions on an AKR/J genetic background were created.[29] *Lith1* and *Lith2* congenic strains showed gallstone formation comparable with the C57L/J parent, confirming that the *Lith1* and the *Lith2* QTL regions can cause gallstones.[29] It was found that (1) *Lith1* plays a predominant role in determining biliary cholesterol hypersecretion and cholesterol gallstone formation because the gallstone and biliary phenotypes in the *Lith1* congenic strain are similar to those in the C57L/J parent; and (ii) *Lith2*, but not *Lith1*, influences bile salt–independent bile flow.

## CANDIDATE GENES FOR CHOLESTEROL GALLSTONES IN MICE

On the basis of the pathophysiology of cholesterol gallstones, **Table 1** summarizes major classes of candidate genes for *Lith* genes,[7] which could have an important effect on gallstone formation in mice. Lithogenic actions of some candidate genes have not yet been identified, and their roles in cholelithogenesis need to be investigated further. Genetic factors contributing to cholesterol gallstones include candidate genes that encode (1) hepatic and intestinal lipid transporters on the apical and basolateral membranes; (2) hepatic and intestinal lipid regulatory enzymes; (3) hepatic and intestinal intracellular lipid transporters; (4) hepatic and intestinal lipid regulatory transcription factors; (5) hepatic lipoprotein receptors and related proteins; (6) nuclear receptors in the liver and small intestine; (7) hormone receptors in the gallbladder; and (8) biliary mucins. **Fig. 2** illustrates the locations of *Lith* genes and the candidate genes on mouse chromosomes.

The liver is a main organ regulating cholesterol and bile salt metabolism. Although the source of cholesterol destined for biliary secretion is not fully known, increased biliary cholesterol secretion may result from increases in hepatic cholesterol biosynthesis, and the uptake of high-density lipoprotein (HDL) and low-density lipoprotein (LDL) from plasma, as well as decreases in the conversion of cholesterol into bile salts, and the esterification of cholesterol.[5] The amount of phospholipids and bile salts, as well as the composition of secreted bile salts, are important for the regulation of cholesterol secretion into bile, suggesting that any alterations in these factors may induce cholesterol saturation of bile and the formation of cholesterol gallstones.[2]

Cholesterol gallstones are more common in women than men, and exposure to oral contraceptive steroids and conjugated estrogens increases the risk for gallstones.[30–34] Wang and colleagues[35] observed that estrogen enhances cholesterol cholelithogenesis by augmenting functions of hepatic estrogen receptor α (ERα), but not ERβ. In the liver there is a possible estrogen-ERα-SREBP-2 pathway promoting cholesterol biosynthesis and hepatic secretion of biliary cholesterol.[36] The negative-feedback regulation of cholesterol biosynthesis is inhibited by ERα, which is activated by estrogen, mostly through stimulating the activity of sterol regulatory element-binding protein-2 (SREBP-2) with the resulting activation of the SREBP-2–responsive genes for the cholesterol biosynthetic pathway. Consequently, these alterations induce excess secretion of newly synthesized cholesterol and supersaturation of bile that predisposes to cholesterol precipitation and gallstone formation. The hepatic ERα activated by estrogen could stimulate the activity of ATP-binding cassette (ABC) transporter ABCG5 and ABCG8 on the canalicular membrane of the hepatocyte, and promote biliary cholesterol secretion.[37] These lithogenic effects of estrogen are inhibited by the antiestrogenic compound ICI 182,780. In addition, the estrogen effects on increasing cholesterol biosynthesis and promoting gallstone formation are, in part, blocked by deletion of the *ERα* gene. These findings may offer a new approach to treat gallstones by inhibiting hepatic ER activity with a liver-specific, ERα-selective antagonist.

**Table 1**
**The candidate gallstone genes in the mouse**

| Gene Symbol[a] | Gene Name | Mouse Chr[b] | cM | Human Ortholog |
|---|---|---|---|---|
| **A. Liver** | | | | |
| **(i) Lipid membrane transporters** | | | | |
| ABCG5 and ABCG8 | ATP-binding cassette sterol transporters G5 and G8 | 17 | 54.5 | 2p21 |
| ABCB4 (MDR2) | Phosphatidylcholine transporter (multiple drug resistance 2) | 5 | 1.0 | 7q21.1 |
| ABCB11 (BSEP, SPGP) | Bile salt export pump (Sister of P-glycoprotein) | 2 | 38.4 | 2q24 |
| ABCC2 (CMOAT, MRP2) | Canalicular multispecific organic anion transporter (multidrug resistance-related protein 2) | 19 | 43.0 | 10q24 |
| SLC10A1 (NTCP) | Sodium/taurocholate cotransporting polypeptide | 12 | 37.0 | 14q24.1 |
| SLC21A1 (OATP1) | Organic anion transporting polypeptide 1 | 6 | A3-A5 | ND |
| SLC22A1 (OCT1, ORCT) | Organic cation transporter 1 | 17 | 7.34 | 6q26 |
| ATP8B1 (FIC1) | Familial intrahepatic cholestasis type 1 | 18 | ND | 18q21-q22 |
| NPC1L1 | Niemann-Pick C1 like 1 protein | 11 | ND | 7p13 |
| **(ii) Lipid regulatory enzymes** | | | | |
| CYP7A1 | Cholesterol 7α-hydroxylase | 4 | ND | 8q11-q12 |
| CYP7B1 | Oxysterol 7α-hydroxylase | 3 | 1.0 | 8q21.3 |
| CYP27A1 | Sterol 27-hydroxylase | 1 | 43.1 | 2q33 |
| HMGCR | 3-Hydroxy-3-methyglutaryl-coenzyme A reductase | 13 | 49.0 | 5q13.3-q14 |
| SOAT2 (ACAT2) | Sterol O-acyltransferase 2 (acyl-coenzyme A:cholesterol acyltransferase 2) | 15 | 61.7 | 12q13.13 |
| **(iii) Intracellular lipid transporters** | | | | |
| CAV1 | Caveolin 1 | 6 | A2[c] | 7q31.1 |
| CAV2 | Caveolin 2 | 6 | A2 | 7q31.1 |
| FABP1 | Fatty acid-binding protein 1, liver | 6 | 30.0 | 2p11 |
| NPC1 | Niemann-Pick type C1 | 18 | 4.0 | 18q11-q12 |
| OSBP | Oxysterol-binding protein | 19 | 7.0 | 11q12-q13 |
| PCTP | Phosphatidylcholine transfer protein | 11 | 52.0 | 17q21-q24 |
| SCP2 | Sterol carrier protein 2 | 4 | 52.0 | 1p32 |

**(iv) Lipid regulatory transcription factors**

| | | | | |
|---|---|---|---|---|
| *NR2B1 (RXRα)* | Retinoid X receptor α | 2 | 17.0 | 9q34.3 |
| *NR1H3 (LXRα)* | Liver X receptor α | 2 | 40.4 | 11p11.2 |
| *NR1H2 (LXRβ)* | Liver X receptor β | 7 | ND | 19q13.3 |
| *NR1H4 (FXR)* | Farnesoid X receptor | 10 | 50.0 | 12q23.1 |
| *NR1C1 (PPARα)* | Peroxisomal proliferator activated receptor α | 15 | 48.8 | 22q13.31 |
| *NR1C2 (PPARδ)* | Peroxisomal proliferator activated receptor δ | 17 | 13.5 | 6p21.2-p21.1 |
| *NR1C3 (PPARγ)* | Peroxisomal proliferator activated receptor γ | 6 | 52.7 | 3p25 |
| *NR0B2 (SHP)* | Small heterodimer partner | 4 | 60.0 | 1p36.1 |
| *NR1I3 (CAR)* | Constitutive androstane receptor | 1 | 92.6 | 1q23.3 |
| *SREBF1* | Sterol regulatory element binding transcription factor 1 | 11 | ND | 17p11.2 |
| *SREBF2* | Sterol regulatory element binding transcription factor 2 | 15 | ND | 22q13 |
| *SCAP* | SREBF cleavage activating protein | 9 | 58.0 | 3p21.3 |
| *ESR1 (ERα)* | Estrogen receptor α | 10 | 12.0 | 6q25.1 |
| *ESR2 (ERβ)* | Estrogen receptor β | 12 | 33.0 | 14q23.2 |

**(v) Lipoprotein receptors and related genes**

| | | | | |
|---|---|---|---|---|
| *APOB100* | Apolipoprotein B100 | 12 | 2.0 | 2p24-p23 |
| *APOE* | Apolipoprotein E | 7 | 4.0 | 19q13.2 |
| *LRP1* | LDLR-related protein 1 | 10 | B2-D1 | 12q13-q14 |
| *LRP2 (GP330)* | LDLR-related protein 2 (Megalin, Glycoprotein 330) | 2 | 40.0 | 2q24-q31 |
| *LDLR* | Low density lipoprotein receptor | 9 | 5.0 | 19p13.3 |
| *SRB1* | Scavenger receptor class B type I | 5 | 68.0 | 12q24.31 |
| *LPL* | Lipoprotein lipase | 8 | 33.0 | 8p22 |
| *LIPC (HPL)* | Hepatic lipase | 9 | 39.0 | 15q21-q23 |
| *LCAT* | Lecithin cholesterol acyltransferase | 8 | 53.0 | 16q22.1 |
| *LRPAP1* | LRP-associated protein 1 | 5 | 20.0 | 4p16.3 |
| *PLTP* | Phospholipid transfer protein | 2 | 93.0 | 20q12-q13.1 |

*(continued on next page)*

**Table 1**
*(continued)*

| Gene Symbol[a] | Gene Name | Mouse Chr[b] | cM | Human Ortholog |
|---|---|---|---|---|
| **B. Gallbladder** | | | | |
| (i) Hormone receptors | | | | |
| CCK | Cholecystokinin | 9 | 71.0 | 3p22-p21.3 |
| CCK1R (CCKAR) | Cholecystokinin-1 receptor (CCK-A receptor) | 5 | 34.0 | 4p15.1-p15.2 |
| ESR1 (ERα) | Estrogen receptor α | 10 | 12.0 | 6q25.1 |
| ESR2 (ERβ) | Estrogen receptor β | 12 | 33.0 | 14q23.2 |
| PGR | Progesterone receptor | 9 | ND | 11q22-q23 |
| (ii) Mucin | | | | |
| MUC1 | Mucin 1 | 3 | 44.8 | 1q21 |
| MUC3 | Mucin 3 | 5 | 75 | 7q22 |
| MUC4 | Mucin 4 | 16 | ND | 3q29 |
| MUC5AC | Mucin 5ac | 7 | 69.0 | 11p15.5 |
| MUC5B | Mucin 5b | 7 | 69.0 | 11p15.5 |
| MUC6 | Mucin 6 | 7 | 69.0 | 11p15.5 |
| (iii) Lipid membrane transporters | | | | |
| ABCG5 and ABCG8 | ATP-binding cassette sterol transporters G5 and G8 | 17 | 54.5 | 2p21 |
| SRB1 | Scavenger receptor class B type I | 5 | 68.0 | 12q24.31 |
| (iv) Lipid regulatory enzymes | | | | |
| HMGCR | 3-Hydroxy-3-methylglutaryl-coenzyme A reductase | 13 | 49.0 | 5q13.3-q14 |
| SOAT2 (ACAT2) | Sterol O-acyltransferase 2 (acyl-coenzyme A:cholesterol acyltransferase 2) | 15 | 61.7 | 12q13.13 |
| **C. Small intestine** | | | | |
| (i) Lipid membrane transporters | | | | |
| ABCG5 and ABCG8 | ATP-binding cassette sterol transporters G5 and G8 | 17 | 54.5 | 2p21 |
| SRB1 | Scavenger receptor class B type I | 5 | 68.0 | 12q24.31 |
| SLC10A2 (IBAT) | Ileal (apical) sodium/bile salt transporter | 8 | 20 | 13q33 |

| | | Chr | cM | Human location |
|---|---|---|---|---|
| **(ii) Lipid regulatory enzymes** | | | | |
| HMGCR | 3-Hydroxy-3-methylglutaryl-coenzyme A reductase | 13 | 49.0 | 5q13.3-q14 |
| SOAT2 (ACAT2) | Sterol O-acyltransferase 2 (acyl-coenzyme A:cholesterol acyltransferase 2) | 15 | 61.7 | 12q13.13 |
| **(iii) Intracellular lipid transporters** | | | | |
| CAV1 | Caveolin 1 | 6 | A2 | 7q31.1 |
| CAV2 | Caveolin 2 | 6 | A2 | 7q31.1 |
| FABP6 (ILLBP) | Fatty acid-binding protein 6, ileal | 11 | 24.0 | 5q33.3-q34 |
| OSBP | Oxysterol-binding protein | 19 | 7.0 | 11q12-q13 |
| SCP2 | Sterol carrier protein 2 | 4 | 52.0 | 1p32 |
| NPC1L1 | Niemann-Pick C1 like 1 protein | 11 | ND | 7p13 |
| APOB48 | Apolipoprotein B48 | 12 | 2.0 | 2p24-p23 |
| APOAI | Apolipoprotein AI | 9 | 27.0 | 11q23-q24 |
| APOAIV | Apolipoprotein AIV | 9 | 27.0 | 11q23 |
| APOCIII | Apolipoprotein CIII | 9 | 27.0 | 11q23.1-q23.2 |
| **(iv) Lipid regulatory transcription factors** | | | | |
| NR2B1 (RXRα) | Retinoid X receptor α | 2 | 17.0 | 9q34.3 |
| NR1H3 (LXRα) | Liver X receptor α | 2 | 40.4 | 11p11.2 |
| NR1H2 (LXRβ) | Liver X receptor β | 7 | ND | 19q13.3 |
| NR1H4 (FXR) | Farnesoid X receptor | 10 | 50.0 | 12q23.1 |
| NR1C1 (PPARα) | Peroxisomal proliferator activated receptor α | 15 | 48.8 | 22q13.31 |
| NR1C2 (PPARδ) | Peroxisomal proliferator activated receptor δ | 17 | 13.5 | 6p21.2-p21.1 |
| NR1C3 (PPARγ) | Peroxisomal proliferator activated receptor γ | 6 | 52.7 | 3p25 |
| ESR1 (ERα) | Estrogen receptor α | 10 | 12.0 | 6q25.1 |
| ESR2 (ERβ) | Estrogen receptor β | 12 | 33.0 | 14q23.2 |

*Abbreviations:* Chr, chromosome; cM, centimorgan; p, short arm of the Chr; q, long arm of the Chr.

[a] Former gene symbols and names are given in the parentheses.

[b] Map position is based on conserved homology between mouse and human genomes and assigned indirectly from localization in other species. Information on homologous regions was retrieved from the mouse/human homology databases maintained at the Jackson Laboratory (http://www.informatics.jax.org/searches/marker_form.shtml) and the National Center for Biotechnology Information (http://www.ncbi.nlm.nih.gov/HomoloGene).

[c] As inferred from conserved map locations in mouse and human genomes, the mouse gene might be localized on proximal Chr 2 band A2.

*Adapted from* Wang DQ-H, Afdhal NH. Genetic analysis of cholesterol gallstone formation: searching for Lith (gallstone) genes. Curr Gastroenterol Rep 2004;6(2):140–50; with permission.

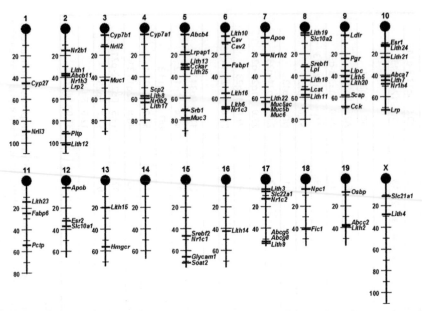

**Fig. 2.** Quantitative trait loci (QTLs) for *Lith* genes, as well as candidate gallstone genes for cholesterol gallstone formation on chromosomes representing the entire mouse genome. A vertical line represents each chromosome, with the centromere at the top; genetic distances from the centromere (*horizontal black lines*) are indicated to the left of the chromosomes in centimorgans (cM). Gallstone QTLs (*Lith* genes) and candidate gene locations are indicated by horizontal black lines with the gene symbols to the right (see **Table 2** for list of gene symbols and names). (*From* Wang DQ-H, Afdhal NH. Genetic analysis of cholesterol gallstone formation: searching for Lith (gallstone) genes. Curr Gastroenterol Rep 2004; 6(2):140–50; with permission.)

Deletion of the farnesoid X receptor (*Fxr*) gene increases susceptibility to the formation of gallstones in mice.[38] In contrast, treatment with a synthetic FXR agonist could prevent gallstones, even in gallstone-susceptible C57L/J mice that recapitulate human gallstone disease. These antilithogenic effects are mediated by FXR-dependent increases in biliary bile salt and phospholipid concentrations, which restore cholesterol solubility and thereby prevent gallstone formation.[38] Furthermore, the loss of small heterodimer partner (SHP) repression of CYP7A1 expression significantly increases hepatic bile salt synthesis, resulting in a significant reduction in hepatic secretion of biliary cholesterol and bile cholesterol content by greatly converting the cholesterol molecules of hepatic and intestinal sources into bile salts, even in challenge to the lithogenic diet.[39] All of these changes prevent the formation of cholesterol gallstones in SHP knockout mice. Taken together, these results indicate that FXR and SHP are promising therapeutic targets for treating or preventing cholesterol gallstone disease.

Because gallbladder biles of ABCB4 knockout mice on chow contain only trace amounts of phospholipid,[40] biles become supersaturated with cholesterol and plot in the left 2-phase zone of the ternary phase diagram, consistent with anhydrous cholesterol crystallization.[41] Spontaneous gallstone formation is a new consistent feature of the ABCB4 phenotype. The ABCB4 knockout mouse is therefore a model of low phospholipid-associated cholelithiasis, recently described in humans with a dysfunctional mutation in the orthologous ABCB4 gene.[42,43] The mouse model supports the concept that this gene is a monogenic risk factor for cholesterol gall-stones and a target for novel therapeutic strategies. More recently, it was found increased susceptibility to diet-induced gallstones in liver fatty-acid binding protein (L-FABP) knockout mice, suggesting that hepatic intracellular lipid transporters could have an important effect on gallstone formation.[44]

The term metabolic syndrome implies the coexistence of multiple metabolic risk factors associated with the development of visceral obesity and increased risk of atherosclerotic cardiovascular disease.[45] The well-documented association between gallstones and the metabolic syndrome suggests that persons with the metabolic syndrome may be susceptible to cholesterol gallstones.[46–51] Biddinger and colleagues[52] found that liver-specific disruption of the insulin receptor results solely in hepatic insulin resistance. This alteration induces a significant predisposition toward cholesterol gallstone formation by at least 2 distinct mechanisms: (1) activation of the forkhead transcription factor FoxO1 upregulates expression of the biliary cholesterol transporters ABCG5 and ABCG8 and promotes biliary cholesterol secretion; and (2) suppression of expression of the bile salt synthetic enzymes leads to a lithogenic bile salt profile. These results show a crucial link between the metabolic syndrome and increased cholesterol gallstone susceptibility, and indicate that cholesterol gallstones could indeed be a "fellow traveler" with the metabolic syndrome.[53]

Cholecystokinin (CCK) is synthesized by proximal small-intestinal I cells and is released postprandially by fatty acids and amino acids, inducing gallbladder contraction and sphincter of Oddi relaxation. Many studies have found enlarged fasting and residual gallbladder volumes in patients with cholesterol gallstones.[54] Gallbladder hypomotility may result from absorption of cholesterol from supersaturated bile by the gallbladder wall. Excess cholesterol in smooth muscle cells stiffens sarcolemmal membranes and thereby decouples normal signal transduction via G proteins when CCK binds to CCK-1 receptor (CCK-1R), thus paralyzing gallbladder contractile function.[55–57] Stasis of cholesterol-supersaturated bile in the gallbladder favors retardation of crystallization, as well as growth and agglomeration of cholesterol monohydrate crystals. Recently, it was observed that lack of endogenous CCK induces gallbladder hypomotility that prolongs the residence time of excess cholesterol in the gallbladder, leading to rapid crystallization and precipitation of solid cholesterol crystals.[58] Moreover, during the early stage of gallstone formation, there are 2 pathways of liquid and polymorph anhydrous crystals evolving to monohydrate crystals, and 3 modes for cholesterol crystal growth.[58] Targeted deletion of the *Cck-1r* gene results in larger gallbladder volumes (predisposing to bile stasis), significant retardation of small-intestinal transit times (resulting in increased cholesterol absorption), and increased biliary cholesterol secretion rates; this sequence of events in turn induces a significantly higher prevalence of cholesterol gallstones in mice.[59]

Accumulated evidence shows that hypersecretion of gallbladder mucins is a prerequisite for gallstone formation because gallbladder mucins are potent pronucleating/crystallizing agents for accelerating cholesterol crystallization in native and model biles.[22,60–65] Gallbladder mucin hypersecretion may be induced in part by cholesterol supersaturation or hydrophobic bile salts. Although the gel-forming mucins play an important role in the early stage of gallstone formation, it is unclear whether the gallbladder epithelial mucin influences susceptibility to gallstones. Increased gallbladder epithelial MUC1 mucin significantly enhances cholelithogenesis by promoting gallbladder cholesterol absorption and impairing gallbladder motility in C57BL/6 J mice transgenic for the human *MUC1* gene.[66] This opens the way for research into whether the epithelial mucins contribute to cholesterol cholelithogenesis, and it constitutes the basic framework for investigating how individual mucin genes influence the various cholesterol gallstone phenotypes.

The small intestine provides dietary and reabsorbed biliary cholesterol to the body,[67] and also plays an important regulatory role in enterohepatic circulation of bile salts. The factors regulating intestinal membrane lipid transporters, lipid regulatory enzymes, intracellular lipid transporters, and lipid regulatory transcription factors could influence the amount of cholesterol of intestinal origin contributing to the liver for biliary secretion. Genetic variations in cholesterol absorption efficiency are associated with cholesterol gallstone formation in inbred mice, and cholesterol absorbed from the intestine could provide an important source for biliary hypersecretion. Differential metabolism of the chylomicron remnant cholesterol between C57L/J and AKR/J mice could play a crucial role in the formation of lithogenic bile and gallstones.[28] Direct evidence for the role of intestinal factors in mouse gallstones came from Buhman and colleagues.[68] They found that the absence of intestinal cholesterol ester synthesis due to deletion of the acyl-CoA:cholesterol acyltransferase gene 2 (Acat2) causes a remarkable decrease in intestinal cholesterol absorption and complete resistance to diet-induced gallstones in mice. The absence of expression of intestinal APO-B48, but not APO-B100, reduces biliary cholesterol secretion and cholelithogenesis, possibly by decreasing intestinal absorption and hepatic bioavailability.[69] Reduced gallstone prevalence in lithogenic diet-fed APO-E knockout mice may be explained by decreased availability of chylomicron-derived cholesterol in the liver for biliary secretion.[70] These studies support the notion that high dietary cholesterol through the chylomicron pathway could provide an important source of excess cholesterol molecules for secretion into bile, thereby inducing cholesterol-supersaturated bile and enhancing cholelithogenesis.

Because ezetimibe significantly suppresses intestinal cholesterol absorption via the Niemann-Pick C1-like 1 (NPC1L1) pathway,[71] possibly a transporter-facilitated mechanism, this should diminish the cholesterol content of the liver, which in turn decreases bioavailability of cholesterol for biliary secretion. Ezetimibe induces a significant dose-dependent reduction in intestinal cholesterol absorption efficiency, coupled with a significant dose-dependent decrease in biliary cholesterol outputs and gallstone prevalence rates.[72,73] In particular, cholesterol gallstones can be prevented in C57L/J mice treated with ezetimibe. It seems reasonable to assume that reduced cholesterol absorption and hepatic chylomicron remnant uptake may induce a decrease in biliary cholesterol secretion and saturation.[72–74] Therefore, ezetimibe could be a novel approach to reduce biliary cholesterol content and a promising strategy for preventing or treating cholesterol gallstones by inhibiting intestinal cholesterol absorption.

## EPIDEMIOLOGIC EVIDENCE AND GENETIC CONSIDERATION OF CHOLESTEROL GALLSTONES IN HUMANS

Because cholesterol cholelithiasis is likely to result from a complex interaction of environmental factors and the effects of multiple undetermined genes, the genetic evidence of this disease in humans is mostly indirect and is based on geographic and ethnic differences, as well as on family and twin studies.[75–83] Epidemiologic investigations have found that a genetic predisposition is clearly present in the Pima Indians, certain other North and South American Indians, and Chileans, all of whom display the highest age-adjusted incidences of gallstones (48%) in the world.[76–79] By contrast, the overall age-adjusted incidences in other American (white) and European populations are approximately 20%.[48,84–86] The lowest incidences (<5%) are observed in African populations, and intermediate rates (5%–20%) are found in Asian populations. Because American and European populations seem to have an Amerindian or Viking genetic inheritance, it is interesting to hypothesize that apparently "thrifty" genes that emerged during the last glacial epoch may cause a higher incidence rate of cholesterol gallstones in American and European countries than in African and Asian countries.[87] Although some independent risk factors such as aging, gender, parity, obesity, some drugs, diet, and rapid weight loss for gallstone formation have been found,[4,5] none of these can explain the striking differences in incidences of gallstones among different populations, thereby suggesting a genetic contribution to the cause of the disease. To examine the influence of the genetic factors more rigorously, a study of populations with different incidences of gallstones but living in the same environment should provide important insights into genetic mechanisms of the disease. However, intermarriages between 2 populations result in a rapid loss of the original genetic background within a few generations, thereby making such a study impossible.

Cholesterol gallstones are more frequent by a ratio of 3:1 in siblings and other family members of affected persons than in spouses or unrelated controls.[88] Using ultrasonography to detect gallstones in first-degree relatives of index patients, Gilat and colleagues[75] found a 21% frequency in first-degree relatives compared with 9% in matched controls, and Sarin and coworkers[81] also observed a frequency that was 5 times higher in relatives of patients with gallstones than in gallstone-free controls. Cholesterol supersaturation is higher in fasting duodenal bile of older sisters of patients with gallstones compared with controls.[82] Cholesterol synthesis rates, bile saturation levels, and gallstone frequency rates are also remarkably higher on pairwise correlations in monozygotic than in dizygotic male twins.[83] Despite these critical clinic observations, a mode of inheritance that fits a Mendelian pattern cannot be found in most cases.

In 1999, Duggirala and colleagues[89] used pedigree data to explore the genetic susceptibility to symptomatic gallstone in 32 Mexican American families and estimated a heritability of 44% ($\pm$18%) for the proportion of the phenotypic variance of the trait that is due to genetic effects. In another family study from the United States, a variance component analysis was performed in 1038 individuals taken from 358 families, and the heritability of symptomatic gallstone disease was calculated to be 29% ($\pm$14%).[90]

Twin studies have been a valuable source of information on the genetic epidemiology of complex traits, and have been used to dissect complex genetics by analyzing the interaction of genotypes and phenotypes with age, gender, and lifestyle factors. Contrary to family studies, comparisons of the concordance rates of symptomatic gallstone disease between monozygotic and dizygotic pairs of twins could determine whether the familial pattern is due to hereditary or environmental factors. Antero Kesaniemi and colleagues[83] investigated 35 Finnish twin pairs and found pairwise correlations within the monozygotic, but not the dizygotic, pairs for biliary cholic and deoxycholic acids and serum precursor sterols, highlighting the importance of genetic contributions to biliary lipid compositions. A large study in Swedish twins estimated the contribution of genetic factors to the development of symptomatic gallstone disease. Katsika and colleagues[91] found that concordance rates (12%) in monozygotic twins of both genders were significantly higher than those (6%) in dizygotic twins in 43,141 twin pairs. The low concordance rates in monozygotic twins indicate the importance of environmental factors. Structural equation modeling has been used to estimate the contributions of genetic as well as shared and nonshared environmental factor effects. Further study revealed that concordance rates are significantly higher in monozygotic twins than in dizygotic twins, with genetic factors accounting for

**Table 2**
Human *LITH* genes that were identified and updated in 2008

| Genes | Gene Symbols | Databases | | Inheritance Pattern (Countries Where Reported) | | | | Gene Variants | Potential Mechanisms |
|---|---|---|---|---|---|---|---|---|---|
| | | OMIM[a] | Genecards[b] | Rare Monogenic | Familial Oligogenic | Common Polygenic | | | |
| ATP-binding cassette transporter B4 | *ABCB4* | 171060 and 600803 | GC07M086676 | (−) | (+) | (−) | | Multiple | Biliary phospholipid secretion ↓ |
| ATP-binding cassette transporter B11 | *ABCB11* | 603201 | GC02M169604 | (+) | (−) | (−) | | Multiple | Biliary bile salt secretion ↓ |
| ATP-binding cassette transporters G5/G8 | *ABCG5/G8* | 605459/605460 and 611465 | GC02P 043951/ GC02P043977 | (−) | (−) | (+) (Germany, Chile, China) | | *ABCG8p.D19H* (*rs1188753*) | Biliary cholesterol secretion ↑ |
| β₃ Adrenergic receptor | *ARDB3* | 109691 | GC08M037939 | (−) | (−) | (+) (Germany) | | p.R64 W (*rs4944*) | Gallbladder hypomotility |
| Apolipoprotein A1 | *APO-A1* | 107680 | GC11M116211 | (−) | (−) | (+) (China, India) | | −75G>A, RFLP | Biliary cholesterol secretion ↑ secondary to reverse cholesterol transport ↑ |
| Apolipoprotein B | *APO-B* | 107730 | GC02M021135 | (+) | (−) | (+) (China, Poland) | | c.2488C>T, c.4154G>A | Biliary cholesterol secretion ↑ secondary to hepatic VLDL synthesis ↓ and intestinal cholesterol absorption ↑ |

| | | OMIM | GeneCards | | | | | |
|---|---|---|---|---|---|---|---|---|
| Apolipoprotein C1 | *APO-C1* | 107710 | GC19P050109 | (−) | (−) | (+) (India) | RFLP | APO-C1 ↑ remnant-like particle cholesterol ↑ |
| Androgen receptor | *AR* | 313700 | GC0XP066680 | (−) | (−) | (+) (Greece) | c.172(CAG)$_n$ | |
| Cholecystokinin 1 receptor | *CCK1R* | 118444 | GC04M026159 | (+) | (−) | (+) (India) | RFLP | Gallbladder and small-intestinal hypomotility |
| Cholesterol ester transfer protein | *CETP* | 118470 | GC16P055553 | (−) | (−) | (+) (Finland) | RFLP | Hepatic cholesterol uptake ↑ from HDL catabolism ↑ |
| Cytochrome P450 7A1 | *CYP7A1* | 118470 | GC08M059565 | (+) | (−) | (+) (China) | Promoter SNP −204A>C | Bile salt synthesis ↓ |
| Estrogen receptor 2 | *ESR2* | 601663 | GC14M063621 | (−) | (−) | (+) (Greece) | c.1092+3607(CA)$_n$ | Cholesterol synthesis ↑ |
| LRP associated protein 1 | *LRPAP1* | 104225 | GC04M003551 | (−) | (−) | (+) (India) | Intron 5 insertion/ deletion (*rs11267919*) | Hepatic cholesterol uptake ↑ from chylomicron remnants via LRP ↑ |

*Abbreviations:* LRP, low-density lipoprotein receptor related protein; OMIM, Online Mendelian inheritance in man; RFLP, restriction fragment length polymorphism; SNP, single nucleotide polymorphism.

ᵃ http://www.ncbi.nim.nih.gov/entrez.

ᵇ http://www.genecards.org.

*Modified from* Lammert F, Sauerbruch T. Pathogenesis of gallstone formation: updated inventory of human lithogenic genes. In: Carey MC, Dité P, Gabryelewicz A, et al, editors. Future perspectives in gastroenterology (Falk Symposium 161). Dordrect: Springer; 2008. p. 99–107; with permission.

25% of the phenotypic variation between the twins, as well as shared environmental effects for 13%, and unique environmental effects for 62% of the phenotypic variance among twins.[91]

Although rare, the first evidence that human gallstones might be caused by a single-gene defect came from a study by Lin and colleagues,[92] who found that among 232 Mexican Americans, a variant of the cholesterol 7α-hydroxylase (CYP7A1) gene was associated with gallstones in men but not in women. A homozygous deletion mutation in the CYP7A1 gene could result in loss of enzyme function. Thus, CYP7A1 is an attractive candidate gene because it encodes the rate-limiting enzyme in the neutral pathway for bile salt synthesis in the liver and because bile salts are essential for forming bile and for keeping cholesterol molecules solubilized in simple and mixed micelles in bile. Pullinger and colleagues[93] found a new link between another single-gene defect of CYP7A1 and cholesterol gallstones associated with hypercholesterolemia resistant to HMG-CoA reductase inhibitors in 2 male homoyzgotes.

These epidemiologic investigations underscore the importance of genetic contributions to the formation of cholesterol gallstones in humans.

## SEARCHING FOR HUMAN *LITH* GENES

Because of its multifactorial pathogenesis, it is difficult to identify human gene abnormalities that are responsible for the formation of cholesterol gallstones. Monogenic predisposition for cholelithiasis has only been ascribed to mutations in the genes in specific subgroups of patients. **Table 2** summarizes human *LITH* genes that have been identified and updated in 2008. Missense mutations in the *ABCB4* gene, which encodes the phospholipid transporter in the canalicular membrane of hepatocytes, are the basis for a particular type of cholelithiasis. The disorder is characterized by intrahepatic sludge, gallbladder cholesterol gallstones, mild chronic cholestasis, a high cholesterol/phospholipid ratio in bile, and recurrent symptoms after cholecystectomy.[42,43] A defect in the *ABCB4* gene could constitute the basis for this highly symptomatic and recurrent form of gallstone disease. In patients with hepatolithiasis, a common disease in Asia, low expression levels of *ABCB4* and phosphatidylcholine transfer protein occur together with markedly reduced phospholipid concentrations in bile.[94] In this disorder, HMG-CoA reductase activity is increased and CYP7A1 activity is reduced in gallstone patients compared with controls. Furthermore, the formation of cholesterol-rich intrahepatic stones could be induced by decreased biliary secretion of phospholipids in the setting of increased cholesterol synthesis and decreased bile salt synthesis.

Because gallbladder hypomotility favors gallstone formation, the genes for CCK and CCK-1R, which regulate gallbladder motility, are attractive candidates.[54,58,59] Genetic variation in the *CCK-1R* gene is associated with gallstone risk, and an aberrant splicing of *CCK-1R*, which is predicted to result in a nonfunctional receptor, is found in a few obese patients with gallstones.[95,96] However, a search for mutations or polymorphisms in the *CCK-1R* gene in patients with gallstones has been unsuccessful.[97]

Some studies have reported that certain polymorphisms of the *APO-E* and *APO-B* genes and the cholesteryl ester transfer protein, all of which are involved in carrying cholesterol in the plasma, are associated with gallstones.[98–102] Although the polymorphisms in the *APO-E* gene have been extensively studied in patients with gallstones, results concerning the protective role of the ε4 allele against gallstones have been inconsistent. The ε2 allele seems to protect against gallstones, and the degree of intestinal cholesterol absorption varies with the *APO-E* isoform (ε4>ε3>ε2).[103] Also, the fecal excretion of cholesterol tends to be higher in persons with the APO-E2 phenotype than in those with the APO-E3 or APO-E4 phenotypes. In a study of poly-morphisms at the *APO-B*, *APO-A1*, and cholesteryl ester transfer protein gene loci in patients with gallbladder disease, a polymorphism of the cholesteryl ester transfer protein gene, in relation to another HDL-lowering factor, was found to be associated with cholesterol gallstones.[102] Also, there is a link between the *X+* allele of the *APO-B* gene and an increased risk of cholesterol gallstones. A genome-wide association study in a large cohort of patients with gallstones from Germany and a linkage study in affected sib pairs identified a common variant (D19H) of the sterol transporters *ABCG5* and *ABCG8* on the canalicular membrane of hepatocytes as a risk factor for gallstones.[104,105] It was shown to confer odds ratios of 2 to 3 in heterozygotes and 7 in homozygous carriers. This variant is also a susceptibility factor for gallstones in Chilean Hispanics, and other *ABCG8* variants (T400 K, D19H, A632 V, M429 V, and C54Y) as well as *ABCG5* variants (Q604E) may be important risk factors for gallstone formation in Chinese and Canadian Caucasians.[106–108] This first common suscepti-bility gene has been predicted by QTL mapping studies in inbred mice.[109]

## FUTURE RESEARCH DIRECTIONS

A new concept has been proposed that interactions of 5 defects could play an impor-tant role in the formation of cholesterol gallstones (see **Fig. 1**), which are considered in terms of *LITH* genes (genetic defect), thermodynamics (solubility defect), kinetics (nucleation defect), stasis (residence time defect), and lipid sources (metabolic defect). Growing evidence from pathophysiological, physical-chemical, and genetic studies shows that disposition to the formation of cholesterol gallstones is multifacto-rial, and the overarching pathogenetic factor is hepatic hypersecretion of cholesterol into bile, and no mode of inheritance fitting to the Mendelian pattern could be found in most cases. Similar to atherosclerosis, the risk for cholesterol gallstone formation increases with aging, dyslipidemia, hyperinsulinemia, obesity, diabetes, and seden-tary lifestyle. All these conditions are risk factors for the metabolic syndrome, of which cholesterol gallstone formation is just another pathogenic facet.

Rapid advances in techniques for genetic analysis and the availability of the nucle-otide sequence of the human genome will lead to the identification and characteriza-tion of *LITH* genes in the coming years. The identification of *LITH* genes responsible for cholesterol gallstone formation by a positional cloning approach in humans is pre-dicted to be elucidated in the near future, which should lead to the discovery of path-ophysiological functions of all *LITH* genes, and yield new insights into the molecular mechanisms that potentially influence gallstone formation. With such knowledge of all the genetic and environmental factors involved in gallstone pathogenesis, it will be possible to investigate multiple avenues of gallstone prevention in humans.

## REFERENCES

1. Liver Disease Subcommittee of the Digestive Disease Interagency Coordinating Committee. Action plan for liver disease research. Bethesda (MD): NIH; 2004. 145–50.
2. Wang DQ, Cohen DE, Carey MC. Biliary lipids and cholesterol gallstone disease. J Lipid Res 2009;50(Suppl):S406–11.
3. Russo MW, Wei JT, Thiny MT, et al. Digestive and liver diseases statistics, 2004. Gastroenterology 2004;126(5):1448–53.
4. Portincasa P, Moschetta A, Palasciano G. Cholesterol gallstone disease. Lancet 2006;368(9531):230–9.

5. Wang HH, Portincasa P, Wang DQ. Molecular pathophysiology and physical chemistry of cholesterol gallstones. Front Biosci 2008;13:401–23.

6. Wang DQ-H, Afdhal NH. Gallstone disease. In: Feldman M, Friedman LS, Brandt LJ, editors. Sleisenger and Fordtran's gastrointestinal and liver disease. 9th edition. Philadelphia: Elsevier; 2010, in press.

7. Wang DQ, Afdhal NH. Genetic analysis of cholesterol gallstone formation: searching for *Lith* (gallstone) genes. Curr Gastroenterol Rep 2004;6(2):140–50.

8. Khanuja B, Cheah YC, Hunt M, et al. *Lith1*, a major gene affecting cholesterol gallstone formation among inbred strains of mice. Proc Natl Acad Sci U S A 1995;92(17):7729–33.

9. Tepperman J, Caldwell FT, Tepperman HM. Induction of gallstones in mice by feeding a cholesterol-cholic acid containing diet. Am J Physiol 1964;206: 628–34.

10. Fujihira E, Kaneta S, Ohshima T. Strain difference in mouse cholelithiasis and the effect of taurine on the gallstone formation in C57BL/C mice. Biochem Med 1978;19(2):211–7.

11. Alexander M, Portman OW. Different susceptibilities to the formation of cholesterol gallstones in mice. Hepatology 1987;7(2):257–65.

12. Lammert F, Carey MC, Paigen B. Chromosomal organization of candidate genes involved in cholesterol gallstone formation: a murine gallstone map. Gastroenterology 2001;120(1):221–38.

13. Lyons MA, Wittenburg H. Cholesterol gallstone susceptibility loci: a mouse map, candidate gene evaluation, and guide to human *LITH* genes. Gastroenterology 2006;131(6):1943–70.

14. Korstanje R, Paigen B. From QTL to gene: the harvest begins. Nat Genet 2002; 31(3):235–6.

15. Lander ES, Schork NJ. Genetic dissection of complex traits. Science 1994; 265(5181):2037–48.

16. Darvasi A. Experimental strategies for the genetic dissection of complex traits in animal models. Nat Genet 1998;18(1):19–24.

17. Cornall RJ, Aitman TJ, Hearne CM, et al. The generation of a library of PCR-analyzed microsatellite variants for genetic mapping of the mouse genome. Genomics 1991;10(4):874–81.

18. Hearne CM, McAleer MA, Love JM, et al. Additional microsatellite markers for mouse genome mapping. Mamm Genome 1991;1(4):273–82.

19. Aitman TJ, Hearne CM, McAleer MA, et al. Mononucleotide repeats are an abundant source of length variants in mouse genomic DNA. Mamm Genome 1991;1(4):206–10.

20. Gregory SG, Sekhon M, Schein J, et al. A physical map of the mouse genome. Nature 2002;418(6899):743–50.

21. Waterston RH, Lindblad-Toh K, Birney E, et al. Initial sequencing and comparative analysis of the mouse genome. Nature 2002;420(6915):520–62.

22. Wang DQ, Paigen B, Carey MC. Phenotypic characterization of *Lith* genes that determine susceptibility to cholesterol cholelithiasis in inbred mice: physical-chemistry of gallbladder bile. J Lipid Res 1997;38(7):1395–411.

23. Wittenburg H, Lyons MA, Li R, et al. QTL mapping for genetic determinants of lipoprotein cholesterol levels in combined crosses of inbred mouse strains. J Lipid Res 2006;47(8):1780–90.

24. Paigen B, Carey MC. Gallstones. In: King RA, Rotter JI, Motulsky AG, editors. The genetic basis of common diseases. 2nd edition. New York: Oxford University Press; 2002. p. 298–335.

25. Wang DQ, Lammert F, Paigen B, et al. Phenotypic characterization of *Lith* genes that determine susceptibility to cholesterol cholelithiasis in inbred mice. Pathophysiology of biliary lipid secretion. J Lipid Res 1999;40(11):2066–79.

26. Lammert F, Wang DQ, Paigen B, et al. Phenotypic characterization of *Lith* genes that determine susceptibility to cholesterol cholelithiasis in inbred mice: integrated activities of hepatic lipid regulatory enzymes. J Lipid Res 1999;40(11): 2080–90.

27. van Erpecum KJ, Wang DQ, Lammert F, et al. Phenotypic characterization of *Lith* genes that determine susceptibility to cholesterol cholelithiasis in inbred mice: soluble pronucleating proteins in gallbladder and hepatic biles. J Hepatol 2001;35(4):444–51.

28. Wang DQ, Zhang L, Wang HH. High cholesterol absorption efficiency and rapid biliary secretion of chylomicron remnant cholesterol enhance cholelithogenesis in gallstone-susceptible mice. Biochim Biophys Acta 2005;1733(1):90–9.

29. Paigen B, Schork NJ, Svenson KL, et al. Quantitative trait loci mapping for cholesterol gallstones in AKR/J and C57L/J strains of mice. Physiol Genomics 2000;4(1):59–65.

30. Diehl AK. Epidemiology and natural history of gallstone disease. Gastroenterol Clin North Am 1991;20(1):1–19.

31. Bennion LJ, Ginsberg RL, Gernick MB, et al. Effects of oral contraceptives on the gallbladder bile of normal women. N Engl J Med 1976;294(4):189–92.

32. Grodstein F, Colditz GA, Hunter DJ, et al. A prospective study of symptomatic gallstones in women: relation with oral contraceptives and other risk factors. Obstet Gynecol 1994;84(2):207–14.

33. Grodstein F, Colditz GA, Stampfer MJ. Postmenopausal hormone use and cholecystectomy in a large prospective study. Obstet Gynecol 1994; 83(1):5–11.

34. Simon JA, Hunninghake DB, Agarwal SK, et al. Effect of estrogen plus progestin on risk for biliary tract surgery in postmenopausal women with coronary artery disease. The Heart and Estrogen/progestin Replacement Study. Ann Intern Med 2001;135(7):493–501.

35. Wang HH, Afdhal NH, Wang DQ. Estrogen receptor alpha, but not beta, plays a major role in 17beta-estradiol-induced murine cholesterol gallstones. Gastroenterology 2004;127(1):239–49.

36. Wang HH, Afdhal NH, Wang DQ. Overexpression of estrogen receptor alpha increases hepatic cholesterogenesis, leading to biliary hypersecretion in mice. J Lipid Res 2006;47(4):778–86.

37. Wang HH, Liu M, Clegg DJ, et al. New insights into the molecular mechanisms underlying effects of estrogen on cholesterol gallstone formation. Biochim Biophys Acta 2009;1791(11):1037–47.

38. Moschetta A, Bookout AL, Mangelsdorf DJ. Prevention of cholesterol gallstone disease by FXR agonists in a mouse model. Nat Med 2004;10(12):1352–8.

39. Wang HH, Evans MJ, Portincasa P, et al. Increased hepatic bile acid synthesis prevents cholesterol gallstones in small heterodimer partner (SHP) knockout mice. Gastroenterology 2009;136:A281.

40. Smit JJ, Schinkel AH, Oude Elferink RP, et al. Homozygous disruption of the murine mdr2 P-glycoprotein gene leads to a complete absence of phospholipid from bile and to liver disease. Cell 1993;75(3):451–62.

41. Lammert F, Wang DQ, Hillebrandt S, et al. Spontaneous cholecysto- and hepatolithiasis in Mdr2-/- mice: a model for low phospholipid-associated cholelithiasis. Hepatology 2004;39(1):117–28.

42. Rosmorduc O, Hermelin B, Boelle PY, et al. ABCB4 gene mutation-associated cholelithiasis in adults. Gastroenterology 2003;125(2):452–9.

43. Rosmorduc O, Hermelin B, Poupon R. MDR3 gene defect in adults with symptomatic intrahepatic and gallbladder cholesterol cholelithiasis. Gastroenterology 2001;120(6):1459–67.

44. Xie Y, Newberry EP, Kennedy SM, et al. Increased susceptibility to diet-induced gallstones in liver fatty acid binding protein knockout mice. J Lipid Res 2009; 50(5):977–87.

45. Eckel RH, Grundy SM, Zimmet PZ. The metabolic syndrome. Lancet 2005; 365(9468):1415–28.

46. Tsai CJ, Leitzmann MF, Willett WC, et al. Prospective study of abdominal adiposity and gallstone disease in US men. Am J Clin Nutr 2004;80(1):38–44.

47. Ruhl CE, Everhart JE. Association of diabetes, serum insulin, and C-peptide with gallbladder disease. Hepatology 2000;31(2):299–303.

48. Everhart JE, Khare M, Hill M, et al. Prevalence and ethnic differences in gallbladder disease in the United States. Gastroenterology 1999;117(3):632–9.

49. Everhart JE. Contributions of obesity and weight loss to gallstone disease. Ann Intern Med 1993;119(10):1029–35.

50. Diehl AK, Schwesinger WH, Holleman DR Jr, et al. Gallstone characteristics in Mexican Americans and non-Hispanic whites. Dig Dis Sci 1994;39(10):2223–8.

51. Stampfer MJ, Maclure KM, Colditz GA, et al. Risk of symptomatic gallstones in women with severe obesity. Am J Clin Nutr 1992;55(3):652–8.

52. Biddinger SB, Haas JT, Yu BB, et al. Hepatic insulin resistance directly promotes formation of cholesterol gallstones. Nat Med 2008;14(7):778–82.

53. Grundy SM. Cholesterol gallstones: a fellow traveler with metabolic syndrome? Am J Clin Nutr 2004;80(1):1–2.

54. Portincasa P, Di Ciaula A, Wang HH, et al. Coordinate regulation of gallbladder motor function in the gut-liver axis. Hepatology 2008;47(6):2112–26.

55. Yu P, Chen Q, Harnett KM, et al. Direct G protein activation reverses impaired CCK signaling in human gallbladders with cholesterol stones. Am J Physiol 1995;269(5 Pt 1):G659–65.

56. Yu P, De Petris G, Biancani P, et al. Cholecystokinin-coupled intracellular signaling in human gallbladder muscle. Gastroenterology 1994;106(3):763–70.

57. Xiao ZL, Chen Q, Amaral J, et al. Defect of receptor-G protein coupling in human gallbladder with cholesterol stones. Am J Physiol 2000;278(2):G251–8.

58. Wang HH, Portincasa P, Liu M, et al. Effect of gallbladder hypomotility on cholesterol crystallization and growth in CCK-deficient mice. Biochim Biophys Acta 2010;180(2):138–46.

59. Wang DQ, Schmitz F, Kopin AS, et al. Targeted disruption of the murine cholecystokinin-1 receptor promotes intestinal cholesterol absorption and susceptibility to cholesterol cholelithiasis. J Clin Invest 2004;114(4):521–8.

60. Lee SP, Nicholls JF. Nature and composition of biliary sludge. Gastroenterology 1986;90(3):677–86.

61. Lee SP, LaMont JT, Carey MC. Role of gallbladder mucus hypersecretion in the evolution of cholesterol gallstones. J Clin Invest 1981;67(6):1712–23.

62. Shiffman ML, Shamburek RD, Schwartz CC, et al. Gallbladder mucin, arachidonic acid, and bile lipids in patients who develop gallstones during weight reduction. Gastroenterology 1993;105(4):1200–8.

63. Pemsingh RS, MacPherson BR, Scott GW. Mucus hypersecretion in the gallbladder epithelium of ground squirrels fed a lithogenic diet for the induction of cholesterol gallstones. Hepatology 1987;7(6):1267–71.

64. Levy PF, Smith BF, LaMont JT. Human gallbladder mucin accelerates nucleation of cholesterol in artificial bile. Gastroenterology 1984;87(2):270–5.
65. Afdhal NH, Gong D, Niu N, et al. Cholesterol cholelithiasis in the prairie dog: role of mucin and nonmucin glycoproteins. Hepatology 1993;17(4):693–700.
66. Wang HH, Afdhal NH, Gendler SJ, et al. Evidence that gallbladder epithelial mucin enhances cholesterol cholelithogenesis in MUC1 transgenic mice. Gastroenterology 2006;131(1):210–22.
67. Wang DQ. Regulation of intestinal cholesterol absorption. Annu Rev Physiol 2007;69:221–48.
68. Buhman KK, Accad M, Novak S, et al. Resistance to diet-induced hypercholesterolemia and gallstone formation in ACAT2-deficient mice. Nat Med 2000;6(12):1341–7.
69. Wang HH, Wang DQ. Reduced susceptibility to cholesterol gallstone formation in mice that do not produce apolipoprotein B48 in the intestine. Hepatology 2005;42(4):894–904.
70. Amigo L, Quinones V, Mardones P, et al. Impaired biliary cholesterol secretion and decreased gallstone formation in apolipoprotein E-deficient mice fed a high-cholesterol diet. Gastroenterology 2000;118(4):772–9.
71. Altmann SW, Davis HR Jr, Zhu LJ, et al. Niemann-Pick C1 Like 1 protein is critical for intestinal cholesterol absorption. Science 2004;303(5661):1201–4.
72. Wang HH, Portincasa P, Mendez-Sanchez N, et al. Effect of ezetimibe on the prevention and dissolution of cholesterol gallstones. Gastroenterology 2008;134(7):2101–10.
73. Zuniga S, Molina H, Azocar L, et al. Ezetimibe prevents cholesterol gallstone formation in mice. Liver Int 2008;28(7):935–47.
74. Valasek MA, Repa JJ, Quan G, et al. Inhibiting intestinal NPC1L1 activity prevents diet-induced increase in biliary cholesterol in Golden Syrian hamsters. Am J Physiol 2008;295(4):G813–22.
75. Gilat T, Feldman C, Halpern Z, et al. An increased familial frequency of gallstones. Gastroenterology 1983;84(2):242–6.
76. Sampliner RE, Bennett PH, Comess LJ, et al. Gallbladder disease in Pima Indians. Demonstration of high prevalence and early onset by cholecystography. N Engl J Med 1970;283(25):1358–64.
77. Thistle JL, Schoenfield LJ. Lithogenic bile among young Indian women. N Engl J Med 1971;284(4):177–81.
78. Everhart JE, Yeh F, Lee ET, et al. Prevalence of gallbladder disease in American Indian populations: findings from the Strong Heart Study. Hepatology 2002;35(6):1507–12.
79. Weiss KM, Ferrell RE, Hanis CL, et al. Genetics and epidemiology of gallbladder disease in New World native peoples. Am J Hum Genet 1984;36(6):1259–78.
80. van der Linden W, Simonson N. Familial occurrence of gallstone disease. Incidence in parents of young patients. Hum Hered 1973;23(2):123–7.
81. Sarin SK, Negi VS, Dewan R, et al. High familial prevalence of gallstones in the first-degree relatives of gallstone patients. Hepatology 1995;22(1):138–41.
82. Danzinger RG, Gordon H, Schoenfield LJ, et al. Lithogenic bile in siblings of young women with cholelithiasis. Mayo Clin Proc 1972;47(10):762–6.
83. Antero Kesaniemi Y, Koskenvuo M, Vuoristo M, et al. Biliary lipid composition in monozygotic and dizygotic pairs of twins. Gut 1989;30(12):1750–6.
84. Lammert F, Sauerbruch T. Mechanisms of disease: the genetic epidemiology of gallbladder stones. Nat Clin Pract Gastroenterol Hepatol 2005;2(9):423–33.

85. Everhart JE. Gallstones and ethnicity in the Americas. J Assoc Acad Minor Phys 2001;12(3):137–43.
86. Kratzer W, Mason RA, Kachele V. Prevalence of gallstones in sonographic surveys worldwide. J Clin Ultrasound 1999;27(1):1–7.
87. Carey MC, Paigen B. Epidemiology of the American Indians' burden and its likely genetic origins. Hepatology 2002;36(4 Pt 1):781–91.
88. van der Linden W. Genetic factors in gallstone disease. Clin Gastroenterol 1973; 2:603–14.
89. Duggirala R, Mitchell BD, Blangero J, et al. Genetic determinants of variation in gallbladder disease in the Mexican-American population. Genet Epidemiol 1999;16(2):191–204.
90. Nakeeb A, Comuzzie AG, Martin L, et al. Gallstones: genetics versus environment. Ann Surg 2002;235(6):842–9.
91. Katsika D, Grjibovski A, Einarsson C, et al. Genetic and environmental influences on symptomatic gallstone disease: a Swedish study of 43,141 twin pairs. Hepatology 2005;41(5):1138–43.
92. Lin JP, Hanis CL, Boerwinkle E. Genetic epidemiology of gallbladder disease in Mexican-Americans and cholesterol 7alpha-hydroxylase gene variation. Am J Hum Genet 1994;55:A48.
93. Pullinger CR, Eng C, Salen G, et al. Human cholesterol 7alpha-hydroxylase (CYP7A1) deficiency has a hypercholesterolemic phenotype. J Clin Invest 2002;110(1):109–17.
94. Shoda J, Oda K, Suzuki H, et al. Etiologic significance of defects in cholesterol, phospholipid, and bile acid metabolism in the liver of patients with intrahepatic calculi. Hepatology 2001;33(5):1194–205.
95. Miller LJ, Holicky EL, Ulrich CD, et al. Abnormal processing of the human cholecystokinin receptor gene in association with gallstones and obesity. Gastroenterology 1995;109(4):1375–80.
96. Schneider H, Sanger P, Hanisch E. In vitro effects of cholecystokinin fragments on human gallbladders. Evidence for an altered CCK-receptor structure in a subgroup of patients with gallstones. J Hepatol 1997;26(5):1063–8.
97. Nardone G, Ferber IA, Miller LJ. The integrity of the cholecystokinin receptor gene in gallbladder disease and obesity. Hepatology 1995;22(6):1751–3.
98. Juvonen T, Kervinen K, Kairaluoma MI, et al. Gallstone cholesterol content is related to apolipoprotein E polymorphism. Gastroenterology 1993;104(6):1806–13.
99. Bertomeu A, Ros E, Zambon D, et al. Apolipoprotein E polymorphism and gallstones. Gastroenterology 1996;111(6):1603–10.
100. Van Erpecum KJ, Van Berge-henegouwen GP, Eckhardt ER, et al. Cholesterol crystallization in human gallbladder bile: relation to gallstone number, bile composition, and apolipoprotein E4 isoform. Hepatology 1998;27(6):1508–16.
101. Fischer S, Dolu MH, Zundt B, et al. Apolipoprotein E polymorphism and lithogenic factors in gallbladder bile. Eur J Clin Invest 2001;31(9):789–95.
102. Juvonen T, Savolainen MJ, Kairaluoma MI, et al. Polymorphisms at the apoB, apoA-I, and cholesteryl ester transfer protein gene loci in patients with gallbladder disease. J Lipid Res 1995;36(4):804–12.
103. Kesaniemi YA, Ehnholm C, Miettinen TA. Intestinal cholesterol absorption efficiency in man is related to apoprotein E phenotype. J Clin Invest 1987;80(2): 578–81.
104. Buch S, Schafmayer C, Volzke H, et al. A genome-wide association scan identifies the hepatic cholesterol transporter ABCG8 as a susceptibility factor for human gallstone disease. Nat Genet 2007;39(8):995–9.

105. Grunhage F, Acalovschi M, Tirziu S, et al. Increased gallstone risk in humans conferred by common variant of hepatic ATP-binding cassette transporter for cholesterol. Hepatology 2007;46(3):793–801.
106. Kuo KK, Shin SJ, Chen ZC, et al. Significant association of ABCG5 604Q and ABCG8 D19H polymorphisms with gallstone disease. Br J Surg 2008;95(8): 1005–11.
107. Wang Y, Jiang ZY, Fei J, et al. ATP binding cassette G8 T400K polymorphism may affect the risk of gallstone disease among Chinese males. Clin Chim Acta 2007;384(1–2):80–5.
108. Rudkowska I, Jones PJ. Polymorphisms in ABCG5/G8 transporters linked to hypercholesterolemia and gallstone disease. Nutr Rev 2008;66(6):343–8.
109. Wittenburg H, Lyons MA, Li R, et al. FXR and ABCG5/ABCG8 as determinants of cholesterol gallstone formation from quantitative trait locus mapping in mice. Gastroenterology 2003;125(3):868–81.

# Endoscopic Management of Biliary Ductal Stones

Kyo-Sang Yoo, MD, Glen A. Lehman, MD*

**KEYWORDS**

• Biliary calculi • Endoscopic management

In Western countries, most stones in the common bile duct (CBD) result from passage of gallbladder stones into the CBD. Stones in the common duct are found in 8% to 18% of patients with symptomatic gallbladder stones.[1] At least 3% to 10% of patients undergoing cholecystectomy have CBD stones.[2] Patients with symptomatic bile duct stones are at high risk of experiencing further symptoms or complications if left untreated. Given the potential serious complications of bile duct stones, specific therapy generally is indicated regardless of symptoms.[3]

Introduction of endoscopic retrograde cholangiopancreatography (ERCP) with biliary sphincterotomy in 1974 opened a new era in the nonsurgical treatment of CBD stones. Such endoscopic management is now the mainstay in the management of bile duct stones. Multiple supplemental techniques are now available.

This article discusses the current state of endoscopic treatment of extrahepatic bile duct stones. This includes conventional endoscopic management of CBD stones and alternative strategies for stones that are more difficult to remove. Gallstone pancreatitis, intrahepatic stones (mostly seen in Asians), and postliver transplant problems are not discussed.

## ROUTINE COMMON BILE DUCT STONES

Stones less than 1 cm in diameter with normal terminal CBD/sphincter anatomy are considered routine because more than 85% can be managed by standard biliary endoscopic sphincterotomy (BES) and extraction (**Fig. 1**).

## BILIARY ENDOSCOPIC SPHINCTEROTOMY

Enlargement of the biliary sphincter is necessary for luminal passage and endoscopic stone removal. This is mostly commonly done via electrocautery sphincterotomy.

Division of Gastroenterology/Hepatology, Department of Medicine, Indiana University Hospital, 550 North University Boulevard, Suite 4100, Indianapolis, IN 46202, USA
* Corresponding author.
*E-mail address:* glehman@iupui.edu

Gastroenterol Clin N Am 39 (2010) 209–227
doi:10.1016/j.gtc.2010.02.008
0889-8553/10/$ – see front matter © 2010 Published by Elsevier Inc.

gastro.theclinics.com

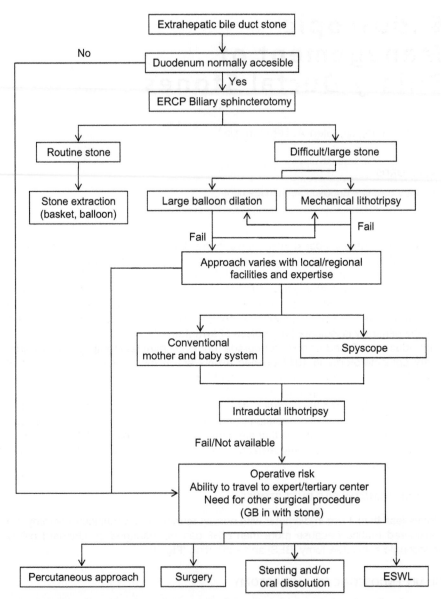

**Fig. 1.** Proposed algorithm for management of extrahepatic duct stones. (Spyglass Spyscope system; Boston Scientific, Natrick, MA, USA.)

Routine pre-ERCP coagulation assessment is probably unnecessary unless there is history of liver disease or kidney disease, family history of bleeding disorder, or anticoagulation medicine use.

The procedure is performed with a sphincterotome, which consists of a Teflon catheter with a cautery wire exposed for a length of 20 to 35 mm near the tip. After deep bile duct cannulation is achieved, the sphincterotome is retracted until only 5 to 8 mm remain in the duct/papilla. The cutting wire of sphincterotome is then bowed so that it comes in greater contact with the roof of the papilla. The orientation of the cutting wire should be between the 11:30 and 12:30 positions to reduce the likelihood of retroperitoneal perforation. Applying intermittent bursts of diathermic current from the electrosurgical generator makes the incision through the sphincter. The length of the incision may range from 7 to 15 mm, depending on the size of the stone to be extracted and size of papilla. The combination of cutting current blended with coagulation current is most frequently used. Attempts to decrease postsphincterotomy pancreatitis by decreased coagulation current have resulted in more bleeding. One cautery option is use of a microprocessor-controlled system, which automatically alternates cutting and coagulation current by intrinsic software, the so-called ENDO CUT mode of the ERBE electrosurgical generator (ERBE Elektromedizin GmbH, Tubingen, Germany).[4] An advantage of this method is a stepwise cutting action, which avoids a rapid uncontrolled incision. Additionally, it may also reduce the bleeding after BES.[5,6] A large retrospective analysis suggested that the microprocessor-controlled BES is associated with a significantly lower frequency of intraprocedural bleeding but had no impact on clinically relevant postprocedure bleeding.[7]

After a successful BES, 85% to 90% of CBD stones can be retrieved by a basket or balloon catheter. The choice between a basket or balloon catheter is largely one of personal preference and size of the stone to be extracted. The extractor basket provides greater mechanical forces than the balloon catheter and is preferable for stones larger than 8 mm.[4] Endoscopists should be prepared to use a needle knife to remove the distally impacted CBD stone, which shows characteristic bulging papilla (**Fig. 2**).

Most prospective series report an overall short-term complication rate for ERCP or sphincterotomy of approximately 4% to 10%.[8–13] In a large, prospective US multicenter trial, the overall complication rate of BES was 9.8% in 2347 patients, including pancreatitis in 5.4%, bleeding in 2%, procedure-related cholangitis in 1%, cholecystitis in 0.5%, and perforation in 0.3%.[8] In the subgroup of 1600 patients who had common duct stones, the overall complication rate was 8%.

## BALLOON SPHINCTEROPLASTY

To potentially decrease the rate of complications of BES, balloon sphincteroplasty (BSP) was introduced as a sphincter-preserving alternative.[4] In addition to the lower

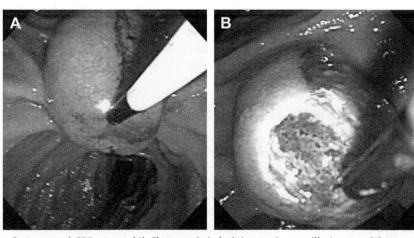

**Fig. 2.** Impacted CBD stone. (*A*) Characteristic bulging major papilla is seen. (*B*) Impacted stone is exposed by the incision on the papillary roof with a needle knife.

risk of bleeding and perforation, another apparent advantage of the procedure is that the sphincter of Oddi function can be preserved. This could avoid the lifelong reflux of duodenal contents into the bile duct through the opened sphincter. BSP was first described by Staritz and colleagues[14] in 1983 but was then nearly abandoned as a treatment of bile duct stones after reports of serious postprocedure pancreatitis.[15] In the mid-1990s, its use was revived with the more favorable results from several groups.[16,17]

For balloon dilation, a standard guide wire is inserted into the bile duct after selective bile duct cannulation. After removing the catheter, usually a 6- to 10-mm hydrostatic balloon-tipped catheter is passed over the guide wire and positioned across the papilla. The balloon is expanded with contrast medium until ablation of the waistline of the balloon occurs. The dilation is maintained for 15 to 30 seconds. The optimal size of the balloon in BES has not been established. Most studies have reported results with 8-mm diameter dilation balloons, although some studies have used balloons up to 15 mm in diameter.[14]

The drawback of sphincteroplasty compared with sphincterotomy is the more limited size of the papillary opening. Mechanical lithotripsy assistance was more frequently required in the patients undergoing BSP.[18] Stones measuring more than 8 mm often require mechanical lithotripsy to enable extraction across the papilla.

Overall success rate for BSP is comparable with that of BES. The reported success rates of stones removal are 81% to 99% for BSP and 85% to 98% for BES.[17,19-21] Randomized trials comparing BSP with BES suggest that BSP is at least as effective as BES in patients with small to moderate-sized bile duct stones. Although sphincteroplasty has decreased rates of bleeding and probably perforation, higher rates of postprocedure pancreatitis are reported. In a US multicenter study by DiSario and colleagues,[22] which randomized patients with suspected biliary stone to endoscopic balloon dilation or endoscopic sphincterotomy, pancreatitis occurred at a rate 2 times greater in the balloon dilation group compared with the sphincterotomy group (15.4% vs 8%, $P<.001$). The meta-analysis of randomized controlled trials by Baron and Harewood[20] showed an early complication rate of BSP comparable with BES for removing CBD stones during ERCP. Overall, the early complication rates for BSP and BES were 10.5% vs 10.3% ($P = .9$). The bleeding rate was higher in the BES group (2.0% vs 0, $P = .001$) whereas the rate of pancreatitis was higher in the BSP group (7.4% vs 4.3%, $P = .05$). Another recent meta-analysis demonstrated that the procedure carries significant higher risk of pancreatitis (RR = 1.96) over sphincterotomy.[18] Therefore, in the Western world, BSP is reserved for patients who have uncorrectable coagulopathy and possibly older patients who are less prone to post-ERCP pancreatitis.[18]

## DIFFICULT/LARGE COMMON BILE DUCT STONES

Approximately 10% to 15% of patients have bile duct stones that cannot be removed using standard BES and balloon/basket extraction techniques. These stones generally are larger than 1.0 cm, impacted, located proximal to strictures, or associated with duodenal diverticulua.[23] Such factors make adequate sphincterotomy and extraction difficult. Ultimately, the stone must be (1) extracted from above (ie, bile duct exploration), (2) made smaller (ie, lithotripsy), or (3) have a larger passage way (ie, large balloon dilation). All transpapillary intraductal approaches can also be performed via a percutaneous access with similar success rates[24] but added complications of the transhepatic approach (see **Fig. 1**).

## MECHANICAL LITHOTRIPSY

Mechanical lithotripsy was first introduced in 1982 by Riemann and colleagues[25] from Erlangen, Germany, and is now the most widely used technique for fragmentation of stones. The lithotripter unit is a strong-wired basket, which entraps the stone and is then pulled slowly via wench back through a metal sheath. The sheath can go through the scope or be applied after stone capture. The latter requires that the basket handle be cut off, the scope withdrawn, and the spiral metal sheath passed over the basket shaft wire. A lithotripter handle with a large screw or wench is used to pull the basket stepwise into the metal coil. The stone is broken into several pieces as the basket filaments cut through the stone (**Fig. 3**).

The combination of BES and mechanical lithotripsy has a stone removal success rate of 90% to 97% if the papilla is accessible and the stone can be captured by a basket.[26] In 2 studies, mechanical lithotripsy successfully removed 85% to 90% of difficult bile duct stones.[27,28] Mechanical lithotripsy usually is successful only in stones smaller than 3 cm. The most common reason for unsuccessful mechanical lithotripsy is inability to capture the stones (eg, inadequate space to open the basket).[3] Densely calcified stones are also more likely to fail lithotripsy.

The complication rate of mechanical lithotripsy has been reported as 3.6% in a recent multicenter comprehensive review. The most frequent complication was trapped or broken basket, and the others were wire fracture, broken handle, or perforation/duct injury.[29] To avoid breakage of the traction wire during procedure, only lithotripsy compatible baskets should be used.[26]

## ELECTROHYDRAULIC LITHOTRIPSY

An electrohydraulic lithotripsy (EHL) system consists of a bipolar lithotripsy probe and a charge generator. Initiation of a high-voltage spark discharged across the tip of the

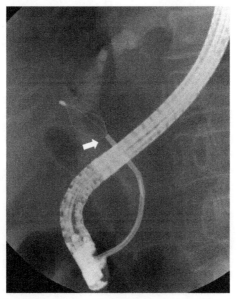

**Fig. 3.** Mechanical lithotripsy. Stone capturing basket is drawing into the metal sheath (*arrow*).

EHL probe causes expansion of the surrounding fluid that generates shock waves to fragment stones. Although EHL can be performed under fluoroscopic or direct cholangioscopic guidance, direct visualization is strongly preferred to enable proper deployment of the probe at the surface of the stone to avoid ductal injury (**Fig. 4**). This technique has the advantage of not requiring stone capture before applying energy. Disadvantages of using cholangioscopy for EHL are the need for 2 operators, the use of a fragile intraductal miniscope, and need for simultaneous nasobiliary tube (in some patients) to flush out fragments. Recently, single-operator cholangioscopy has been used to direct EHL therapy for bile duct stones; preliminary results have been encouraging.[30]

## LASER LITHOTRIPSY

In laser lithotripsy, laser light at a particular wavelength is focused on the surface of a stone to achieve stone fragmentation. An oscillating plasma, consisting of a gaseous collection of ions and free electrons, is created to induce wave-mediated fragmentation of stones. Laser lithotripsy is performed under direct visualization using the cholangioscope or under fluoroscopic guidance. The latter has greater potential to damage the bile duct wall. A recent-generation device can differentiate between the light reflection patterns of the bile duct wall and those of stones. The laser pulses are automatically interrupted when readings indicate that the probe is aimed at tissue rather than stone. Experience with this modality is limited, however. The success rates of bile duct stone clearance with laser lithotripsy have been reported at 64% to 97%.[31,32]

A new pulsed, solid-state laser system equipped with higher laser energy, double-pulse neodymium:YAG laser (FREDDY) (World of Medicine, Berlin, Germany), has been developed in Germany. This system promises to combine the advantages of

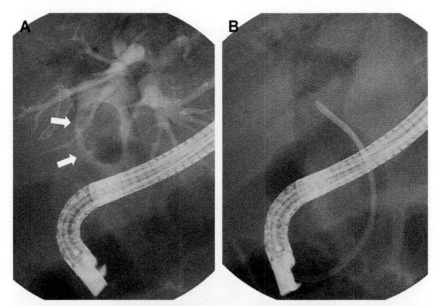

**Fig. 4.** EHL under direct cholangioscopic guidance. (*A*) Large stone (*arrows*) is noted in the bile duct. (*B*) Baby scope is introduced through the working channel of mother scope for fragmentation of stone.

dye and solid state lasers, such as reliability, effectiveness, and low cost.[26] Complete stone removal is achieved in 88% to 94%. Transient hemobilia occurred in 15% of the patients, mostly those who underwent the procedure with fluoroscopic guidance alone.[33,34]

## EXTRACORPOREAL SHOCK WAVE LITHOTRIPSY

Extracorporeal shock wave lithotripsy (ESWL) generates a shock wave originating outside the body using piezoelectric, electrohydraulic, or electromagnetic systems. A liquid or tissue medium is required to prevent energy attenuation. Because ESWL is painful, general anesthesia or, less frequently, epidural or conscious sedation is required. Because most bile duct stones are not radiopaque and are not visualized by fluoroscopy alone, a nasobiliary tube with contrast injection is required before ESWL. Complete stone clearance rates of 83% to 90% have been reported.[35,36] A large prospective study reported that overall clearance rate with successful fragmentation was 84.5%, but a single session of ESWL cleared the stones in only 16% of 283 patients with large CBD stones. In 25% of the patients, 4 to 7 sessions of ESWL were needed.[37] Complications of ESWL have been minimal.[35–37] A limitation is the considerable recurrence rate of bile duct stones after ESWL reported in 12.7% to 28% of patients on 1- to 3-year follow-up.[38–40]

## MOTHER AND BABY CHOLEDOCHOSCOPY AND INTRADUCTAL LITHOTRIPSY

Intraductal EHL or laser lithotripsy is best performed under direct visual control using the mother and baby scope system. An older system consisted of a jumbo size duodenoscope with a 5.5-mm working channel and a baby scope of 4.7 mm in diameter. The EHL or laser probe is passed into the bile duct through the instrument channel of a baby scope for fragmenting stones. Newer baby scopes are smaller, with a 3.2-mm diameter and a 1-mm instrument channel. Such small diameter scopes can be inserted through a standard therapeutic duodenoscope with a 4.2-mm instrument channel. The mother and baby endoscopic system has several limitations, such as its technical difficulty, its time-consuming nature, and the need for an additional endoscopic unit and 2 skilled endoscopists.

SpyGlass SpyScope (Boston Scientific, Natick, MA, USA) is a new partially disposable, less-expensive, single-operator endoscope that has been recently introduced into the endoscopic arena.[30] It includes a baby scope, which is 10F in diameter, has a 4-way tip deflection, and has a 1.2-mm working channel. The baby scope houses the SpyGlass optical fiber, an independent accessory channel, and a separate channel for water irrigation (**Fig. 5**). It can be used perorally or percutaneously. EHL can be readily applied by this system.[41] Recent studies showed rate of stone clearance at 87% to 100% as well as usefulness in histologic diagnosis of bile duct stricture.[30,41]

## DIRECT PERORAL CHOLANGIOSCOPY

The goal of this most recent stone management tool, direct peroral cholangioscopy, is to avoid mother and baby scope system limitations. Direct peroral cholangioscopy uses an ultraslim upper endoscope with a 4.9- to 6-mm tip diameter and greater than 140 cm length and is conducted by a single endoscopist. The procedure generally requires a large sphincterotomy, a terminal CBD greater than 10 mm diameter, placement of a guide wire or anchoring balloon into a peripheral bile duct via standard ERCP, passage of the direct cholangioscope over the anchoring balloon/wire, removal

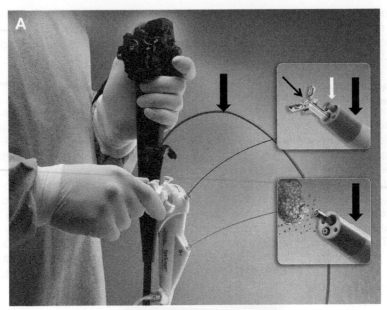

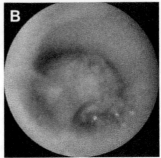

**Fig. 5.** Spyglass Spyscope system (*A*) and the cholangioscopic image (*B*).

of the anchoring wire, and then use of intraductal lithotripsy. A nasobiliary drain for flushing out fragments may be needed. An overtube may be needed to prevent intragastric bowing. Experience is limited, but recent studies show feasibility and clinical usefulness.[42,43] Limitations of the technique included limited availability of such prototype endoscopes, limited experience to date, and tendency for the endoscope to fall back into the duodenum.

## SUPPLEMENTAL ENDOSCOPIC PAPILLARY LARGE BALLOON DILATION

Use of a large-diameter (12 to 20 mm) dilation balloon after near-maximal or limited BES has been introduced as an adjunctive tool to enlarge a papillary orifice for the removal of large or difficult bile duct stones (**Fig. 6**). The concept is to combine the advantages of sphincterotomy with those of balloon dilation. Theoretically, risk of perforation or bleeding would be reduced by performing a less than maximal sphincterotomy, and risk of pancreatitis from balloon dilation would be reduced by first separating the biliary and pancreatic orifices with biliary sphincterotomy.[44]

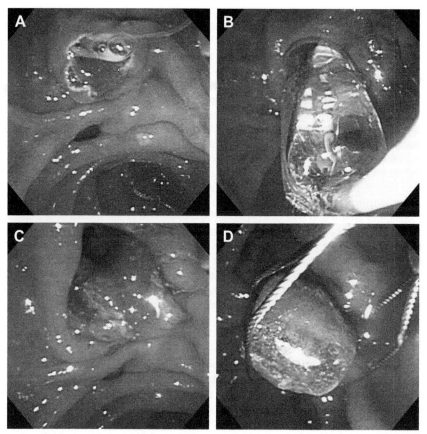

**Fig. 6.** Supplemental EPLBD. (*A*) Partial biliary sphincterotomy. (*B*) Papillary orifice is dilated with 12-mm–diameter balloon. (*C*) Large orifice is noted after the dilation. (*D*) The 12-mm–sized stone is easily removed through the orifice.

Data regarding supplemental endoscopic papillary large balloon dilation (EPLBD) are relatively limited. Most of the studies regarding EPLBD are retrospective analyses or have limited numbers of patients enrolled. In a multicenter study, Attasaranya and colleagues[45] reported efficacy of EPLBD using large-diameter balloons (≥ 12 mm) after sphincterotomy in 103 patients with large CBD stones at 5 ERCP referral centers in the United States. The combined technique had a success rate of 95% and a complication rate of 6%. Failure of complete stone clearance occurred in 5 procedures (5%). Short-term complications were documented in 6 patients (5.4%), including a single case of cystic duct perforation. Two patients had complications of hemorrhage, including 1 patient who had severe bleeding requiring vascular coil embolization, but none had procedure-related pancreatitis. Heo and colleagues[46] from Korea randomized 200 consecutive patients with bile duct stones of mean 15 mm in diameter in equal numbers to partial BES plus large balloon dilation (12- to 20-mm balloon diameter) or full BES alone. Outcomes were similar in terms of overall successful stone removal, large (>15 mm) stone removal, and need for mechanical lithotripsy assistance. Overall complications were also similar between the 2 groups. Pancreatitis occurred in 4% of the large balloon dilation group whereas none of the patients developed perforation or bleeding.

Other recent studies have reported similar results for large/difficult bile duct stones with a complete stone removal rate at 95% to 100%, overall complication rate at 3.8% to 8.3%, and low incidence of pancreatitis.[47–49] A preliminary report from Korea noted 2 fatal complications, 1 due to perforation and the other from massive bleeding, in a series of 166 patients.[50] Although their multivariate analysis could not identify clear risk factors for complications, the size of balloons used in this study was likely larger than in other studies and may have been larger than the native duct in some cases.

Details of the method not yet standardized include optimal size of balloon, duration of dilation, and extent of sphincterotomy.[51] Use of a balloon that is equal to or smaller in diameter than the native distal bile duct seems logical, because use of a larger balloon might be expected to tear the sphincter and possibly the duct as well, resulting in the cases of bleeding and perforation that have been observed. Additionally, it seems logical that achieving best results would require adapting a balance of size of sphincterotomy and balloon dilation to each patient's anatomy, the size and burden of stones, the shape and size of the papilla, and presence of the papilla in or adjacent to diverticula.[44] Patients with distal CBD stenosis or a relatively narrow "normal" CBD are probably at higher risk of complications after balloon dilation. Therefore, it seems prudent to limit dilation to 2 to 3 mm larger than the native duct diameter.

This technique may be helpful in patients with difficult papillary anatomy, such as those with small papilla or intra- or peridiverticular papilla. Its role in patients with coagulopathy, however, or other risks for bleeding remain to be investigated.[44]

## MIRIZZI SYNDROME

Mirizzi syndrome (MS) is an atypical presentation of gallstone disease in which the impaction of a gallstone in the cystic duct or the gallbladder neck causes stenosis of the extrahepatic bile duct by extrinsic compression or fibrosis.[52] Bile duct wall necrosis and subsequent cholecystobiliary fistula caused by chronic inflammation are rare sequelae of the disease. The syndrome was first described by the Argentinean surgeon Pablo Mirizzi in 1948. It is reported to occur in 0.7% to 2.5% of all US patients undergoing cholecystectomy.[53,54]

Patients have the same presenting signs and symptoms as CBD stones. CT and magnetic resonance cholangiopancreatography have 80% to 90% sensitivity to detect MS. Transabdominal ultrasound is less sensitive. MS is of particular importance to surgeons because the diagnosis may not be appreciated preoperatively and because the surgical treatment of this condition is associated with a significantly increased risk of bile duct injury.[52] ERCP is probably the most effective preoperative test to diagnose MS and can provide good localization and characterization of the source of the biliary obstruction.

Surgical intervention remains the definitive treatment for the majority of patients.[52] Currently, laparoscopic treatment is technically feasible in highly selected patients but is associated with a high rate of conversion to open cholecystectomy and increased morbidity and mortality rates.[55,56]

Endoscopic treatment of MS can consist of establishing biliary ductal drainage by stent insertion or definitive gallstone removal from the gallbladder neck or cystic duct. Direct basketing of the stone and mechanical lithotripsy are usually not possible. Intraductal lithotripsy is most effective. Because gallbladder surgery is nearly always indicated, other alternatives, such as dissolution therapy[55,57] and percutaneous transhepatic management, are infrequently considered.[58,59]

The success rate of endoscopic therapy in the management of MS has been reported in 2 series. Seitz and colleagues[60] achieved successful fragmentation and clearance of stones in 38 cases using EHL delivered via cholangioscopy with a mother and baby endoscope system. Tsuyuguchi and colleagues[61] used a similar approach in 25 patients with MS. They were able to clear the obstructing stone in all 23 patients with cholecystocholedochal fistula (type II). Four of the patients required rehospitalization for acute cholangitis when residual gallbladder stones migrated into the CBD. Cholangioscopy was unsuccessful in 2 patients. Similar success has been reported with the SpyGlass system and has made the technique more widely available. The limitations of nonsurgical treatment include the need of special expertise, time-consuming procedures, multiple sessions of treatment, cost of equipment, and risk of complications. Complications of nonsurgical treatment occurring in 5% to 15% of cases include bile leakage and focal perforation, sepsis, and residual stones. Decision for surgical versus nonsurgical treatment of MS should be made on local expertise. Stenting of the CBD or cystic duct can also be used as a temporary measure during the preparation of patients for an elective operation.[57,62]

## CYSTIC DUCT STONES AFTER CHOLECYSTECTOMY

Patients with retained cystic duct stones may present at any time, from a few days to many years, after cholecystectomy. The estimated incidence of retained stones within the cystic duct remnant after cholecystectomy is less than 2.5%. In a series of 322 patients explored for postcholecystectomy syndrome, Rogy and colleagues[63] found only 8 patients with a stone in the cystic duct stump/gallbladder remnant. Similarly, Zhou and colleagues[64] reported 4 patients with stone in the cystic duct remnant in a series of 371 patients. To date, there does not seem to be an increased risk of cystic duct remnant stones in patients who have undergone laparoscopic cholecystectomy (and presumably have a longer cystic duct remnant) compared with patients who have undergone open cholecystectomy.

ERCP and endoscopic removal of stones in the cystic duct remnant can be attempted with the same techniques (discussed previously) as for routine or difficult stones. Case reports of cystic duct stones after cholecystectomy show variable success rates with regard to interventions using ERCP alone.[65–68] Usually 2 or 3 ERCP sessions involving stenting, balloon dilation of the cystic duct, or mother and baby lithotripsy are required.

Surgical options may involve open and laparoscopic exploration,[66,67,69–71] including redo cholecystectomy with shortening of the cystic duct remnant or cystic duct treatment just like with MS. Decisions on use of endoscopy or surgery should be individualized based on local expertise and patients' preference.

## SURGICALLY ALTERED ANATOMY

ERCP may be performed for a variety of clinical indications in patients with surgically altered gastrointestinal anatomy. Such procedures can be more technically challenging, time consuming, and often require a significant level of expertise to optimize success.[72] Moreover, the obesity epidemic has led to further increases in bariatric surgery and increased the patient population with difficult to access pancreaticobiliary anatomy.

Several significant challenges to performance of ERCP in a patient with surgically altered gastrointestinal anatomy exist.[73] First, access to the ampulla of Vater or biliary-enteric anastomosis may require an endoscopist to traverse a significant length of small intestine. The length of small intestine that must be traversed to access the major papilla dictates the type and length of endoscope that can be used. The use of forward-viewing endoscopes in a retrograde fashion for cannulation presents its own set of challenges. The papillary orifice is not always visible using a forward-viewing instrument. Attempt of cannulation of the major papilla with a forward-viewing endoscope may be challenging due to the alignment of the working channel and lack of an elevator. The use of an enteroscope for the performance of therapeutic ERCP requires the use of enteroscope-length accessory tools, the availability of which is limited in many markets.

Patients with Billroth II gastrectomy/jejunostomy are seen worldwide but in Asian countries, they are more frequent due to higher incidence of gastric cancer and peptic ulcer. Cases of Billroth II are some of the more difficult ERCP procedures. In a study involving 185 Billroth II ERCP procedures, the failure rate was 34%.[74]

When using a duodenoscope, the difficulty starts with gaining entry into the afferent lumen. Tips to traversing the afferent limb include (1) rolling patients in supine position if afferent limb orifice unclear, (2) using fluoroscopy frequently to aid scope passage, (3) passing stiff guide wire ahead in the lumen under fluoroscopy guidance, (4) using an end-view scope first and exchanging for a side-view scope over a stiff guide wire, (5) limiting air inflation to decrease gut wall rigidity, and (6) reducing intragastric looping frequently. In cases of retrocolic Billroth II anastomosis, the major papilla is usually accessible using a standard duodenoscope because the length of bowel that must be traversed can be as short as 30 cm. In cases of antecolic anastomosis, the afferent limb may be longer and a more tortuous route to reach the papilla.

Once the papilla is in view, tips to successful biliary cannulation and sphincterotomy with a side-view scope include (1) remembering the papilla is truly upside down; (2) putting the papilla in the lower portion of endoscope viewing screen; (3) using a straight catheter for straight guidance; (4) directing biliary cannulation toward the maximal 6 o'clock position; (5) if the pancreas is entered repeatedly, placing a 3- to 4-F pancreatic stent then precutting with a needle knife over stent; (6) if the papilla is large or with bulging stone, considering precut earlier; and (7) if the cutting space is limited or direction is uncertain, performing a small sphincterotomy followed by hydrostatic balloon dilation.

ERCP in Billroth II predisposes to a higher risk of jejunal and periampullary perforation and should be done only by an endoscopist with a record of acceptable safety. Patients who have a Roux-en-Y anastomosis typically require the use of a long forward-viewing endoscope to access the major papilla for the performance of ERCP. The longest roux limbs are encountered in patients who have undergone a standard Roux-en-Y gastric bypass for bariatric indications or in those individuals in whom bowel resection proximal to the ligament of Treitz has not been performed. Performance of ERCP in these patients may require the use of specialized enteroscopes designed for deep enteral access, such as the double-balloon,[75] single-balloon,[76] or spiral enteroscopy systems.[77]

The rate of reaching the papilla or the bilioenteric anastomosis was 86% to 94%, and the success rate of diagnostic/therapeutic ERCP was lower, at 55% to 89%.[78–81] Using these long tools, pancreatic studies are more difficult to perform than biliary ones; such procedures commonly require 90 to 120 minutes.

For elective cases, the authors prefer to have a surgical 30- to 36-F gastrostomy tube placed and then perform ERCP after maturation of the tract.[82] This method offers better biliary and pancreatic access. Additionally, the gastrostomy tube can be left in situ for several months until complete therapeutic response of the patient is evaluated, and more therapeutic intervention undertaken if needed. The authors' experience with 27 such cases resulted in full desired therapeutic success in more than 90%. It is also possible to perform surgical gastrostomy and ERCP in 1 setting.[83] This requires intraoperative ERCP with lesser-quality fluoroscopy.

A similar alternative is to have a percutaneous endoscopic gastrostomy by inserting double-balloon enteroscope retrograde into the stomach. After the maturation of large bore fistula, a duodenoscope can be inserted through the gastric fistula to perform ERCP.[84] Studies comparing the surgery-assisted techniques with laparoscopy or open laparotomy are needed.

Preprocedure planning with knowledge of the operation performed and the resultant anatomy and use of appropriate accessories are as important as good endoscopic skills in achieving success for ERCP in patients with surgically altered gastrointestinal anatomy.

## LONG-TERM BILIARY STENTING

A practical approach to difficult stones refractory to endoscopic retrieval is to place a biliary stent as a temporizing measure to maintain biliary drainage and to prevent stone impaction, pending more definitive management.[4] Alternatively, long-term biliary stenting is used in patients who have severe comorbid medical conditions that preclude surgery or have failed repeated endoscopic interventions for definitive therapy of bile duct stones.[85–88]

Stones may partially disintegrate or decrease in size because of a mechanical effect of the placement of stent.[89] It has been shown in several prospective series that elderly patients with difficult stones may remain symptom-free after insertion of a plastic stent. In a Hong Kong study, 46 patients with large CBD stones received plastic stents.[89] Twenty-eight patients had repeated ERCP for stone extraction after a median of 63 days. The size of the stones was significantly reduced, from 11 to 46 mm (mean 24.9 mm) to 5 to 46 mm (mean 20.1 mm), and duct clearance was achieved in 25 patients (89%) during the repeated procedure. Similar results have also been reported by Maxton and colleagues and Jain and colleagues.[85,88] Attempts to leave plastic biliary stents intraductally for more than 18 months often leads to further stone formation attached to the stent, cholangitis, and occasional deaths.

The oral administration of ursodeoxycholic acid (UDCA) (Actigall, Ursosan, Ursofalk, or Urso) may further enhance softening or disintegration of the stone.[4] One report showed good results in 9 of 10 patients who became stone-free with the use of stenting plus orally administered UDCA compared with none of the 40 patients with stents alone.[90] Terpene preparation (Rowachol), a well-tolerated oil preparation containing 6 cyclic monoterpenes, was also reported to have an inhibitory effect on hepatic hydroxymethylglutaryl coenzyme A reductase, altering biliary cholesterol saturation, thus dissolving gallstones.[91] In recent study, biliary stenting with combined UDCA and terpene preparation administration for 6 months significantly reduced the stone size, and the endoscopic stone removal was successful in 92.8%.[92] Another study reported that UDCA did not contribute to reduction in stone size or stone fragmentation in addition to long-term biliary stenting.[93]

## PERCUTANEOUS INTERVENTION

The percutaneous approach uses the percutaneous access to intrahepatic duct through the transhepatic route. There are 2 methods for removal of the bile duct stones: percutaneous transhepatic cholangioscopic stone removal (PTCS) and interventional radiologic stone removal under fluoroscopic guidance. PTCS is performed using the short, thin (diameter ranges from 3.0 to 5.2 mm) cholangioscope direct visual guidance. This method is more useful for intrahepatic stones or the tissue acquisition for bile duct strictures. Smaller stone retrieval basket or stone fragmentation methods, such as EHL or laser, can be also used as a transpapillary approach. Irrigating and flushing the fragments of stone with saline into the duodenal lumen is often helpful for the ductal clearance. The recently introduced SpyGlass Spyscope can be also used as conventional cholangioscope.[41]

## SURGERY

For stones that have failed endoscopic removal or those with limited access to the major papilla, surgical intervention can be considered. Open CBD exploration with stone removal has been the standard treatment, although laparoscopic approaches are increasingly used. Laparoscopic transcystic CBD exploration seems the safest and most effective (90%) approach to the CBD.[94] Transcystic CBD stone extraction has the advantage of avoiding choledochotomy and subsequent suture repair.[70,94,95] Studies have demonstrated success with extracting larger stones, from 10 to 15 mm, with an associated dilated CBD through this approach.[70,95,96] Laparoscopic choledochotomy and CBD exploration require advanced laparoscopic skills, and local expertise is variable.

## SUMMARY

Bile duct stone management has greatly changed in the past 2 decades. Open surgical techniques have mostly been replaced by transoral endoscopic techniques. Advanced transoral techniques can also manage most difficult ductal stones. In skilled centers, laparoscopic ductal stone management has assumed a back-up role.

## REFERENCES

1. Ko CW, Lee SP. Epidemiology and natural history of common bile duct stones and prediction of disease. Gastrointest Endosc 2002;56:S165–9.
2. Freitas ML, Bell RL, Duffy AJ. Choledocholithiasis: evolving standards for diagnosis and management. World J Gastroenterol 2006;12:3162–7.
3. Attasaranya S, Fogel EL, Lehman GA. Choledocholithiasis, ascending cholangitis, and gallstone pancreatitis. Med Clin North Am 2008;92:925–60.
4. Binmoeller KF, Schafer TW. Endoscopic management of bile duct stones. J Clin Gastroenterol 2001;32:106–18.
5. Norton ID, Petersen BT, Bosco J, et al. A randomized trial of endoscopic biliary sphincterotomy using pure-cut versus combined cut and coagulation waveforms. Clin Gastroenterol Hepatol 2005;3:1029–33.
6. Verma D, Kapadia A, Adler DG. Pure versus mixed electrosurgical current for endoscopic biliary sphincterotomy: a meta-analysis of adverse outcomes. Gastrointest Endosc 2007;66:283–90.
7. Perini RF, Sadurski R, Cotton PB, et al. Post-sphincterotomy bleeding after the introduction of microprocessor-controlled electrosurgery: does the new technology make the difference? Gastrointest Endosc 2005;61:53–7.
8. Freeman ML, Nelson DB, Sherman S, et al. Complications of endoscopic biliary sphincterotomy. N Engl J Med 1996;335:909–18.
9. Freeman ML, DiSario JA, Nelson DB, et al. Risk factors for post-ERCP pancreatitis: a prospective, multicenter study. Gastrointest Endosc 2001;54:425–34.
10. Masci E, Toti G, Mariani A, et al. Complications of diagnostic and therapeutic ERCP: a prospective multicenter study. Am J Gastroenterol 2001;96:417–23.
11. Loperfido S, Angelini G, Benedetti G, et al. Major early complications from diagnostic and therapeutic ERCP: a prospective multicenter study. Gastrointest Endosc 1998;48:1–10.

12. Vandervoort J, Soetikno RM, Tham TC, et al. Risk factors for complications after performance of ERCP. Gastrointest Endosc 2002;56:652–6.
13. Cheng CL, Sherman S, Watkins JL, et al. Risk factors for post-ERCP pancreatitis: a prospective multicenter study. Am J Gastroenterol 2006;101:139–47.
14. Staritz M, Ewe K, Meyer zum Buschenfelde KH. Endoscopic papillary dilation (EPD) for the treatment of common bile duct stones and papillary stenosis. Endoscopy 1983;15(Suppl 1):197–8.
15. Kozarek RA. Balloon dilation of the sphincter of Oddi. Endoscopy 1988;20(Suppl 1):207–10.
16. MacMathuna PM, White P, Clarke E, et al. Endoscopic balloon sphincteroplasty (papillary dilation) for bile duct stones: efficacy, safety, and follow-up in 100 patients. Gastrointest Endosc 1995;42:468–74.
17. Minami A, Nakatsu T, Uchida N, et al. Papillary dilation vs sphincterotomy in endoscopic removal of bile duct stones. A randomized trial with manometric function. Dig Dis Sci 1995;40:2550–4.
18. Weinberg BM, Shindy W, Lo S. Endoscopic balloon sphincter dilation (sphincteroplasty) versus sphincterotomy for common bile duct stones. Cochrane Database Syst Rev 2006;(18):CD004890.
19. Bergman JJ, Rauws EA, Fockens P, et al. Randomised trial of endoscopic balloon dilation versus endoscopic sphincterotomy for removal of bileduct stones. Lancet 1997;349:1124–9.
20. Baron TH, Harewood GC. Endoscopic balloon dilation of the biliary sphincter compared to endoscopic biliary sphincterotomy for removal of common bile duct stones during ERCP: a metaanalysis of randomized, controlled trials. Am J Gastroenterol 2004;99:1455–60.
21. Vlavianos P, Chopra K, Mandalia S, et al. Endoscopic balloon dilatation versus endoscopic sphincterotomy for the removal of bile duct stones: a prospective randomised trial. Gut 2003;52:1165–9.
22. DiSario JA, Freeman ML, Bjorkman DJ, et al. Endoscopic balloon dilation compared with sphincterotomy for extraction of bile duct stones. Gastroenterology 2004;127:1291–9.
23. McHenry L, Lehman G. Difficult bile duct stones. Curr Treat Options Gastroenterol 2006;9:123–32.
24. Lammert F, Miquel JF. Gallstone disease: from genes to evidence-based therapy. J Hepatol 2008;48(Suppl 1):S124–35.
25. Riemann JF, Seuberth K, Demling L. Clinical application of a new mechanical lithotripter for smashing common bile duct stones. Endoscopy 1982;14:226–30.
26. Hochberger J, Tex S, Maiss J, et al. Management of difficult common bile duct stones. Gastrointest Endosc Clin N Am 2003;13:623–34.
27. Shaw MJ, Mackie RD, Moore JP, et al. Results of a multicenter trial using a mechanical lithotripter for the treatment of large bile duct stones. Am J Gastroenterol 1993;88:730–3.
28. Hintze RE, Adler A, Veltzke W. Outcome of mechanical lithotripsy of bile duct stones in an unselected series of 704 patients. Hepatogastroenterology 1996;43:473–6.
29. Thomas M, Howell DA, Carr-Locke D, et al. Mechanical lithotripsy of pancreatic and biliary stones: complications and available treatment options collected from expert centers. Am J Gastroenterol 2007;102:1896–902.
30. Chen YK, Pleskow DK. SpyGlass single-operator peroral cholangiopancreatoscopy system for the diagnosis and therapy of bile-duct disorders: a clinical feasibility study (with video). Gastrointest Endosc 2007;65:832–41.

31. Caddy GR, Tham TC. Gallstone disease: symptoms, diagnosis and endoscopic management of common bile duct stones. Best Pract Res Clin Gastroenterol 2006;20:1085–101.

32. Hochberger J, Bayer J, May A, et al. Laser lithotripsy of difficult bile duct stones: results in 60 patients using a rhodamine 6G dye laser with optical stone tissue detection system. Gut 1998;43:823–9.

33. Kim TH, Oh HJ, Choi CS, et al. Clinical usefulness of transpapillary removal of common bile duct stones by frequency doubled double pulse Nd:YAG laser. World J Gastroenterol 2008;14:2863–6.

34. Cho YD, Cheon YK, Moon JH, et al. Clinical role of frequency-doubled double-pulsed yttrium aluminum garnet laser technology for removing difficult bile duct stones (with videos). Gastrointest Endosc 2009;70:684–9.

35. Sackmann M, Holl J, Sauter GH, et al. Extracorporeal shock wave lithotripsy for clearance of bile duct stones resistant to endoscopic extraction. Gastrointest Endosc 2001;53:27–32.

36. Ellis RD, Jenkins AP, Thompson RP, et al. Clearance of refractory bile duct stones with extracorporeal shockwave lithotripsy. Gut 2000;47:728–31.

37. Tandan M, Reddy DN, Santosh D, et al. Extracorporeal shock wave lithotripsy of large difficult common bile duct stones: efficacy and analysis of factors that favor stone fragmentation. J Gastroenterol Hepatol 2009;24:1370–4.

38. Kratzer W, Mason RA, Grammer S, et al. Difficult bile duct stone recurrence after endoscopy and extracorporeal shockwave lithotripsy. Hepatogastroenterology 1998;45:910–6.

39. Adamek HE, Kudis V, Jakobs R, et al. Impact of gallbladder status on the outcome in patients with retained bile duct stones treated with extracorporeal shockwave lithotripsy. Endoscopy 2002;34:624–7.

40. Conigliaro R, Camellini L, Zuliani CG, et al. Clearance of irretrievable bile duct and pancreatic duct stones by extracorporeal shockwave lithotripsy, using a transportable device: effectiveness and medium-term results. J Clin Gastroenterol 2006;40:213–9.

41. Fishman DS, Tarnasky PR, Patel SN, et al. Management of pancreaticobiliary disease using a new intra-ductal endoscope: the Texas experience. World J Gastroenterol 2009;15:1353–8.

42. Larghi A, Waxman I. Endoscopic direct cholangioscopy by using an ultra-slim upper endoscope: a feasibility study. Gastrointest Endosc 2006;63:853–7.

43. Moon JH, Ko BM, Choi HJ, et al. Direct peroral cholangioscopy using an ultra-slim upper endoscope for the treatment of retained bile duct stones. Am J Gastroenterol 2009;104:2729–33.

44. Attam R, Freeman ML. Endoscopic papillary large balloon dilation for large common bile duct stones. J Hepatobiliary Pancreat Surg 2009;16:618–23.

45. Attasaranya S, Cheon YK, Vittal H, et al. Large-diameter biliary orifice balloon dilation to aid in endoscopic bile duct stone removal: a multicenter series. Gastrointest Endosc 2008;67:1046–52.

46. Heo JH, Kang DH, Jung HJ, et al. Endoscopic sphincterotomy plus large-balloon dilation versus endoscopic sphincterotomy for removal of bile-duct stones. Gastrointest Endosc 2007;66:720–6 [quiz: 68, 71].

47. Maydeo A, Bhandari S. Balloon sphincteroplasty for removing difficult bile duct stones. Endoscopy 2007;39:958–61.

48. Itoi T, Itokawa F, Sofuni A, et al. Endoscopic sphincterotomy combined with large balloon dilation can reduce the procedure time and fluoroscopy time for removal of large bile duct stones. Am J Gastroenterol 2009;104:560–5.

49. Draganov PV, Evans W, Fazel A, et al. Large size balloon dilation of the ampulla after biliary sphincterotomy can facilitate endoscopic extraction of difficult bile duct stones. J Clin Gastroenterol 2009;43:782–6.

50. Yoo B, Kim J, Jung J, et al. Large balloon sphincteroplasty along with or without sphincterotomy in patients with large extrahepatic bile duct stones—multi center study. Gastrointest Endosc 2007;66:720–6.

51. Carr-Locke DL. Difficult bile-duct stones: cut, dilate, or both? Gastrointest Endosc 2008;67:1053–5.

52. Mithani R, Schwesinger WH, Bingener J, et al. The Mirizzi syndrome: multidisciplinary management promotes optimal outcomes. J Gastrointest Surg 2008;12:1022–8.

53. Pemberton M, Wells AD. The Mirizzi syndrome. Postgrad Med J 1997;73:487–90.

54. Shah OJ, Dar MA, Wani MA, et al. Management of Mirizzi syndrome: a new surgical approach. ANZ J Surg 2001;71:423–7.

55. Lai EC, Lau WY. Mirizzi syndrome: history, present and future development. ANZ J Surg 2006;76:251–7.

56. Antoniou SA, Antoniou GA, Makridis C. Laparoscopic treatment of Mirizzi syndrome: a systematic review. Surg Endosc 2010;24:33–9.

57. England RE, Martin DF. Endoscopic management of Mirizzi's syndrome. Gut 1997;40:272–6.

58. Cairns SR, Watson GN, Lees WR, et al. Percutaneous lithotripsy and endoprosthesis: a new treatment for obstructive jaundice in Mirizzi's syndrome. Br Med J (Clin Res Ed) 1987;295:1448.

59. Oxtoby JW, Yeong CC, West DJ. Mirizzi syndrome treated by percutaneous stone removal. Cardiovasc Intervent Radiol 1994;17:207–9.

60. Seitz U, Bapaye A, Bohnacker S, et al. Advances in therapeutic endoscopic treatment of common bile duct stones. World J Surg 1998;22:1133–44.

61. Tsuyuguchi T, Saisho H, Ishihara T, et al. Long-term follow-up after treatment of Mirizzi syndrome by peroral cholangioscopy. Gastrointest Endosc 2000;52:639–44.

62. Hazzan D, Golijanin D, Reissman P, et al. Combined endoscopic and surgical management of Mirizzi syndrome. Surg Endosc 1999;13:618–20.

63. Rogy MA, Fugger R, Herbst F, et al. Reoperation after cholecystectomy. The role of the cystic duct stump. HPB Surg 1991;4:129–34.

64. Zhou PH, Liu FL, Yao LQ, et al. Endoscopic diagnosis and treatment of postcholecystectomy syndrome. Hepatobiliary Pancreat Dis Int 2003;2:117–20.

65. Mergener K, Clavien PA, Branch MS, et al. A stone in a grossly dilated cystic duct stump: a rare cause of postcholecystectomy pain. Am J Gastroenterol 1999;94:229–31.

66. Shaw C, O'Hanlon DM, Fenlon HM, et al. Cystic duct remnant and the 'postcholecystectomy syndrome'. Hepatogastroenterology 2004;51:36–8.

67. Walsh RM, Ponsky JL, Dumot J. Retained gallbladder/cystic duct remnant calculi as a cause of postcholecystectomy pain. Surg Endosc 2002;16:981–4.

68. Lum YW, House MG, Hayanga AJ, et al. Postcholecystectomy syndrome in the laparoscopic era. J Laparoendosc Adv Surg Tech A 2006;16:482–5.

69. Chowbey PK, Bandyopadhyay SK, Sharma A, et al. Laparoscopic reintervention for residual gallstone disease. Surg Laparosc Endosc Percutan Tech 2003;13:31–5.

70. Petelin JB. Laparoscopic approach to common duct pathology. Am J Surg 1993;165:487–91.

71. Phillips EH. Laparoscopic transcystic duct common bile duct exploration. Surg Endosc 1998;12:365–6.

72. Ross AS. Endoscopic retrograde cholangiopancreatography in the surgically modified gastrointestinal tract. Gastrointest Endosc Clin N Am 2009;19:497–507.
73. Haber GB. Double balloon endoscopy for pancreatic and biliary access in altered anatomy (with videos). Gastrointest Endosc 2007;66:S47–50.
74. Faylona JM, Qadir A, Chan AC, et al. Small-bowel perforations related to endoscopic retrograde cholangiopancreatography (ERCP) in patients with Billroth II gastrectomy. Endoscopy 1999;31:546–9.
75. Sunada K, Yamamoto H. Double-balloon endoscopy: past, present, and future. J Gastroenterol 2009;44:1–12.
76. Kawamura T, Yasuda K, Tanaka K, et al. Clinical evaluation of a newly developed single-balloon enteroscope. Gastrointest Endosc 2008;68:1112–6.
77. Akerman PA, Agrawal D, Chen W, et al. Spiral enteroscopy: a novel method of enteroscopy by using the Endo-Ease Discovery SB overtube and a pediatric colonoscope. Gastrointest Endosc 2009;69:327–32.
78. Aabakken L, Bretthauer M, Line PD. Double-balloon enteroscopy for endoscopic retrograde cholangiography in patients with a Roux-en-Y anastomosis. Endoscopy 2007;39:1068–71.
79. Moreels TG, Roth B, Vandervliet EJ, et al. The use of the double-balloon enteroscope for endoscopic retrograde cholangiopancreatography and biliary stent placement after Roux-en-Y hepaticojejunostomy. Endoscopy 2007;39(Suppl 1): E196–7.
80. Ryozawa S, Iwamoto S, Iwano H, et al. ERCP using double-balloon endoscopes in patients with Roux-en-Y anastomosis. J Hepatobiliary Pancreat Surg 2009;16:613–7.
81. Koornstra JJ, Fry L, Monkemuller K. ERCP with the balloon-assisted enteroscopy technique: a systematic review. Dig Dis 2008;26:324–9.
82. Baron TH, Vickers SM. Surgical gastrostomy placement as access for diagnostic and therapeutic ERCP. Gastrointest Endosc 1998;48:640–1.
83. Pimentel RR, Mehran A, Szomstein S, et al. Laparoscopy-assisted transgastrostomy ERCP after bariatric surgery: case report of a novel approach. Gastrointest Endosc 2004;59:325–8.
84. Baron TH. Double-balloon enteroscopy to facilitate retrograde PEG placement as access for therapeutic ERCP in patients with long-limb gastric bypass. Gastrointest Endosc 2006;64:973–4.
85. Jain SK, Stein R, Bhuva M, et al. Pigtail stents: an alternative in the treatment of difficult bile duct stones. Gastrointest Endosc 2000;52:490–3.
86. Bowrey DJ, Fligelstone LJ, Solomon A, et al. Common bile duct stenting for choledocholithiasis: a district general hospital experience. Postgrad Med J 1998;74: 358–60.
87. Cotton PB, Forbes A, Leung JW, et al. Endoscopic stenting for long-term treatment of large bile duct stones: 2- to 5-year follow-up. Gastrointest Endosc 1987;33:411–2.
88. Maxton DG, Tweedle DE, Martin DF. Retained common bile duct stones after endoscopic sphincterotomy: temporary and longterm treatment with biliary stenting. Gut 1995;36:446–9.
89. Chan AC, Ng EK, Chung SC, et al. Common bile duct stones become smaller after endoscopic biliary stenting. Endoscopy 1998;30:356–9.
90. Johnson GK, Geenen JE, Venu RP, et al. Treatment of non-extractable common bile duct stones with combination ursodeoxycholic acid plus endoprostheses. Gastrointest Endosc 1993;39:528–31.
91. Doran J, Keighley MR, Bell GD. Rowachol—a possible treatment for cholesterol gallstones. Gut 1979;20:312–7.

92. Han J, Moon JH, Koo HC, et al. Effect of biliary stenting combined with ursodeox-ycholic acid and terpene treatment on retained common bile duct stones in elderly patients: a multicenter study. Am J Gastroenterol 2009;104:2418–21.

93. Katsinelos P, Kountouras J, Paroutoglou G, et al. Combination of endoprostheses and oral ursodeoxycholic acid or placebo in the treatment of difficult to extract common bile duct stones. Dig Liver Dis 2008;40:453–9.

94. Lyass S, Phillips EH. Laparoscopic transcystic duct common bile duct explora-tion. Surg Endosc 2006;20(Suppl 2):S441–5.

95. Hunter JG, Soper NJ. Laparoscopic management of bile duct stones. Surg Clin North Am 1992;72:1077–97.

96. Cuschieri A, Croce E, Faggioni A, et al. EAES ductal stone study. Preliminary findings of multi-center prospective randomized trial comparing two-stage vs single-stage management. Surg Endosc 1996;10:1130–5.

# Surgical Treatment of Gallstones

Kurinchi S. Gurusamy, MRCS*, Brian R. Davidson, FRCS

**KEYWORDS**

- Gallstones • Cholelithiasis • Choledocholithiasis
- Cholecystectomy • Surgical procedures • Operative
- Postoperative complications

About 5% to 25% of the adult western population have gallstones.[1–4] About 2% to 4% become symptomatic each year.[3,5,6] Most common symptoms are upper abdominal pain, biliary colic, and dyspepsia.[7,8] Biliary colic is defined as "a steady right upper quadrant abdominal pain lasting for more than half an hour," which may be associated with radiation to the back and nausea and may force patients to stop their activities.[7] Dyspepsia is defined as the presence of three or more of the following symptoms: belching, flatulence, nausea, intolerance to fatty food, bloating of the abdomen, epigastric discomfort, and acid regurgitation.[8] The complications of gallstones include acute cholecystitis (including empyema, when the gallbladder is filled with pus), acute gallstone pancreatitis, obstructive jaundice,[9] and rarely small bowel obstruction (gallstone ileus).[10] The relationship between gallstones and gallbladder cancer is controversial. Some studies suggest a strong association between gallstones and gallbladder cancer.[11,12] Other studies have questioned this association, as only a small proportion of patients (11%) with gallbladder cancer had gallstones for more than 1 year.[13]

Cholecystectomy (removal of gallbladder) is the preferred option in the treatment of gallstones. Medical treatment (bile acid dissolution therapy) or extracorporeal shock wave lithotripsy (ESWL) has a low rate of cure and high rate of recurrent gallstones.[14] In patients not suitable for cholecystectomy because of their general medical condition, percutaneous cholecystostomy (temporary drainage of gallbladder through a tube inserted under radiological guidance) may be considered in an emergency situation. When the patient's condition has improved, cholecystectomy,[15] medical treatment, or ESWL may be considered. The role of nonsurgical management in the treatment of gallstones is discussed elsewhere in this issue.

Cholecystectomy can be performed by a key-hole operation (laparoscopic cholecystectomy), by a small-incision cholecystectomy (incision <8 cm in length), or by

Department of Surgery, Royal Free Campus, University College London Medical School, 9th Floor, Royal Free Hospital, Pond Street, London NW3 2QG, UK
* Corresponding author.
*E-mail address:* kurinchi2k@hotmail.com

Gastroenterol Clin N Am 39 (2010) 229–244
doi:10.1016/j.gtc.2010.02.004
0889-8553/10/$ – see front matter © 2010 Elsevier Inc. All rights reserved.

gastro.theclinics.com

traditional open operation (incision >8 cm in length)[16–18]. There is considerable controversy in the indications, timing, and the route of access for the removal of gallbladder. In this article, these controversies are presented. The strength of evidence has been graded as grade A for randomized controlled trials and meta-analyses and grade B for other evidence such as well-designed controlled and uncontrolled studies as recommended by the manuscript guidelines for authors of *Gastroenterology Clinics of North America*.

## APPROACHES AND RISKS OF CHOLECYSTECTOMY

Cholecystectomy can be performed by a key-hole operation (laparoscopic cholecystectomy), by a small-incision cholecystectomy (incision <8 cm in length), or by traditional open operation (incision >8 cm in length).[16–18] The complications after cholecystectomy depend on the clinical presentation. The overall perioperative mortality varies between 0% and 0.3%.[19–21] The overall incidence of bile duct injuries requiring corrective surgery varies between 0.1% and 0.3%.[19–21] Corrective surgery for bile duct injury carries its own risks including perioperative mortality (1% to 4%),[22–24] secondary biliary cirrhosis (11%),[22] anastomotic stricture (9% to 20%),[22,24] and cholangitis (5%).[23] The quality of life can be poor several years after the corrective surgery.[25] Apart from the serious complications of perioperative mortality and bile duct injury and its sequelae, other complications of cholecystectomy include

- Bile leak treated conservatively (0.1% to 0.2%),[19,20] radiologically (0% to 0.1%)[19,20] or endoscopically (0.05% to 0.1%)[19,20] or by operation (0% to 0.05%)[19,20]
- Peritonitis requiring reoperation (0.2%)[19]
- Postoperative bleeding requiring operation (0.1% to 0.5%)[19,20]
- Intra-abdominal abscesses requiring operation (0.1%)[19]
- Other minor complications such as wound infection.[16–18]

In addition to these complications, in laparoscopic cholecystectomy, there is an additional 0.02% risk of major bowel or vessel injury during insertion of the trocar.[26,27] Currently, there is no evidence to suggest that there is any difference between the different techniques (open or Hassan's method vs closed or Veress needle method) of laparoscopic entry[27] (grade A). The choice of route of access (laparoscopic vs small-incision vs open cholecystectomy) varies with the indications for cholecystectomy and is discussed under the different indications for cholecystectomy.

## PRIMARY PREVENTION

Certain groups of patients have a high risk of development of gallstones. These include patients undergoing gastrectomy for gastric malignancy (14% to 26% of patients develop gallstones within 5 years)[28,29] and patients undergoing gastric bypass procedures for morbid obesity (22% to 28% of patients develop gallstones within 1 year).[30,31] Some surgeons perform routine prophylactic cholecystectomy because of the high incidence of gallstones in these patients.[28] Other surgeons, however, do not recommend routine prophylactic cholecystectomy, because most patients developing gallstones are asymptomatic.[31–33] Currently, a randomized controlled trial is underway to investigate whether prophylactic cholecystectomy is indicated in patients undergoing gastrectomy for gastric cancer.[34] Currently, prophylactic cholecystectomy to prevent gallstone formation is not recommended in any group of patients (grade B).

## ASYMPTOMATIC GALLSTONES

The distinction between symptomatic and asymptomatic gallstones can be difficult, as symptoms can be mild and varied. The different symptoms attributable to gall-stones include upper abdominal pain, biliary colic, and dyspepsia.[7,8] About 92% of patients with biliary colic, 72% of patients with upper abdominal pain, and 56% of patients with dyspepsia have relief of symptoms after cholecystectomy.[8] Cholecys-tectomy for asymptomatic gallstones is a matter of frequent debate in the manage-ment of gallstones. The annual incidence of complications of gallstones in asymptomatic patients is 0.3% acute cholecystitis, 0.2% obstructive jaundice, 0.04% to 1.5% of acute pancreatitis,[9] and rarely gallstone ileus.[10] As mentioned previously, the causative association between gallstones and gallbladder cancer has not been proven. As gallbladder surgery can be associated with life-threatening or life-changing postoperative complications, cholecystectomy for asymptomatic gallstones is not recommended routinely in any group of patients. This includes patients at risk of gallstone-related complications such as diabetic patients,[6,35] chil-dren with sickle cell disease,[36] children in general, and patients undergoing organ transplantation[37] (grade B). The controversies surrounding routine cholecystectomy for asymptomatic gallstones is far from resolved. Some surgeons recommend that routine prophylactic cholecystectomy is indicated in children with sickle cell disease because of the proportion and severity of complications related to gallstones in chil-dren with sickle cell disease (more than 70% of children required cholecystectomy because of gallstone symptoms or complications after a mean period of 3 years).[38] Other surgeons recommend cholecystectomy in all children with gallstones irrespec-tive of whether they have sickle disease or not, as the natural history of gallstones in children is not known.[39] It should be noted, however, that the complications related to cholecystectomy such as bile duct injury are present in the pediatric age group also.[40] There were two bile duct injuries in 109 children in this study.[40] Although other studies with more than 100 patients each did not report any bile duct injury,[41,42] the risk of bile duct injury and its consequences should not be neglected in the pediatric age group.

One special situation is the presence of asymptomatic gallstones in patients under-going major abdominal surgery for other pathologies. Concomitant cholecystectomy along with the major abdominal procedure does not appear to significantly increase the postoperative morbidity or hospital stay,[43,44] and some surgeons advocate routine cholecystectomy.[43] Considering that adhesions related to a major operation may make further minimal access surgeries difficult or impossible, it appears reasonable to offer cholecystectomy to patients with asymptomatic gallstones undergoing major abdominal operations (grade B).

## SYMPTOMATIC PATIENTS WITHOUT COMPLICATIONS

Patients with symptomatic gallstones are generally offered cholecystectomy. This is based on several longitudinal studies on the natural history of symptomatic gall-stones without complications (grade B). These studies assess the hospital admis-sions and the complications that patients with symptomatic gallstones developed. The number of hospital admissions varied from 2.5 hospital admissions per 100 patients per month to 23 hospital admissions per 100 patients per month,[45–47] possibly because of the severity of the symptoms at inclusion in the study. By

1 year, 14% of patients develop acute cholecystitis; 5% of patients develop gallstone pancreatitis, and 5% of patients develop obstructive jaundice.[45] Other studies report an annual complication risk of 1% in patients with mild symptoms.[48,49] Of the later studies, one was a randomized controlled trial comparing cholecystectomy and observation.[49] In this trial, in a mean follow-up period of 4 years, 50% of the patients in the observation group had undergone cholecystectomy.[49] The timing of cholecystectomy for patients with biliary colic is controversial. There is no reason to delay cholecystectomy in these patients other than for resource implications. One randomized controlled trial of urgent versus elective laparoscopic cholecystectomy for biliary colic showed a decrease in the hospital stay and complications related to gallstones in the urgent group.[50] Another randomized controlled trial of the same comparison did not show any difference in the hospital stay or complications related to gallstones.[51] Considering that urgent cholecystectomy needs prioritization ahead of other surgeries, with no evidence for additional benefit of urgent cholecystectomy over elective cholecystectomy, elective cholecystectomy appears sufficient in patients with biliary colic (grade B). Systematic reviews of randomized controlled trials show that there is no difference in the complication rates between laparoscopic, small-incision, and open cholecystectomy performed for symptomatic uncomplicated gallstones.[16–18] However, laparoscopic and small-incision cholecystectomies have a significantly shorter post-operative hospital stay and are hence preferable to open cholecystectomy (grade A).

## ACUTE CHOLECYSTITIS

Most surgeons recommend surgery after a complication of gallstone. This is because of the high risk of recurrence of the cholecystitis, non-resolution of the cholecystitis, and other complications during the waiting period[45,46,52–54] (grade B). There has been one randomized controlled trial comparing delayed cholecystectomy (conservative treatment followed by elective cholecystectomy) and observation in patients with mild cholecystitis. Gallstone related events and hospital admissions occurred in 19% and 10% of the patients belonging to the delayed cholecystectomy group, and these events occurred in 36% and 12% of patients belonging to the observation group. This difference was not statistically significant. After a mean follow-up period of 60 months, 24% of the patients in the observation group had undergone cholecystectomy. There was no difference in the number of gallstone related complications. However, the study was underpowered to measure even a 17% difference in the gallstone complication rate. Besides, delayed cholecystectomy is not the optimal option in the treatment of acute cholecystitis. Systematic reviews with meta-analysis of randomized controlled trials have shown that early cholecystectomy (performed within 1 week of onset of symptoms) is superior to delayed cholecystectomy in terms of reduction in the gallstone-related complications during the waiting time.[54] Earlier fears that early laparoscopic cholecystectomy was not safe and resulted in increased conversion to open cholecystectomy are unfounded.[52,53] Early cholecystectomy is the treatment of choice for acute cholecystitis. It shortens hospital stay and results in considerable cost savings[52,53,55] (grade A). Evidence from randomized controlled trials show that early laparoscopic cholecystectomy for acute cholecystitis has similar morbidity as compared with early mini-incision cholecystectomy[56] and early open cholecystectomy[57,58] for acute cholecystitis but is associated with a shorter hospital stay.[56–58] Early laparoscopic cholecystectomy performed within 1 week of onset of symptoms is the treatment of choice for patients with acute cholecystitis (grade A).

## PANCREATITIS

Gallstone pancreatitis is caused by migration of stones into the common bile duct with subsequent obstruction to the bile duct, the pancreatic duct, or both.[59] This causes increase in pancreatic duct pressure, resulting in unregulated activation of trypsin and pancreatitis.[59] Gallstones are the most common cause for acute pancreatitis.[60,61] The overall mortality of acute pancreatitis is between 3% and 10%.[60,61] The role of early endoscopic sphincterotomy in the management of gallstone pancreatitis is controversial. Although the total number of complications is fewer after early endoscopic sphincterotomy for predicted severe pancreatitis,[62] there is no reduction in either the local pancreatic complications or the overall mortality for predicted mild or severe pancreatitis.[63] There is of no benefit of early endoscopic sphincterotomy for patients with acute gallstone pancreatitis without cholangitis.[64] Irrespective of the role of endoscopic sphincterotomy in pancreatitis, endoscopic sphincterotomy alone is not a definitive treatment for common bile duct stones. In a systematic review of randomized controlled trials, a policy of observation alone after endoscopic sphincterotomy increased the risk of mortality and gallstone-related complications compared with prophylactic cholecystectomy.[65] Hence, cholecystectomy is recommended after an attack of gallstone pancreatitis (grade A). There have been two randomized controlled trials investigating the timing of cholecystectomy.[66,67] In one trial, the mortality and morbidity were higher when the cholecystectomy was performed within 48 hours of admission compared with cholecystectomy performed after 48 hours of surgery but within the same hospital admission.[66] In the other trial, the patients were operated between 3 days and 14 days after hospital admission for pancreatitis in the early group and after 3 months in the delayed group.[67] There was no difference in the postoperative mortality or morbidity between the two groups. Of the nine patients allocated to the delayed group, however, one patient (11%) developed another attack of pancreatitis, and two patients developed abdominal pain while waiting for surgery.[67] Both these studies were conducted in the era of open cholecystectomy and were underpowered to detect reasonable differences in mortality and morbidity. There has been no trial on the timing of surgery in the laparoscopic surgery. For those patients who undergo pancreatic necrosectomy or debridement after failed percutaneous drainage for infected pancreatic necrosis,[68,69] it is reasonable to perform cholecystectomy at the same time.[68] For the remaining patients who do not require surgical interventions on the pancreas, laparoscopic cholecystectomy can be performed safely when the general condition improves and can be completed laparoscopically in 85% to 90% of patients with mild pancreatitis[68,70] and in about 60% of patients with severe pancreatitis.[68] Cholecystectomy is completed in the remaining patients by conversion to an open procedure. Some authors recommend laparoscopic cholecystectomy as soon as the serum amylase and the abdominal tenderness start to decrease[70] rather than waiting for amylase to return to normal and for the patient to be free from abdominal pain. This approach was based on their observation that such an approach was safe, did not result in a high rate of conversion to open cholecystectomy, and resulted in a shorter hospital stay compared with the traditional early cholecystectomy group (ie, waiting for amylase to return to normal and relief from abdominal symptoms).[70] Considering that early laparoscopic cholecystectomy is safe and can be completed successfully in most patients with mild acute pancreatitis, delaying laparoscopic cholecystectomy seems unnecessary and can expose the patient to further gallstone-related complications. Thus, cholecystectomy in the same admission appears to be the preferable option in patients with mild gallstone pancreatitis (grade B). The general condition and the severity of the pancreatic disease will determine the timing of the cholecystectomy in patients with severe pancreatitis. Cholecystectomy appears safe as soon as the general condition of the patient improves and the pancreatic necrosis becomes sterile if infected (or remains sterile if not infected)[68] (grade B). Considering that laparoscopic cholecystectomy is safe and seems to be the preferred option (most cholecystectomies in the United Kingdom and the United States are performed laparoscopically),[71,72] laparoscopic cholecystectomy can be recommended as the preferred approach in patients with gallstone pancreatitis (grade B).

## OBSTRUCTIVE JAUNDICE

Patients with gallstones develop obstructive jaundice if stones migrate into the common bile duct. Although common bile duct stones can be removed endoscopically,[73] subsequent cholecystectomy is recommended based on a systematic review of randomized controlled trials in which a policy of observation after endoscopic sphincterotomy increased the risk of mortality and gallstone-related complications compared with routine cholecystectomy[65] (grade A). There are no studies investigating the natural history of patients with obstructive jaundice caused by common bile duct stones. Considering that obstructive jaundice can lead to complications such as cholangitis, renal dysfunction, cardiovascular dysfunction, and coagulopathy,[74,75] obstructive jaundice caused by common bile duct stones needs to be treated as an emergency (grade B). The various options for the treatment of common bile duct stones include open cholecystectomy with open common bile duct exploration, laparoscopic cholecystectomy with laparoscopic common bile duct exploration, and laparoscopic cholecystectomy with endoscopic sphincterotomy (performed preoperatively, intraoperatively, or postoperatively).[76,77] A systematic review of randomized controlled trials has shown that open cholecystectomy with open common bile duct exploration has the lowest incidence of retained stones[76] but is associated with high morbidity and mortality, particularly in elderly patients.[78] There was no difference in the incidence of retained stones between preoperative and postoperative endoscopic retrograde cholangiopancreatography (ERCP) and laparoscopic common bile duct clearance at the time of laparoscopic cholecystectomy.[76] The total hospital stay was shorter in the laparoscopic exploration group.[76] One randomized controlled trial has shown that there is no difference in any of the important outcomes between laparoscopic cholecystectomy with laparoscopic common bile duct exploration and laparoscopic cholecystectomy with intraoperative endoscopic sphinterotomy.[77] Three trials have shown that intraoperative endoscopic sphincterotomy is at least as safe and effective as preoperative endoscopic sphincterotomy followed by laparoscopic cholecystectomy[79–81] and shortens hospital stay.[79–81] There was no significant difference in the success rates between preoperative endoscopic sphincterotomy and intraoperative endoscopic sphincterotomy.[79–81] There are no trials comparing open cholecystectomy and common bile duct exploration with laparoscopic cholecystectomy and laparoscopic common bile duct exploration. There is also no randomized controlled trial comparing open cholecystectomy with open common bile exploration to laparoscopic cholecystectomy with intraoperative endoscopic sphincterotomy. Considering that laparoscopic cholecystectomy is preferred to open cholecystectomy (a significant majority of the cholecystectomies in the United Kingdom and in the United States are performed laparoscopically),[71,72] laparoscopic cholecystectomy along with laparoscopic common bile duct exploration or intraoperative endoscopic sphincterotomy can be recommended as the preferred method of treatment of patients with obstructive jaundice due to gallstones where the expertise and infrastructure are available (grade B). When these are not available, laparoscopic cholecystectomy with preoperative endoscopic sphincterotomy or post-operative endoscopic sphincterotomy may be the preferred treatment for common bile duct stones. For patients with impacted common bile duct stone not amenable to laparoscopic or endoscopic clearance, lithotripsy[82] or open common bile duct exploration can be the other options (grade B).

## SPECIAL SITUATIONS
### High-Risk Individuals

If patients are at high risk of surgery because of pancreatitis, jaundice, or sepsis, cholecystectomy should be offered once their general condition improves. This is because of evidence from a systematic review of randomized controlled trials, which shows leaving the gallbladder in situ after endoscopic sphinterotomy results in an increased overall mortality[65] (grade A). In a randomized controlled trial, percutaneous cholecystostomy followed by early laparoscopic cholecystectomy (in 3 to 4 days after the percutaneous cholecystostomy) resulted in a considerable decrease in the hospital stay compared with delayed laparoscopic cholecystectomy.[15] It is not possible, however, to assess the effect of percutaneous cholecystostomy alone from this trial. It appears that percutaneous cholecystostomy with early laparoscopic cholecystectomy is an effective option in patients who are temporarily unwell because of gallbladder sepsis. The only trial that assessed whether percutaneous cholecystostomy in addition to antibiotic therapy (but without early laparoscopic cholecystectomy) was of any benefit in high-risk surgical individuals showed that there was no benefit in performing percutaneous cholecystostomy in patients with acute choleystitis.[83] This study, however, was not powered to measure the difference in mortality, which was 9.1% in the percutaneous cholecystostomy group and 17.7% in the antibiotics-alone group. Further studies are necessary to assess the role of percutaneous cholecystostomy as a temporary measure in the treatment of high-risk surgical individuals with acute cholecystitis. In patients who are at high risk of surgery because of comorbidities that will not improve with the treatment of sepsis, surgery cannot be recommended (grade B).

### Cirrhotic

There are few studies that report the natural history of gallstones in cirrhotic patients.[84,85] The frequency of symptoms or complications does not appear to be any different from other groups of patients with gallstones. When patients develop complications, however, they can be more severe.[85] Cholecystectomy is recommended for symptomatic gallstones (grade B). There are no differences in the timing of surgery for various indications between compensated cirrhotic patients and other patients with symptomatic gallstones. For compensated cirrhotic patients with symptomatic gallstones, laparoscopic cholecystectomy appears better than open cholecystectomy, as randomized controlled trials have shown that the laparoscopic cholecystectomy has similar morbidity as open cholecystectomy[86,87] but results in lower blood loss,[86,87] transfusion requirements,[86] and hospital stay.[86,87] The overall morbidity and mortality after cholecystectomy, however, are higher in cirrhotic patients than in noncirrhotic patients.[88]

### Pregnancy

Most pregnant women with gallstones remain asymptomatic during their pregnancy,[89] and there is no indication for cholecystectomy. Patients with symptomatic gallstones

**Table 1**
Summary of recommendations

| Patient Population | Dilemma | Recommendation (Grade of Recommendation) | Grade | Remarks |
|---|---|---|---|---|
| Patients at high risk of developing gallstones but currently do not have gallstones | Is surgery required? | No | B | Applicable in all patients including those undergoing gastrectomy for gastric cancer and gastric bypass for obesity |
| | When? | Not applicable | | - |
| | How? | Not applicable | | - |
| Asymptomatic gallstones (except those undergoing major abdominal surgery) | Is surgery indicated? | No | B | Applicable in all patients with asymptomatic gallstones including diabetics, sickle cell disease, and children |
| | When? | Not applicable | | - |
| | How? | Not applicable | | - |
| Asymptomatic gallstones and undergoing major abdominal surgery | Is surgery indicated? | Yes | B | Applicable in patients undergoing major abdominal operations such as gastrectomy, gastric bypass, and splenectomy. |
| | When? | At the same time as the major procedure | B | - |
| | How? | By the same route of access as the major procedure | B | - |
| Symptomatic gallstones without complications | Is surgery indicated? | Yes | B | - |
| | When? | Elective surgery is acceptable | B | - |
| | How? | Laparoscopic and small-incision cholecystectomies are preferable to open cholecystectomy | A | - |
| Acute cholecystitis | Is surgery indicated? | Yes | B | - |
| | When? | Within 1 week of onset of symptoms | A | - |
| | How? | Laparoscopic cholecystectomy | A | - |
| Pancreatitis | Is surgery indicated? | Yes | A | - |

| Condition | | Answer | Grade | |
|---|---|---|---|---|
| | When? | In the same hospital admission for mild pancreatitis | B | - |
| | | As soon as the general condition improves and pancreatic necrosis becomes sterile in severe pancreatitis | B | - |
| | How? | Laparoscopic cholecystectomy | B | - |
| Obstructive jaundice | Is surgery indicated? | Yes | A | |
| | When? | Obstructive jaundice needs to be treated immediately | B | |
| | How? | Laparoscopic cholecystectomy with laparoscopic bile duct exploration or laparoscopic cholecystectomy with intraoperative endoscopic sphincterotomy if expertise and infrastructure are available. If these are not available, laparoscopic cholecystectomy in combination with preoperative or postoperative ERCP is a suitable alternative. | B | |
| High-risk patients with temporary deterioration of general condition due to acute cholecystitis | Is surgery indicated? | Yes | A | Temporary percutaneous cholecystostomy followed by cholecystectomy once the patient improves |
| High-risk patients who are unlikely to become fit for surgery | Is surgery indicated? | No | B | |
| Compensated cirrhosis | Is surgery indicated? | Yes | B | |
| | When? | Same as other patients with symptomatic gallstones | - | |
| | How? | Laparoscopic cholecystectomy | A | |
| Pregnancy (requiring hospitalization for biliary disease or biliary pancreatitis) | Is surgery indicated? | Yes | B | |
| | When? | Second trimester | B | |
| | How? | Laparoscopic cholecystectomy | B | |

present a great dilemma, however. Traditionally, cholecystectomy was performed only in the presence of severe or nonresolution of symptoms. This is because of the risk of perioperative fetal complications. A recent large retrospective case–control study on pregnant women requiring admission with biliary disease or biliary pancreatitis compared those pregnant women (with biliary disease or biliary pancreatitis) who underwent cholecystectomy with those pregnant women (with biliary disease or biliary pancreatitis) who did not undergo surgery.[90] Over a 10-year period, 36,929 pregnant women with biliary disease or biliary pancreatitis were admitted in the hospital. Of these, 9714 (26%) women underwent cholecystectomy. Of these 9714 women, about 5% underwent endoscopic retrograde cholangiopancreatography; about 3% underwent common bile duct exploration, and 0.1% had placement of a percutaneous cholecystostomy tube in addition to cholecystectomy. The remaining women did not undergo surgery. Patients who underwent surgery had significantly lower maternal complication rates (4.3% vs 16.5%) and fetal complication rates (5.8% vs 16.5%) compared with those who did not undergo surgery. The overall hospital mortality in the surgical group was 0.05%. The cause for mortality was not stated. The hospital mortality in the nonsurgical group was not stated but is likely to be zero. There is likely to be a large selection bias in this study. Patients are more likely to be offered cholecystectomy during pregnancy if the biliary disease or biliary pancreatitis is severe. Many patients who underwent cholecystectomy would have been treated conservatively first[91] before they would have been offered cholecystectomy. Thus the complications in this group of patients who had failed conservative treatment would have been included under the surgery group rather than the nonsurgery group (ie, a treatment-received analysis that can only favor the non-surgery group was performed). The proportion of patients who presented in each trimester and the outcomes of patients stratified by the trimester of presentation were not reported. It is possible that a significant proportion of patients treated conservatively presented in the third trimester, and a significant proportion of patients treated surgically presented in the second trimester, resulting in an apparent but not true benefit of surgery over conservative management. In another study of 63 women, surgical management was compared with nonsurgical management in pregnant women with symptomatic gallstones. The authors of this study recommend surgical management because of the higher risk of fetal and maternal complications in the nonsurgical group.[92] The time of presentation of the pregnant women stratified by the trimester of pregnancy was not reported in this study also. In another study of 126 pregnant women with symptomatic gallstones, the patients were treated conservatively, and surgical management was offered only in patients in whom conservative management failed.[91] Medical management failed in 57% of patients. These patients underwent surgical management without maternal or fetal complications.[91] In this study, only second trimester patients were offered laparoscopic cholecystectomy, while the patients in the first and third trimesters were offered percutaneous gallbladder aspiration. Thus it appears that surgical management by cholecystectomy is safe in selected patients and should be considered in pregnant women with symptomatic cholelithiasis who require hospital admission for symptomatic gallstones or other complications at least in the second trimester of pregnancy (grade B).

The long-term effect of cholecystectomy in pregnant women on fetal and child development has not been reported. Carbon dioxide pneumoperitoneum at 15 mm Hg pressure causes fetal hypercarbia in pregnant ewes.[93] However, another study, a randomized controlled trial of 15 mm Hg pneumoperitoneum in pregnant ewes, did not demonstrate any effect of pneumoperitoneum on fetal acidosis.[94] Thus, it is unlikely that pneumoperitoneum has any effects on fetal acid–base balance. The safety of anesthesia during early pregnancy, however, has not been established.[95] So, it is best to avoid surgery during the first trimester of pregnancy if possible. Another issue of laparoscopic surgery in pregnant women is to gain access without causing injury to the enlarged uterus, particularly in the third trimester. Because of this, a significant proportion of the operations may have to be performed by open cholecystectomy. Thus, the second trimester appears to be the best time for performing cholecystectomy in pregnant women (grade B).

In the study including 9714 pregnant women who underwent cholecystectomy, patients who underwent laparoscopic cholecystectomy had lower surgical morbidity, fewer maternal complications (hysterectomy, caesarean section, and dilation, and curettage), fewer fetal complications (fetal death, loss, or distress), and shorter hospital stay compared with those who underwent open cholecystectomy.[90] There is likely to be a selection bias favoring laparoscopic cholecystectomy however, as surgeons are more likely to opt for the open approach in the presence of complications such as severe inflammation or empyema, particularly if this is during the third trimester. Other studies have shown that laparoscopic cholecystectomy can be done safely with similar morbidity as open cholecystectomy during pregnancy.[96,97]

The overall surgery-related morbidity and hospital stay were higher in the pregnant women undergoing cholecystectomy as compared with nonpregnant women undergoing cholecystectomy.[90] Both maternal and fetal outcomes should be considered in relation to the management of gallstones during pregnancy and further studies are required on the risks and benefits of cholecystectomy.

With certain reservations about obtaining access in the third trimester and the safety of anesthesia and pneumoperitoneum in the first trimester, laparoscopic cholecystectomy appears to be the preferred route for cholecystectomy in pregnant women in the second trimester of pregnancy (grade B).

## SUMMARY

A summary of the recommendations regarding whether surgery is indicated as well as when and how the surgery should be performed can be found in **Table 1**. The major conclusions from this review are as follows. Currently there is no evidence for prophylactic cholecystectomy to prevent gallstone formation. Cholecystectomy cannot be recommended for any group of patients with asymptomatic gallstones except in those undergoing major abdominal operations for other pathologies. Laparoscopic cholecystectomy is the preferred treatment of symptomatic gallstones. Cholecystectomy should be offered even after endoscopic sphincterotomy for common bile duct stones. Laparoscopic cholecystectomy with laparoscopic common bile duct exploration or with intraoperative endoscopic sphincterotomy is the preferred treatment for obstructive jaundice caused by common bile duct stones, when the expertise and infrastructure are available.

## REFERENCES

1. Prevalence of gallstone disease in an Italian adult female population. Rome Group for the Epidemiology and Prevention of Cholelithiasis (GREPCO). Am J Epidemiol 1984;119(5):796–805.
2. The epidemiology of gallstone disease in Rome, Italy. Part I. Prevalence data in men. The Rome Group for Epidemiology and Prevention of Cholelithiasis (GREPCO). Hepatology 1988;8(4):904–6.
3. Halldestam I, Enell EL, Kullman E, et al. Development of symptoms and complications in individuals with asymptomatic gallstones. Br J Surg 2004;91(6):734–8.

4. Bates T, Harrison M, Lowe D, et al. Longitudinal study of gall stone prevalence at necropsy. Gut 1992;33(1):103–7.
5. Attili AF, De Santis A, Capri R, et al. The natural history of gallstones: the GREPCO experience. The GREPCO Group. Hepatology 1995;21(3):655–60.
6. Del Favero G, Caroli A, Meggiato T, et al. Natural history of gallstones in noninsulin-dependent diabetes mellitus. A prospective 5-year follow-up. Dig Dis Sci 1994;39(8):1704–7.
7. Berger MY, van der Velden JJIM, Lijmer JG, et al. Abdominal symptoms: do they predict gallstones? A systematic review. Scand J Gastroenterol 2000;35(1):70–6.
8. Berger MY, Olde Hartman TC, Bohnen AM. Abdominal symptoms: do they disappear after cholecystectomy? Surg Endosc 2003;17(11):1723–8.
9. Venneman NG, van Erpecum KJ. Gallstone disease: primary and secondary prevention. Best Pract Res Clin Gastroenterol 2006;20(6):1063–73.
10. Pavlidis TE, Atmatzidis KS, Papaziogas BT, et al. Management of gallstone ileus. J Hepatobiliary Pancreat Surg 2003;10(4):299–302.
11. Randi G, Franceschi S, La Vecchia C. Gallbladder cancer worldwide: geographical distribution and risk factors. Int J Cancer 2006;118(7):1591–602.
12. Hsing AW, Bai Y, Andreotti G, et al. Family history of gallstones and the risk of biliary tract cancer and gallstones: a population-based study in Shanghai, China. Int J Cancer 2007;121(4):832–8.
13. Broden G, Bengtsson L. Carcinoma of the gallbladder. Its relation to cholelithiasis and to the concept of prophylactic cholecystectomy. Acta Chir Scand Suppl 1980;500:15–8.
14. Strasberg SM, Clavien PA. Overview of therapeutic modalities for the treatment of gallstone diseases. Am J Surg 1993;165(4):420–6.
15. Akyurek N, Salman B, Yuksel O, et al. Management of acute calculous cholecystitis in high-risk patients: percutaneous cholecystotomy followed by early laparoscopic cholecystectomy. Surg Laparosc Endosc Percutan Tech 2005;15(6):315–20.
16. Keus F, de Jong J, Gooszen Hein G, et al. Small-incision versus open cholecystectomy for patients with symptomatic cholecystolithiasis. Cochrane Database Syst Rev 2006;(4):CD004788.
17. Keus F, de Jong J, Gooszen Hein G, et al. Laparoscopic versus small-incision cholecystectomy for patients with symptomatic cholecystolithiasis. Cochrane Database Syst Rev 2006;(4):CD006229.
18. Keus F, de Jong J, Gooszen HG, et al. Laparoscopic versus open cholecystectomy for patients with symptomatic cholecystolithiasis. Cochrane Database Syst Rev 2006;(4):CD006231.
19. Duca S, Bala O, Al-Hajjar N, et al. Laparoscopic cholecystectomy: incidents and complications. A retrospective analysis of 9542 consecutive laparoscopic operations. HPB (Oxford) 2003;5(3):152–8.
20. Tuveri M, Tuveri A. Laparoscopic cholecystectomy: complications and conversions with the 3-trocar technique: a 10-year review. Surg Laparosc Endosc Percutan Tech 2007;17(5):380–4.
21. Giger UF, Michel JM, Opitz I, et al. Risk factors for perioperative complications in patients undergoing laparoscopic cholecystectomy: analysis of 22,953 consecutive cases from the Swiss Association of Laparoscopic and Thoracoscopic Surgery database. J Am Coll Surg 2006;203(5):723–8.
22. Schmidt SC, Settmacher U, Langrehr JM, et al. Management and outcome of patients with combined bile duct and hepatic arterial injuries after laparoscopic cholecystectomy. Surgery 2004;135(6):613–8.

23. Sicklick JK, Camp MS, Lillemoe KD, et al. Surgical management of bile duct injuries sustained during laparoscopic cholecystectomy: perioperative results in 200 patients. Ann Surg 2005;241(5):786–92.
24. Lillemoe KD, Melton GB, Cameron JL, et al. Postoperative bile duct strictures: management and outcome in the 1990s. Ann Surg 2000;232(3):430–41.
25. Moore DE, Feurer ID, Holzman MD, et al. Long-term detrimental effect of bile duct injury on health-related quality of life. Arch Surg 2004;139(5):476–81.
26. Azevedo JL, Azevedo OC, Miyahira SA, et al. Injuries caused by Veress needle insertion for creation of pneumoperitoneum: a systematic literature review. Surg Endosc 2009;23(7):1428–32.
27. Ahmad G, Duffy JM, Phillips K, et al. Laparoscopic entry techniques. Cochrane Database Syst Rev 2008;(2):CD006583.
28. Fukagawa T, Katai H, Saka M, et al. Gallstone formation after gastric cancer surgery. J Gastrointest Surg 2009;13(5):886–9.
29. Kobayashi T, Hisanaga M, Kanehiro H, et al. Analysis of risk factors for the development of gallstones after gastrectomy. Br J Surg 2005;92(11):1399–403.
30. Iglezias Brandao de Oliveira C, Adami Chaim E, da Silva BB. Impact of rapid weight reduction on risk of cholelithiasis after bariatric surgery. Obes Surg 2003;13(4):625–8.
31. Villegas L, Schneider B, Provost D, et al. Is routine cholecystectomy required during laparoscopic gastric bypass? Obes Surg 2004;14(2):206–11.
32. Taylor J, Leitman IM, Horowitz M. Is routine cholecystectomy necessary at the time of Roux-en-Y gastric bypass? Obes Surg 2006;16(6):759–61.
33. Li VK, Pulido N, Fajnwaks P, et al. Predictors of gallstone formation after bariatric surgery: a multivariate analysis of risk factors comparing gastric bypass, gastric banding, and sleeve gastrectomy. Surg Endosc 2009;23(7):1640–4.
34. Farsi M, Bernini M, Bencini L, et al. The CHOLEGAS study: multicentric randomized, blinded, controlled trial of gastrectomy plus prophylactic cholecystectomy versus gastrectomy only, in adults submitted to gastric cancer surgery with curative intent. Trials 2009;10:32.
35. Friedman LS, Roberts MS, Brett AS, et al. Management of asymptomatic gallstones in the diabetic patient. A decision analysis. Ann Intern Med 1988;109(11):913–9.
36. Gumiero AP, Bellomo-Brandao MA, Costa-Pinto EA. Gallstones in children with sickle cell disease followed up at a Brazilian hematology center. Arq Gastroenterol 2008;45(4):313–8.
37. Greenstein SM, Katz S, Sun S, et al. Prevalence of asymptomatic cholelithiasis and risk of acute cholecystitis after kidney transplantation. Transplantation 1997;63(7):1030–2.
38. Curro G, Meo A, Ippolito D, et al. Asymptomatic cholelithiasis in children with sickle cell disease: early or delayed cholecystectomy? Ann Surg 2007;245(1):126–9.
39. Chan S, Currie J, Malik AI, et al. Paediatric cholecystectomy: shifting goalposts in the laparoscopic era. Surg Endosc 2008;22(5):1392–5.
40. Esposito C, Alicchio F, Giurin I, et al. Lessons learned from the first 109 laparoscopic cholecystectomies performed in a single pediatric surgery center. World J Surg 2009;33(9):1842–5.
41. Holcomb GW 3rd, Morgan WM 3rd, Neblett WW 3rd, et al. Laparoscopic cholecystectomy in children: lessons learned from the first 100 patients. J Pediatr Surg 1999;34(8):1236–40.
42. St Peter SD, Keckler SJ, Nair A, et al. Laparoscopic cholecystectomy in the pediatric population. J Laparoendosc Adv Surg Tech A 2008;18(1):127–30.

43. Tucker ON, Fajnwaks P, Szomstein S, et al. Is concomitant cholecystectomy necessary in obese patients undergoing laparoscopic gastric bypass surgery? Surg Endosc 2008;22(11):2450–4.
44. Patel JA, Patel NA, Piper GL, et al. Perioperative management of cholelithiasis in patients presenting for laparoscopic Roux-en-Y gastric bypass: have we reached a consensus? Am Surg 2009;75(6):470–6.
45. Rutledge D, Jones D, Rege R. Consequences of delay in surgical treatment of biliary disease. Am J Surg 2000;180(6):466–9.
46. Somasekar K, Shankar PJ, Foster ME, et al. Costs of waiting for gall bladder surgery. Postgrad Med J 2002;78(925):668–9.
47. Sobolev B, Mercer D, Brown P, et al. Risk of emergency admission while awaiting elective cholecystectomy. CMAJ 2003;169(7):662–5.
48. Friedman GD, Raviola CA, Fireman B. Prognosis of gallstones with mild or no symptoms: 25 years of follow-up in a health maintenance organization. J Clin Epidemiol 1989;42(2):127–36.
49. Vetrhus M, Soreide O, Solhaug JH, et al. Symptomatic, noncomplicated gall-bladder stone disease. Operation or observation? A randomized clinical study. Scand J Gastroenterol 2002;37(7):834–9.
50. Salman B, Yuksel O, Irkorucu O, et al. Urgent laparoscopic cholecystectomy is the best management for biliary colic. A prospective randomized study of 75 cases. Dig Surg 2005;22(1–2):95–9.
51. Macafee DA, Humes DJ, Bouliotis G, et al. Prospective randomized trial using cost–utility analysis of early versus delayed laparoscopic cholecystectomy for acute gallbladder disease. Br J Surg 2009;96(9):1031–40.
52. Gurusamy KS, Samraj K. Early versus delayed laparoscopic cholecystectomy for acute cholecystitis. Cochrane Database Syst Rev 2006;(4):CD005440.
53. Gurusamy KS, Samraj K, Gluud C, et al. Meta-analysis of randomized controlled trials on the safety and effectiveness of early versus delayed laparoscopic chole-cystectomy for acute cholecystitis. Br J Surg 2010;97(2):141–50.
54. Papi C, Catarci M, D'Ambrosio L, et al. Timing of cholecystectomy for acute calculous cholecystitis: a meta-analysis. Am J Gastroenterol 2004;99(1):147–55.
55. Wilson E, Gurusamy KS, Gluud C, et al. A cost utility and value of information analysis of early versus delayed laparoscopic cholecystectomy for acute chole-cystitis. Br J Surg 2010;97(2):210–9.
56. Boo YJ, Kim WB, Kim J, et al. Systemic immune response after open versus lapa-roscopic cholecystectomy in acute cholecystitis: a prospective randomized study. Scand J Clin Lab Invest 2007;67(2):207–14.
57. Kiviluoto T, Siren J, Luukkonen P, et al. Randomised trial of laparoscopic versus open cholecystectomy for acute and gangrenous cholecystitis. Lancet 1998; 351(9099):321–5.
58. Johansson M, Thune A, Nelvin L, et al. Randomized clinical trial of open versus laparoscopic cholecystectomy in the treatment of acute cholecystitis. Br J Surg 2005;92(1):44–9.
59. Frossard JL, Steer ML, Pastor CM. Acute pancreatitis. Lancet 2008;371(9607): 143–52.
60. Frey CF, Zhou H, Harvey DJ, et al. The incidence and case fatality rates of acute biliary, alcoholic, and idiopathic pancreatitis in California, 1994-2001. Pancreas 2006;33(4):336–44.
61. Lowenfels AB, Maisonneuve P, Sullivan T. The changing character of acute pancreatitis: epidemiology, etiology, and prognosis. Curr Gastroenterol Rep 2009;11(2):97–103.

62. Moretti A, Papi C, Aratari A, et al. Is early endoscopic retrograde cholangiopancreatography useful in the management of acute biliary pancreatitis? A meta-analysis of randomized controlled trials. Dig Liver Dis 2008;40(5):379–85.
63. Petrov MS, van Santvoort HC, Besselink MG, et al. Early endoscopic retrograde cholangiopancreatography versus conservative management in acute biliary pancreatitis without cholangitis: a meta-analysis of randomized trials. Ann Surg 2008;247(2):250–7.
64. Petrov MS, Uchugina AF, Kukosh MV. Does endoscopic retrograde cholangiopancreatography reduce the risk of local pancreatic complications in acute pancreatitis? A systematic review and metaanalysis. Surg Endosc 2008;22(11):2338–43.
65. McAlister VC, Davenport E, Renouf E. Cholecystectomy deferral in patients with endoscopic sphincterotomy. Cochrane Database Syst Rev 2007;(4):CD006233.
66. Kelly TR, Wagner DS. Gallstone pancreatitis: a prospective randomized trial of the timing of surgery. Surgery 1988;104(4):600–5.
67. Mackie CR, Wood RA, Preece PE, et al. Surgical pathology at early elective operation for suspected acute gallstone pancreatitis: preliminary report of a prospective clinical trial. Br J Surg 1985;72(3):179–81.
68. Uhl W, Muller CA, Krahenbuhl L, et al. Acute gallstone pancreatitis: timing of laparoscopic cholecystectomy in mild and severe disease. Surg Endosc 1999;13(11):1070–6.
69. Freeny PC, Hauptmann E, Althaus SJ, et al. Percutaneous CT-guided catheter drainage of infected acute necrotizing pancreatitis: techniques and results. AJR Am J Roentgenol 1998;170(4):969–75.
70. Taylor E, Wong C. The optimal timing of laparoscopic cholecystectomy in mild gallstone pancreatitis. Am Surg 2004;70(11):971–5.
71. Dolan JP, Diggs BS, Sheppard BC, et al. The national mortality burden and significant factors associated with open and laparoscopic cholecystectomy: 1997–2006. J Gastrointest Surg 2009;13(12):2292–301.
72. Ballal M, David G, Willmott S, et al. Conversion after laparoscopic cholecystectomy in England. Surg Endosc 2009;23(10):2338–44.
73. Heo JH, Kang DH, Jung HJ, et al. Endoscopic sphincterotomy plus large-balloon dilation versus endoscopic sphincterotomy for removal of bile-duct stones. Gastrointest Endosc 2007;66(4):720–6 [quiz: 68, 71].
74. Green J, Better O. Systemic hypotension and renal failure in obstructive jaundice—mechanistic and therapeutic aspects. J Am Soc Nephrol 1995;5(11):1853–71.
75. Rege R. Adverse effects of biliary obstruction: implications for treatment of patients with obstructive jaundice. Am J Roentgenol 1995;164(2):287–93.
76. Martin DJ, Vernon DR, Toouli J. Surgical versus endoscopic treatment of bile duct stones. Cochrane Database Syst Rev 2006;(2):CD003327.
77. Hong DF, Xin Y, Chen DW. Comparison of laparoscopic cholecystectomy combined with intraoperative endoscopic sphincterotomy and laparoscopic exploration of the common bile duct for cholecystocholedocholithiasis. Surg Endosc 2006;20(3):424–7.
78. Larraz-Mora E, Mayol J, Martinez-Sarmiento J, et al. Open biliary tract surgery: multivariate analysis of factors affecting mortality. Dig Surg 1999;16(3):204–8.
79. Lella F, Bagnolo F, Rebuffat C, et al. Use of the laparoscopic–endoscopic approach, the so-called rendezvous technique, in cholecystocholedocholithiasis: a valid method in cases with patient-related risk factors for post-ERCP pancreatitis. Surg Endosc 2006;20(3):419–23.

80. Morino M, Baracchi F, Miglietta C, et al. Preoperative endoscopic sphincterotomy versus laparoendoscopic rendezvous in patients with gallbladder and bile duct stones. Ann Surg 2006;244(6):889–93.
81. Rabago LR, Vicente C, Soler F, et al. Two-stage treatment with preoperative endoscopic retrograde cholangiopancreatography (ERCP) compared with single-stage treatment with intraoperative ERCP for patients with symptomatic cholelithiasis with possible choledocholithiasis. Endoscopy 2006;38(8):779–86.
82. Swahn F, Edlund G, Enochsson L, et al. Ten years of Swedish experience with intraductal electrohydraulic lithotripsy and laser lithotripsy for the treatment of difficult bile duct stones: an effective and safe option for octogenarians. Surg Endosc 2009. [Epub ahead of print].
83. Hatzidakis AA, Prassopoulos P, Petinarakis I, et al. Acute cholecystitis in high-risk patients: percutaneous cholecystostomy vs conservative treatment. Eur Radiol 2002;12(7):1778–84.
84. Dunnington G, Alfrey E, Sampliner R, et al. Natural history of cholelithiasis in patients with alcoholic cirrhosis (cholelithiasis in cirrhotic patients). Ann Surg 1987;205(3):226–9.
85. Orozco H, Takahashi T, Mercado MA, et al. Long-term evolution of asymptomatic cholelithiasis diagnosed during abdominal operations for variceal bleeding in patients with cirrhosis. Am J Surg 1994;168(3):232–4.
86. El-Awadi S, El-Nakeeb A, Youssef T, et al. Laparoscopic versus open cholecystectomy in cirrhotic patients: a prospective randomized study. Int J Surg 2009; 7(1):66–9.
87. Ji W, Li LT, Wang ZM, et al. A randomized controlled trial of laparoscopic versus open cholecystectomy in patients with cirrhotic portal hypertension. World J Gastroenterol 2005;11(16):2513–7.
88. Sleeman D, Namias N, Levi D, et al. Laparoscopic cholecystectomy in cirrhotic patients. J Am Coll Surg 1998;187(4):400–3.
89. Ko CW, Beresford SA, Schulte SJ, et al. Incidence, natural history, and risk factors for biliary sludge and stones during pregnancy. Hepatology 2005;41(2):359–65.
90. Kuy S, Roman SA, Desai R, et al. Outcomes following cholecystectomy in pregnant and nonpregnant women. Surgery 2009;146(2):358–66.
91. Chiappetta Porras LT, Napoli ED, Canullan CM, et al. Minimally invasive management of acute biliary tract disease during pregnancy. HPB Surg 2009;2009: 829020.
92. Lu EJ, Curet MJ, El-Sayed YY, et al. Medical versus surgical management of biliary tract disease in pregnancy. Am J Surg 2004;188(6):755–9.
93. Hunter JG, Swanstrom L, Thornburg K. Carbon dioxide pneumoperitoneum induces fetal acidosis in a pregnant ewe model. Surg Endosc 1995;9(3):272–9.
94. Cruz AM, Southerland LC, Duke T, et al. Intraabdominal carbon dioxide insufflation in the pregnant ewe. Uterine blood flow, intraamniotic pressure, and cardiopulmonary effects. Anesthesiology 1996;85(6):1395–402.
95. Sylvester GC, Khoury MJ, Lu X, et al. First-trimester anesthesia exposure and the risk of central nervous system defects: a population-based case-control study. Am J Public Health 1994;84(11):1757–60.
96. Abuabara SF, Gross GW, Sirinek KR. Laparoscopic cholecystectomy during pregnancy is safe for both mother and fetus. J Gastrointest Surg 1997;1(1): 48–52.
97. Cosenza CA, Saffari B, Jabbour N, et al. Surgical management of biliary gallstone disease during pregnancy. Am J Surg 1999;178(6):545–8.

# Targets for Current Pharmacologic Therapy in Cholesterol Gallstone Disease

Agostino Di Ciaula, MD[a], David Q.H. Wang, MD, PhD[b],
Helen H. Wang, BS, MS[c], Leonilde Bonfrate, MD[d],
Piero Portincasa, MD, PhD[d],*

KEYWORDS

- Bile salts • Cholesterol absorption • Ezetimibe
- Gallbladder • Nuclear receptors • Statins

Gallstone disease is one of the most frequent and costly digestive diseases in Western countries; its prevalence in adults ranges from 10% to 15%.[1–4] Despite the frequency of the condition, many patients with gallstones remain undiagnosed, although symptoms and/or complications occur in approximately a third of patients. In the United States, medical expenses for the treatment of gallstones exceeded $6 billion in the year 2000. The prevalence of gallstones seems to be rising and approximately 1 million new cases are discovered each year.[5] About 75% of the gallstones in the United States and Westernized countries, including Italy, are cholesterol gallstones.[6–8] The remaining gallstones are pigment stones that contain less than 30% cholesterol by weight, which can be subclassified into 2 groups: black pigment stones (about 20% of all gallstones, found in the gallbladder and/or bile duct, containing mainly insoluble

This work was supported in part by research grants from the Italian Ministry of University and Research (FIRB 2003 RBAU01RANB002), the Italian National Research Council (CNR) (short-term mobility grant 2005), the University of Bari (grants ORBA09XZZT, ORBA08YHKX) (PP), and from the National Institutes of Health (US Public Health Service) (research grants DK54012 and DK73917) (DQ-HW).

[a] Division of Internal Medicine, Hospital of Bisceglie, via Bovio 279, 70052 Bisceglie (Bari), Italy
[b] Liver Center and Gastroenterology Division, Department of Medicine, Beth Israel Deaconess Medical Center, Harvard Medical School and Harvard Digestive Diseases Center, 330 Brookline Avenue, DA 601, Boston, MA 02215, USA
[c] Liver Center and Gastroenterology Division, Department of Medicine, Beth Israel Deaconess Medical Center, Harvard Medical School, 330 Brookline Avenue, DA 601, Boston, MA 02215, USA
[d] Clinica Medica "A. Murri" Department of Internal and Public Medicine, University Medical School, Piazza Giulio Cesare 11, Policlinico, 70124 Bari, Italy
* Corresponding author.
E-mail address: p.portincasa@semeiotica.uniba.it

Gastroenterol Clin N Am 39 (2010) 245–264
doi:10.1016/j.gtc.2010.02.005
0889-8553/10/$ – see front matter © 2010 Elsevier Inc. All rights reserved.

bilirubin pigment polymer mixed with calcium phosphate and carbonate, and cholesterol) and brown pigment stones (about 5% of all gallstones, found mainly in bile ducts, containing calcium bilirubinate, calcium palmitate, and stearate and cholesterol).[9]

Cholesterol gallstones are associated with well-known risk factors, such as obesity, type 2 diabetes, dyslipidemia, and hyperinsulinemia,[1] which are often components of the metabolic syndrome epidemic,[10–14] which has a prevalence greater than 35% in the adult population and which continues to increase in Westernized countries.[15,16] Epidemiologic surveys have observed that cholesterol cholelithiasis is prevalent in populations consuming a Western diet (ie, enriched in saturated fatty acids, cholesterol, and rapidly absorbed refined carbohydrates), rather than a more prudent diet (ie, enriched in monopolyunsaturated fats, fruit, vegetables, and low in refined carbohydrates) associated with physical activity.[17–25] Thus, the prevalence of cholesterol gallstone disease is significantly higher in North and South American as well as European populations than in Asian and African populations.[6] In China, the prevalence of cholesterol gallstones seems to increase with the Westernization of the traditional Chinese diet.[26–28] Even in Japan, the adoption of Western-type dietary habits has resulted in a marked increase of the prevalence of cholesterol cholelithiasis over the past 40 years.[29,30] As discussed later, high efficiency of intestinal cholesterol absorption and high dietary cholesterol seem to be key and independent risk factors for the formation of cholesterol gallstones. The complex pathogenesis of cholesterol gallstones depends on the concurrent existence of hepatic hypersecretion of cholesterol into bile, leading to bile supersaturation with cholesterol, accelerated nucleation/crystallization of cholesterol in gallbladder bile, impaired gallbladder motility leading to gallbladder stasis, and increased cholesterol availability from the small intestine, as well as *LITH* genes and genetic factors.[1,31,32] A complex genetic basis plays a key role in determining individual predisposition to developing cholesterol gallstones in response to environmental factors.[33–37] Some gallstone genes might also play a potential role, including some genes governing the nuclear bile acid receptors such as farnesoid X receptor (FXR). For example, *FXR* variants seem to affect gallbladder motor function and intestinal microflora in Mexicans,[38] whereas functional variants in FXR might account for intrahepatic cholestasis of pregnancy in Whites, as well as being associated with other cholestatic and dyslipidemic disorders.[39]

From a therapeutic point of view, although gallstone disease is frequent in the general population and the costs of therapeutic interventions are high, the natural history of the disease suggests restriction of the medical treatment of gallstones to a subgroup of symptomatic patients.[1,36,40] The selection of patients eligible for medical or surgical therapy, therefore, is of key importance. The onset of biliary pain is the only suggestive marker of symptomatic gallstone disease,[41,42] although it can be difficult to distinguish between symptomatic and asymptomatic patients in a random population of patients with gallstones.[43] The diagnosis can be misleading if patients inadequately describe typical symptoms or suffer from highly atypical symptoms.[44] Previously symptomatic patients who are symptom-free for 5 consecutive years should be included in the group of asymptomatic subjects again. After this time, the risk of pain attacks gradually decreases toward values similar to those of patients with asymptomatic gallstones.[45] Classic drug therapy for cholesterol gallstones (ie, oral litholysis by the bile acid ursodeoxycholic acid [UDCA]) plays a limited role, but novel interesting therapeutic options might arise in the near future, related to the molecular mechanisms responsible for the formation of cholesterol gallstones.[1] Such novel therapeutic approaches might involve subgroups of patients permanently or temporarily at risk for gallstone formation. Recent studies in animal models and humans have found that blocking the intestinal absorption of cholesterol with ezetimibe (EZT), the potent inhibitor of the Niemann-Pick C1-like 1 (NPC1L1) protein,[46] may provide a novel powerful strategy for the medical treatment of cholesterol gallstones.[47] Modification of the expression levels of specific nuclear receptors (NR) in the liver might also provide a clue for novel therapeutic approaches for cholesterol gallstones via manipulation of cholesterol and bile acid homeostasis. Current views and perspectives on medical treatment of cholesterol gallstone disease are discussed in this article.

## GUIDELINES FOR MANAGEMENT OF GALLSTONE DISEASE

Gallbladder stones are frequently found in asymptomatic patients during routine abdominal ultrasonography, because in most cases (60%–80%) gallstones do not generate symptoms.[43,48,49] Previous observations have shown that the average risk of developing symptomatic gallstones is 2.0% to 2.6% per year.[45,50] By contrast, the presence of microstones and sludge in the gallbladder is a major risk factor for the development of biliary pain and complicated gallstone disease, and also plays a main role in the cause of acute otherwise idiopathic pancreatitis.[51–53] Nevertheless, the yearly incidence of complications is low (0.3%), and the annual risk for gallbladder cancer is as low as 0.02%.[54,55] Treatment of asymptomatic patients with gallstones, therefore, is not routinely recommended, as the overall risk of biliary colic, complications, and gallbladder cancer is low.[56–58] Expectant management is considered the appropriate choice in most asymptomatic patients with gallstones (grade A). The decision is different in symptomatic patients with gallstones and should follow the algorithm depicted in **Fig. 1**, in which surgery (namely laparoscopic cholecystectomy) represents the gold standard for treatment; oral litholysis with hydrophilic bile salts plays a limited role.[1,36] Other nonsurgical (nonpharmacologic) therapies include direct contact dissolutions of gallstones using the potent cholesterol solvent methyl tert butyl ether (MTBE),[59] and extracorporeal shock wave lithotripsy.[60] Both options, however, have lost their popularity because of potential side effects (MTBE) and high postdissolution recurrence rate.[1] Available medical treatments for gallstones are discussed in the following paragraphs and include the treatment of biliary colic (all types of stones), oral litholysis by hydrophilic bile acids and novel approaches with statins, EZT, and agonists/antagonists of NR (all for cholesterol gallstones).

## MEDICAL TREATMENTS OF GALLSTONE DISEASE
### Treatment of the Biliary Colic

The presence of a gallstone of any type and size may put the patient at risk of biliary pain. As the intensity of pain is usually high (mean visual analog scale of 9 cm on a 0- to 10-cm scale), patients require immediate medical attention and analgesia. The pain is not exclusively postprandial, and is typically intermittent. The most frequent localization is the right upper quadrant of the abdomen and/or the epigastrium (representative dermatomes T8/9), and the duration is generally longer than 15 to 30 minutes. The pain radiates to the angle of the right scapula and/or shoulder in about 60% of cases. In less than 10% of cases the pain radiates to the retrosternal area. About two-thirds of patients experience an urge to walk,[44] and often are nauseated or vomit.[41,44,49] In biliary colic, the pain is visceral and is caused by the impaction of the stone in the cystic duct or the sphincter of Oddi. Distension of the gallbladder and/or biliary tract with activation of visceral sensory neurons may follow.[41] The pain can last for several hours and be associated with nonspecific symptoms of indigestion. The pain can be relieved if the stone returns into the gallbladder lumen, passes through the sphincter into the duodenum, or migrates back to the common bile duct.[40] The

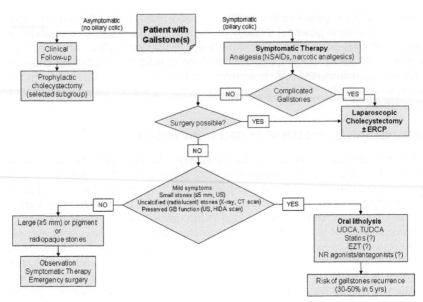

**Fig. 1.** Current therapies of gallstone disease, including cholesterol gallstones. Novel and potentially effective medical therapies are denoted by the symbol (?). See text for details. Results from meta-analyses indicate surgery as the gold standard for treating symptomatic gallstones.[164–166] Laparoscopic cholecystectomy and small-incision cholecystectomy[166] are safe and have similar mortality (from 0.1% to 0.7%).[122,165] Both approaches are cost-effective compared with open cholecystectomy.[165] Compared with open cholecystectomy, convalescence and hospital stay are shorter and total cost is lower for laparoscopic cholecystectomy.[122] Complication rates (including bile duct injuries) are similar for laparoscopic and open cholecystectomy.[122,165] When looking at surgical options, a prophylactic cholecystectomy can be taken into account in a subgroup of asymptomatic patients bearing a high risk of becoming symptomatic: children (who are exposed to long-term physical presence of stones[167]), morbid obese patients undergoing bariatric surgery (who are at high risk of becoming symptomatic during rapid weight loss[168]), patients at increased risk for gallbladder cancer[169] (ie, those with large gallstones, greater than 3 cm,[170,171] a porcelain gallbladder,[172] or gallbladder polyps rapidly growing or larger than 1 cm). Prophylactic cholecystectomy should also be considered in Native Americans with gallstones, who are at increased risk of gallbladder cancer (3%–5%),[173] and asymptomatic patients with gallstones with sickle cell anemia, who form calcium bilirubinate gallstones as a result of chronic hemolysis, and may become symptomatic with recurrent episodes of abdominal pain.[174] Prophylactic cholecystectomy has also been proposed in patients with small gallstones and gallbladder dysmotility, because the coexistence of these conditions increases the risk of pancreatitis.[51] CT, computerized tomography; ERCP, endoscopic retrograde cholangiopancreatography; EZT, ezetimibe; HIDA, 99mTc-N-(2,6-dimethylacetanilide)-iminodiacetic acid; GB, gallbladder; GS, gallstones; NR, nuclear receptors; NSAIDs, nonsteroidal antiinflammatory drugs; TUDCA, tauroursodeoxycholic acid; UDCA, ursodeoxycholic acid; US, abdominal ultrasonography. (*Data from* Portincasa P, Moschetta A, Palasciano G. Cholesterol gallstone disease. Lancet 2006;368(9531):230–39. Portincasa P, Moschetta A, Puglisi F, et al. Medical treatment of gallstone disease. In: Borzellino G, Cordiano C, editors. Biliary lithiasis. Basic science, current diagnosis and management. Milano, Italy: Springer Italia S.r.l.; 2008;149–57. Portincasa P, Di Ciaula A, Wang HH, et al. Medicinal treatments of cholesterol gallstones: old, current and new perspectives. Curr Med Chem 2009;16(12):1531–42.)

biliary pain is rapidly responsive to narcotic analgesics (meperidine[61]) or nonsteroidal anti-inflammatory drugs (NSAIDs) (such as intramuscular or intravenous ketorolac or ibuprofen by mouth), which could also reduce the risk of evolution toward acute cholecystitis.[62–65] A second-line therapy includes the use of antispasmodic (anticholinergic) agents like hyoscine (scopolamine) which are known to be less effective than NSAIDs[62] (grade A). The patient with biliary colic should remain fasting to avoid release of endogenous cholecystokinin and further gallbladder contraction. If a complicated biliary pain is suspected (association of leukocytosis, nausea, jaundice, vomiting, and fever), the patient should be quickly admitted to hospital and treated accordingly. Typical complications of gallstone disease are acute pancreatitis, acute cholecystitis, biliary obstruction and cholangitis, gallbladder perforation, abscess formation, and mucocele of the gallbladder, which may require additional medical therapy with antibiotics or invasive procedures with or without surgery. In mild and moderate acute cholecystitis, early laparoscopic cholecystectomy is recommended at between 2 and 4 days[66] (grade A). The risk of biliary pain in asymptomatic carriers is estimated to be approximately 1% to 2% annually.[67,68] Early studies that were not randomized or placebo-controlled found that UDCA, besides its litholytic effect (see later discussion), might also reduce the risk of biliary colic.[69,70] In a nonrandomized study, Tomida and colleagues[71] treated patients referred for symptomatic or asymptomatic gallstones with 600 mg UDCA per day and used those who refused as a control group. The incidence of biliary pain was apparently reduced by UDCA in asymptomatic patients, although a bias might include a misclassification of symptoms. However, in a large randomized, double-blind, placebo-controlled trial on the effects of UDCA in highly symptomatic patients with gallstones scheduled for cholecystectomy, UDCA did not exert a beneficial effect on biliary colic. The likelihood of remaining colic-free was comparable in patients with strong or weak baseline gallbladder contraction as determined by ultrasonography after a standard mixed meal.[72]

### Dissolution of Cholesterol Gallstones by Oral Bile Acids

About two-thirds of the gallstones in Western countries are composed mainly of cholesterol. However, dissolution therapy by oral administration of the hydrophilic bile acid UDCA, the 7β-epimer of chenodeoxycholate, is suitable only for a small subgroup (about 15%) of symptomatic patients.[1,40] Similar results are reached with the taurine-conjugated UDCA (tauroursodeoxycholic acid [TUDCA]). Chances of dissolution are higher if gallstones are small (less than 0.5 cm in size), not calcified (radiolucent on radiograph, including a computed tomography [CT] scan), cholesterol-enriched (ie, more than 80%), and contained within a functioning gallbladder with a patent cystic duct.[73] Complete dissolution of gallstones by bile acids was first documented by Rewbridge in 1937,[74] although initial reports were published in 1873 and 1876.[75,76] The bile acid chenodeoxycholic acid (CDCA) was first used in the 1970s[77] but was associated with a dose-dependent increase in serum aminotransferases, serum low-density lipoprotein cholesterol levels, and diarrhea. In 1975 Makino and colleagues[78] identified UDCA as a more hydrophilic bile acid that could replace CDCA without side effects. Dissolution of cholesterol gallstones by UDCA following fragmentation by extracorporeal shock wave lithotripsy was introduced first by Sauerbruch and colleagues[60] in Munich in 1986. The bile acid UDCA is currently used for oral dissolution at a dosage of 10 to 14 mg/kg body weight per day. Bedtime administration is suggested because it maintains hepatic bile acid secretion rate overnight, thus reducing secretion of supersaturated bile and increasing the dissolution rate[79,80] (grade A). Oral UDCA (at least 10 mg/kg/d) results in an increased proportion of biliary UDCA in bile (from less than 8%–10% of biliary bile acid pool to about 40%).

Increasing biliary UDCA, in turn, results in a decreased hepatic secretion of biliary cholesterol and the formation of unsaturated gallbladder bile (ie, containing less cholesterol in solution) with a cholesterol saturation index of less than 1 (**Fig. 2**).[81–83] This step represents a key factor in initiating the process of dissolution of cholesterol crystals and gallstones. During UDCA treatment, cholesterol crystallization can be prevented because more cholesterol can be transported within vesicles that contain mainly phospholipids and cholesterol and little bile acid.[84] Also, oral therapy with UDCA is associated with the reduction of intestinal absorption of cholesterol,[85–87] as well as with a better contractility of the stimulated gallbladder smooth muscle, as shown by in vitro studies in animals and patients with gallstones.[88,89] By decreasing

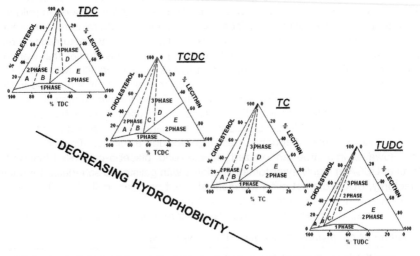

**Fig. 2.** Effects of UDCA on bile composition and cholesterol solubility are explained by using the ternary phase diagram.[175] A group of the equilibrium phase diagram of cholesterol-lecithin-taurine-conjugated bile salt systems (37°C, 0.15 M NaCl, pH 7.0, total lipid concentration 7.5 g/dL) are drawn to display varied positions and configuration of crystallization regions as a result of decreasing bile salt hydrophobicity. The lipid components are expressed in moles percent. The 1-phase micellar zone at the bottom is enclosed by a solid curved line. Above it, 2 solid lines divide the 2-phase zones from a central 3-phase zone. Based on the solid and liquid crystallization sequences present in the bile, the left 2-phase and the central 3-phase regions are divided by dashed lines into regions A to D. The number of phases given represents the equilibrium state. There are cholesterol monohydrate crystals and saturated micelles for crystallization regions A and B, cholesterol monohydrate crystals, saturated micelles, and liquid crystals for regions C and D, and liquid crystals of variable compositions and saturated micelles for region E.[175] As the bile acid hydrophobicity decreases, the maximum micellar cholesterol solubility is reduced and crystallization pathways A to E move to the left. This change results in an enlarged region E that extends to the left and overlaps pathophysiologic compositions as exemplified in the TUDC-lecithin-cholesterol system. This event induces a greatly reduced chance for the formation of solid platelike cholesterol monohydrate crystals in bile. (*Data from* Wang DQH, Carey MC. Complete mapping of crystallization pathways during cholesterol precipitation from model bile: influence of physical-chemical variables of pathophysiologic relevance and identification of a stable liquid crystalline state in cold, dilute and hydrophilic bile salt-containing system. J Lipid Res 1996;37:606–30 and Portincasa P, Di Ciaula A, Wang HH, et al. Medicinal treatments of cholesterol gallstones: old, current and new perspectives. Curr Med Chem 2009;16(12):1531–42.)

cholesterol saturation of bile, UDCA might counteract the impaired contractility caused by incorporation of excessive luminal cholesterol into the plasmalemma of gallbladder smooth muscles.[88–91] UDCA might also counteract the detrimental effects of the hydrophobic bile acid deoxycholate on the gallbladder smooth muscle contractility,[91,92] and have an effect on local oxidative stress[89,93] and risk of acute cholecystitis.[71] Excess biliary cholesterol might provide the basis for stimulation of inflammatory cells in the gallbladder, because cholesterol monohydrate crystals induce expression of T-cell–dependent proinflammatory cytokines in a murine model of cholesterol cholelithogenesis.[94]

Patients suitable for medical dissolution of cholesterol gallstones need to be carefully selected. Well-selected patients are those who have the higher chance for successful oral litholysis alone or after extracorporeal shock wave lithotripsy for stone fragmentation.[95–99] Ultrasonography of the right upper quadrant is still the best and more convenient diagnostic tool for detecting gallstones,[58,100] as well as for assessing gallstone size and burden.[101] Functional ultrasonography, (ie, the study of time-dependent changes of fasting and postprandial gallbladder volumes following a standard test meal), although not routinely used, provides additional information about gallbladder size, emptying, and bile duct patency.[36,95–98,102–105] Abdominal plain radiography (not routinely used) and the CT scan[106,107] detect only calcified stones (as radiopaque bodies) in the right upper quadrant. Such stones are unfit for dissolution because they are either calcified cholesterol stones or stones made of pigment calcium bilirubinate.[9] Oral cholecystography might disclose the presence of floating (cholesterol) stones in the gallbladder and a preserved cystic duct patency. The expected dissolution rate following UDCA at the standard dosage is estimated to be about a 1-mm decrement in stone diameter per month.[108] In patients with a gallstone diameter less than 5 mm, the complete disappearance of stones assessed by ultrasonography is expected to be reached in about 90% of cases by 6 months of UDCA administration.[109] A series of conditions might impede the dissolution of cholesterol gallstones by UDCA or TUDCA. In patients with larger and/or multiple stones the dissolution rate approaches 40% to 50% after 1 year of the treatment,[54,110] whereas the appearance of a surface calcification on cholesterol gallstones during oral dissolution therapy with UDCA, CDCA, or TUDCA has been reported in about 10% to 12% of patients. This event would impede any further dissolution of the calcified stone.[111,112] Another issue is the possibility that gallstones will recur sometime after dissolution with bile acids, and this is a major limitation of oral dissolution therapy. Overall, recurrence might be as high as 10% per year (ie, about 30%–50% of cases) 5 years after bile acid therapy or lithotripsy.[96,113–117] Recurrence rate is higher particularly in patients with multiple gallstones.[116] Whereas recurrent gallstones respond well to retreatment,[107,118] such a high recurrence rate may be dependent on persistent pathogenetic conditions.[1] Oral dissolution therapy for cholesterol gallstones with bile acids might still represent the option in patients who are at minimal risk of gallstone recurrence or have transient risk factors including rapid weight loss (ie, obese patients following bariatric surgery), pregnancy, and convalescence from abdominal surgery.[1,119–121] Major limitations for oral litholysis with bile acids, by contrast, are the small number of suitable patients and the high rate of gallstone recurrence.[37,122,123]

## NOVEL MEDICAL TREATMENTS

The presence of a lithogenic bile is primarily a result of a sustained hypersecretion of biliary cholesterol, which has 2 key components: hepatic and intestinal.[31] In principle, drugs influencing hepatic synthesis and/or secretion of cholesterol (ie, statins) and/or intestinal absorption of cholesterol (ie, EZT) are potentially able to influence the formation of cholesterol gallstones and to promote dissolution of gallstones.

### Inhibition of Hepatic Cholesterol Synthesis by Statins

Statins are competitive inhibitors of 3-hydroxy-3-methylglutaryl coenzyme A (HMG CoA) reductase, the rate-limiting step in cholesterol biosynthesis. They occupy a portion of the binding site of HMG CoA, blocking access of this substrate to the active site on the enzyme.[124] Currently available statins in the United States include lovastatin, pravastatin, simvastatin, fluvastatin, atorvastatin, and rosuvastatin. Statins seem also to reduce cholesterol secretion and concentration in bile independently of their ability to block hepatic cholesterol synthesis.[125–128] Such combined effects of statins on cholesterol homeostasis in the liver and bile might be able to lower the risk of cholesterol gallstones.[129–131] Beneficial effects of statins in preventing gallstone formation have been reported in animal studies.[132,133] In humans the effect of statins on gallstone disease has been controversial; reduced gallstone formation, decreased cholesterol concentration in bile, and gallstone dissolution following therapy with statins have been reported by some,[134–137] but not all, studies.[130,138,139] Another 2 small studies have also been conflicting, with either no association between statin use and the risk of gallstones[140] or with an effect of statin on gallstones, although the statistical power was small.[141] More recently, 2 studies have reassessed the problem of statin use and risk of gallstone disease, and opened new perspectives. In a cohort of US women self-reporting long-term use statins, the risk of cholecystectomy was found to decrease slightly.[142] In a case-control analysis using the United Kingdom–based General Practice Research Database and evaluating incident patients between 1994 and 2004, long-term use of statins (1–1.5 years) was associated with a decreased risk of gallstones followed by cholecystectomy, compared with patients without statin use.[143] Whether statin use will be part of the medical therapeutic armamentarium in a subgroup of patients with gallstone disease or to prevent gallstone disease in selected patients at risk needs to be investigated further by appropriate clinical studies.

### Inhibition of Intestinal Cholesterol Absorption by EZT

The importance of intestinal factors in the pathogenesis of cholesterol gallstones has recently been investigated by several research groups.[1,144] Animal studies have shown that when no dietary cholesterol is available, all biliary cholesterol is mainly derived from hepatic de novo synthesis with a limited contribution (less than 15%) to biliary cholesterol secretion. Rather, the small intestine is the site that solely provides the absorption of dietary cholesterol, as well as reabsorption of biliary cholesterol.[144] The importance of intestinal absorption of cholesterol for gallstone pathogenesis is supported by the positive correlation between the efficiency of intestinal cholesterol absorption and the prevalence of cholesterol gallstone formation in several strains of inbred mice.[34] The protein NPC1L1 is highly expressed in the small intestine and localized along the brush border of the enterocytes in humans and mice.[145,146] There is also a significant amount of NPC1L1 in the human liver but not in the mouse liver.[146,147] Cholesterol is the most effective substrate of NPC1L1,[148] which governs intestinal absorption of cholesterol[146] by recycling between endocytic recycling compartment and plasma membrane (Fig. 3).[148] Thus, inhibition of cholesterol absorption in the intestine or hepatic uptake of chylomicron remnants has become an attractive possibility to decrease biliary cholesterol secretion and saturation.[100] Similar to humans, the abundance of NPC1L1 in the small intestine far exceeded that in other regions of the gastrointestinal tract, liver, and gallbladder in

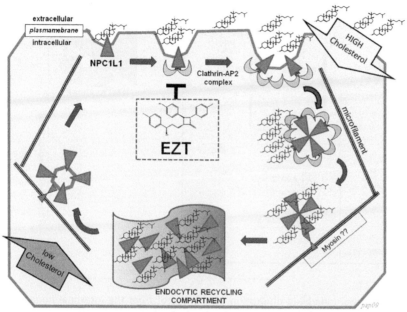

**Fig. 3.** Mechanisms for cholesterol uptake mediated by the NPC1L1 according to the model proposed by Ge and colleagues.[148] The NPC1L1 protein recycles between the plasma membrane facing the extracellular space and the endocytic recycling compartment. If extracellular cholesterol concentration is high, cholesterol is incorporated into the plasma membrane and is sensed by cell surface-localized NPC1L1. NPC1L1 and cholesterol are then internalized together through clathrin/AP2-mediated endocytosis. The clathrin-coated globular vesicles are transported along microfilaments to the endocytic recycling compartment. The role of myosin in this process is unclear. Large quantities of cholesterol and NPC1L1 are subsequently stored within the endocytic recycling compartment. If the intracellular cholesterol level is low, endocytic recycling compartment-localized NPC1L1 moves back to the plasma membrane along microfilaments, and new cholesterol is absorbed. The key role of the NPC1L1 inhibitor EZT is shown at the center of the cell. EZT prevents NPC1L1 from entering the AP2-mediated clathrin-coated vesicles. At this stage, the endocytosis of NPC1L1 is inhibited and cholesterol absorption is decreased. (*Adapted from* Portincasa P, Di Ciaula A, Wang HH, et al. Medicinal treatments of cholesterol gallstones: old, current and new perspectives. Curr Med Chem 2009;16(12):1531–42; with permission.)

the Golden Syrian hamster.[149] EZT-induced reduction in intestinal cholesterol absorption is coupled with a decrease in the absolute and relative cholesterol levels in bile in hamsters fed a high-cholesterol and high-fat diet. These results are consistent with the recent finding that EZT treatment significantly reduced biliary cholesterol saturation in patients with gallstones.[47] EZT belongs to the new class of 2-azetidinones approved as a novel hypocholesterolemic drug[150] with a potent inhibitory effect on intestinal cholesterol absorption by specifically suppressing the NPC1L1. EZT might therefore play a primary role in the medical treatment or prevention of cholesterol gallstones, as suggested by studies from the authors' group (**Fig. 4**). In mice, EZT reduces cholesterol and partly phospholipid but not bile salt content in gallbladder bile; all crystallization pathways and phase boundaries in the bile phase diagram remain similar, with or without EZT.[47] If EZT is increased, the relative lipid compositions of pooled gallbladder bile samples are progressively shifted down and to the left of the phase diagram, and

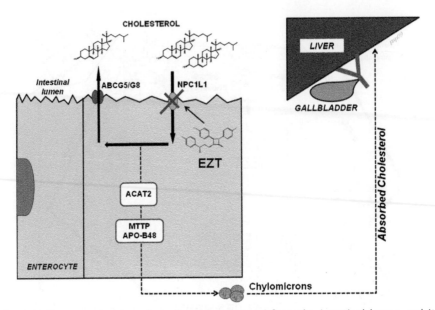

**Fig. 4.** Pathways underlying absorption of cholesterol from the intestinal lumen and its delivery to the liver. High dietary cholesterol through the chylomicron pathway could provide an important source of excess cholesterol molecules for secretion into bile, thereby inducing cholesterol-supersaturated bile and enhancing cholesterol gallstone formation.[31,47] EZT significantly suppresses cholesterol absorption from the small intestine via the NPC1L1 pathway.[47] This effect should diminish the cholesterol content of the liver, which in turn decreases bioavailability of cholesterol for biliary secretion. ABCG5/G8, ATP-binding cassette (transporter); ACAT2, acyl-CoA:cholesterol acyltransferase isoform 2; APO-B48, apolipoprotein B48; MTTP, microsomal triglyceride transfer protein. See text for details.

enter the 1-phase (protective) micellar zone (which contains an abundance of unsaturated micelles but never solid cholesterol crystals or liquid crystals). Thus, the micellar cholesterol solubility is increased in gallbladder bile with more cholesterol molecules transferred from the cholesterol monohydrate surface into unsaturated micelles. In this environment, gallstones can dissolve.[47,151] EZT also protected gallbladder motility function by desaturating bile.[47] The physical-chemical mechanisms underlying the beneficial effects of EZT on supersaturated bile, cholesterol crystals, and cholesterol stones differ from those of hydrophilic bile acids such as UDCA, TUDCA and β-muricholic acid. These hydrophilic bile acids enhance dissolution of cholesterol gallstones by promoting the formation of a vesicle-enriched liquid crystalline mesophase.[152] Translational studies have shown that EZT (20 mg/d by mouth for 1 month) significantly reduced cholesterol concentration and cholesterol saturation index and retarded cholesterol crystallization in patients with gallstones.[47]

Animal and preliminary human studies show that EZT by inhibiting NPC1L1-mediated intestinal cholesterol absorption also lowers biliary cholesterol secretion, desaturates bile, and preserves gallbladder motility function, even under conditions of high dietary cholesterol loads.[47,151,153] Whether EZT will become a novel and effective cholelitholytic agent (alone or combined with statins and/or hydrophilic bile acids), is a matter of research in future well-designed, controlled, long-term clinical studies.

## Agents Effective on NR

Coherent and coordinate activation of sets of genes involved in multiple cellular activities depends on NR, which are ligand-activated transcription factors.[154] Lipid-sensing NR govern lipid homeostasis in the hepatobiliary and gastrointestinal systems. Hepatic and biliary lipid metabolism are involved in lipid secretion by the hepatocytes, and are controlled by the oxysterol receptor LXR (the intracellular sensor of cholesterol[155]) and the bile acid receptor FXR (the intracellular sensor of bile acids[156,157]). The subtle cellular mechanisms governing lipid homeostasis imply that cells synthesize oxysterols under conditions of cholesterol overload, and oxysterols in turn bind and activate LXR, which acts to reduce systemic cholesterol burden.[156–158] In the enterohepatic system FXR is highly expressed and regulates the expression of genes involved in the maintenance of cholesterol, bile acid, and triglyceride homeostasis.[159] Liver FXR might become a pharmacologic target for the treatment of cholestasis and cholelithiasis,[160] because this NR upregulates the expression of bile acid transporters in the canalicular membrane and of enzymes responsible for bile acid detoxification. Manipulation of NR in the animal model has disclosed novel potential approaches to the problem of cholesterol gallstone disease. FXR is a promising therapeutic target for treating or preventing cholesterol gallstone disease. FXR-null mice are susceptible to cholesterol gallstone formation; activating FXR with the compound GW4064, a specific synthetic ligand, by contrast, increases biliary bile salt and phospholipid concentrations.[161] The effect is tightly dependent on FXR-induced regulation of the energy dependent adenosine triphosphate (ATP)-binding cassette (ABC) transporters ABCB11 (for bile salts) and ABCB4 (for phospholipid)[162] and is associated with better solubilization of cholesterol, and prevention of solid platelike crystals and stones. Increased propensity to cholesterol crystallization and stone formation in bile has been described in mice following the activation of hepatic LXR and direct upregulation of the major hepatocyte cholesterol canalicular transporters ABCG5 and ABCG8, which together form a heterodimer.[163] Future studies need to test if liver-specific FXR agonists and LXR antagonists might be safe and effective in human gallstone disease, as is the case for dyslipidemia, type II diabetes, and several cancers.

## SUMMARY

The advent of laparoscopic cholecystectomy has moved the interest away from the pharmacologic treatment of gallstones. Medical therapy is restricted to a scant group of symptomatic (colicky pain) well-selected patients, in which the unfavorable cost-benefit analyses and a high rate of gallstone recurrence play a negative role. Following early cholelitholytic therapies with the oral bile acid UDCA, recent studies indicate that the research agenda should include studies on the role of gallstone (LITH) genes, as well as the mechanisms of intestinal absorption of cholesterol and pathways of liver synthesis-secretion of cholesterol. Promising agents might include, alone or in combination, statins (competitive inhibitors of HMG CoA reductase, the rate-limiting step in cholesterol biosynthesis), EZT (specific inhibitor of the intestinal cholesterol transporter protein NPC1L1), and liver-specific agonists/antagonists of the NR FXR/LXR involved in biliary lipid secretion.

## ACKNOWLEDGMENTS

The authors are grateful to Paola De Benedictis, Rosa De Venuto, and Michele Persichella for their skillful technical assistance.

## REFERENCES

1. Portincasa P, Moschetta A, Palasciano G. Cholesterol gallstone disease. Lancet 2006;368(9531):230–9.
2. Wang DQ, Afdhal NH. Genetic analysis of cholesterol gallstone formation: searching for Lith (gallstone) genes. Curr Gastroenterol Rep 2004;6(2):140–50.
3. Everhart JE, Khare M, Hill M, et al. Prevalence and ethnic differences in gallbladder disease in the United States. Gastroenterology 1999;117(3):632–9.
4. Sandler RS, Everhart JE, Donowitz M, et al. The burden of selected digestive diseases in the United States. Gastroenterology 2002;122(5):1500–11.
5. Liver Disease Subcommittee of the Digestive Disease Interagency Coordinating Committee. Action plan for liver disease research. Bethesda (MD): NIH; 2004. p. 145–50.
6. Diehl AK. Epidemiology and natural history of gallstone disease. Gastroenterol Clin North Am 1991;20(1):1–19.
7. Attili AF, Carulli N, Roda E, et al. Epidemiology of gallstone disease in Italy: prevalence data of the multicenter italian study on cholelithiasis (M.I.C.O.L. Am J Epidemiol 1995;141:158–65.
8. Attili AF, Capocaccia R, Carulli N, et al. Factors associated with gallstone disease in the MICOL experience. Hepatology 1997;26:809–18.
9. Sherlock S, Dooley J. Diseases of the liver and biliary system. Oxford (UK): Blackwell Science; 2002.
10. Grundy SM, Barnett JP. Metabolic and health complications of obesity. Dis Mon 1990;36:641–731.
11. Grundy SM. Metabolic syndrome scientific statement by the American Heart Association and the National Heart, Lung, and Blood Institute. Arterioscler Thromb Vasc Biol 2005;25(11):2243–4.
12. Grundy SM, Cleeman JI, Daniels SR, et al. Diagnosis and management of the metabolic syndrome: an American Heart Association/National Heart, Lung, and Blood Institute Scientific Statement. Circulation 2005;112(17):2735–52.
13. Eckel RH, Grundy SM, Zimmet PZ. The metabolic syndrome. Lancet 2005; 365(9468):1415–28.
14. Tsai CJ, Leitzmann MF, Willett WC, et al. Prospective study of abdominal adiposity and gallstone disease in US men. Am J Clin Nutr 2004;80(1):38–44.
15. Ford ES, Giles WH, Mokdad AH. Increasing prevalence of the metabolic syndrome among US adults. Diabetes Care 2004;27(10):2444–9.
16. Ford ES. Prevalence of the metabolic syndrome defined by the International Diabetes Federation among adults in the US. Diabetes Care 2005;28(11): 2745–9.
17. Tsai CJ, Leitzmann MF, Willett WC, et al. Dietary protein and the risk of cholecystectomy in a cohort of US women: the Nurses' Health Study. Am J Epidemiol 2004;160(1):11–8.
18. Tsai CJ, Leitzmann MF, Hu FB, et al. Frequent nut consumption and decreased risk of cholecystectomy in women. Am J Clin Nutr 2004;80(1):76–81.
19. Tsai CJ, Leitzmann MF, Willett WC, et al. Fruit and vegetable consumption and risk of cholecystectomy in women. Am J Med 2006;119(9):760–7.
20. Tsai CJ, Leitzmann MF, Willett WC, et al. Long-term intake of dietary fiber and decreased risk of cholecystectomy in women. Am J Gastroenterol 2004;99(7): 1364–70.
21. Tsai CJ, Leitzmann MF, Willett WC, et al. Long-term intake of trans-fatty acids and risk of gallstone disease in men. Arch Intern Med 2005;165(9):1011–5.

22. Leitzmann MF, Rimm EB, Willett WC, et al. Recreational physical activity and the risk of cholecystectomy in women. N Engl J Med 1999;341(11):777–84.

23. Tsai CJ, Leitzmann MF, Willett WC, et al. The effect of long-term intake of cis unsaturated fats on the risk for gallstone disease in men: a prospective cohort study. Ann Intern Med 2004;141(7):514–22.

24. Leitzmann MF, Giovannucci EL, Rimm EB, et al. The relation of physical activity to risk for symptomatic gallstone disease in men. Ann Intern Med 1998;128(6): 417–25.

25. Shaffer EA. Gallstone disease: epidemiology of gallbladder stone disease. Best Pract Res Clin Gastroenterol 2006;20(6):981–96.

26. Zhu X, Zhang S, Huang Z. [The trend of the gallstone disease in China over the past decade]. Zhonghua Wai Ke Za Zhi 1995;33(11):652–8 [in Chinese].

27. Huang YC, Zhang XW, Yang RX. Changes in cholelithiasis in Tianjin in the past 30 years. Chin Med J (Engl) 1984;97(2):133–5.

28. Sun H, Tang H, Jiang S, et al. Gender and metabolic differences of gallstone diseases. World J Gastroenterol 2009;15(15):1886–91.

29. Nakayama F, Miyake H. Changing state of gallstone disease in Japan. Composition of the stones and treatment of the condition. Am J Surg 1970;120(6): 794–9.

30. Nagase M, Tanimura H, Setoyama M, et al. Present features of gallstones in Japan. A collective review of 2,144 cases. Am J Surg 1978;135(6):788–90.

31. Wang HH, Portincasa P, Wang DQ. Molecular pathophysiology and physical chemistry of cholesterol gallstones. Front Biosci 2008;13:401–23.

32. Portincasa P, Di Ciaula A, Wang HH, et al. Coordinate regulation of gallbladder motor function in the gut-liver axis. Hepatology 2008;47(6):2112–26.

33. Wittenburg H, Lammert F. Genetic predisposition to gallbladder stones. Semin Liver Dis 2007;27(1):109–21.

34. Wang DQH, Zhang L, Wang HH. High cholesterol absorption efficiency and rapid biliary secretion of chylomicron remnant cholesterol enhance cholelithogenesis in gallstone-susceptible mice. Biochim Biophys Acta 2005;1733(1): 90–9.

35. Lammert F, Sauerbruch T. Mechanisms of disease: the genetic epidemiology of gallbladder stones. Nat Clin Pract Gastroenterol Hepatol 2005;2(9):423–33.

36. Portincasa P, Moschetta A, Puglisi F, et al. Medical treatment of gallstone disease. In: Borzellino G, Cordiano C, editors. Biliary lithiasis. Basic science, current diagnosis and management. Milano (Italy): Springer Italia S.r.l; 2008. p. 149–57.

37. Lammert F, Miquel JF. Gallstone disease: from genes to evidence-based therapy. J Hepatol 2008;48(Suppl 1):S124–35.

38. Kovacs P, Kress R, Rocha J, et al. Variation of the gene encoding the nuclear bile salt receptor FXR and gallstone susceptibility in mice and humans. J Hepatol 2008;48(1):116–24.

39. Van Mil SW, Milona A, Dixon PH, et al. Functional variants of the central bile acid sensor FXR identified in intrahepatic cholestasis of pregnancy. Gastroenterology 2007;133(2):507–16.

40. Portincasa P, Moschetta A, Petruzzelli M, et al. Gallstone disease: symptoms and diagnosis of gallbladder stones. Best Pract Res Clin Gastroenterol 2006; 20(6):1017–29.

41. Diehl AK, Sugarek NJ, Todd KH. Clinical evaluation for gallstone disease: usefulness of symptoms and signs in diagnosis. Am J Med 1990;89(1):29–33.

42. Paumgartner G, Carr-Locke DL, Roda E, et al. Biliary stones: non-surgical therapeutic approach. Gastroenterol Int 1988;1(1):17–24.

43. Jorgensen T. Abdominal symptoms and gallstone disease: an epidemiological investigation. Hepatology 1989;9:856–60.
44. Berhane T, Vetrhus M, Hausken T, et al. Pain attacks in non-complicated and complicated gallstone disease have a characteristic pattern and are accompanied by dyspepsia in most patients: the results of a prospective study. Scand J Gastroenterol 2006;41(1):93–101.
45. Friedman GD, Raviola CA, Fireman B. Prognosis of gallstones with mild or no symptoms: 25 years of follow-up in a health maintenance organization. J Clin Epidemiol 1989;42(2):127–36.
46. Hou R, Goldberg AC. Lowering low-density lipoprotein cholesterol: statins, ezetimibe, bile acid sequestrants, and combinations: comparative efficacy and safety. Endocrinol Metab Clin North Am 2009;38(1):79–97.
47. Wang HH, Portincasa P, Mendez-Sanchez N, et al. Effect of ezetimibe on the prevention and dissolution of cholesterol gallstones. Gastroenterology 2008; 134:2101–10.
48. Gibney EJ. Asymptomatic gallstones. Br J Surg 1990;77(4):368–72.
49. Festi D, Sottili S, Colecchia A, et al. Clinical manifestations of gallstone disease: evidence from the multicenter Italian study on cholelithiasis (MICOL). Hepatology 1999;30(4):839–46.
50. Thistle JL, Cleary PA, Lachin JM, et al. The natural history of cholelithiasis: the National Cooperative Gallstone Study. Ann Intern Med 1984;101(2):171–5.
51. Venneman NG, Renooij W, Rehfeld JF, et al. Small gallstones, preserved gallbladder motility, and fast crystallization are associated with pancreatitis. Hepatology 2005;41(4):738–46.
52. Venneman NG, Buskens E, Besselink MG, et al. Small gallstones are associated with increased risk of acute pancreatitis: potential benefits of prophylactic cholecystectomy? Am J Gastroenterol 2005;100(11):2540–50.
53. Lee SP, Nicholls JF, Park HZ. Biliary sludge as a cause of acute pancreatitis. N Engl J Med 1992;326(9):589–93.
54. Paumgartner G, Carr-Locke DL, Dubois F, et al. Strategies in the treatment of gallstone disease. Working team report. Gastroenterol Int 1993;6:65–75.
55. Brugge WR. The silent gallstone. In: Afdhal NH, editor. Gallbladder and biliary tract diseases. New York, Basel: Marcel Dekker, Inc; 2000. p. 447–53.
56. Tait N, Little JM. The treatment of gall stones. BMJ 1995;311(6997):99–105.
57. Hofmann AF, Amelsberg A, Vansonnenberg E. Pathogenesis and treatment of gallstones. N Engl J Med 1993;328(25):1854–5.
58. Johnston DE, Kaplan MM. Pathogenesis and treatment of gallstones. N Engl J Med 1993;328:412–21.
59. Thistle JL, May GR, Bender CE, et al. Dissolution of cholesterol gallbladder stones by methyl tert-butyl ether administered by percutaneous transhepatic catheter. N Engl J Med 1989;320:633–9.
60. Sauerbruch T, Delius M, Paumgartner G, et al. Fragmentation of gallstones by extracorporeal shock waves. N Engl J Med 1986;314(13):818–22.
61. Elta GH, Barnett JL. Meperidine need not be proscribed during sphincter of Oddi manometry. Gastrointest Endosc 1994;40(1):7–9.
62. Kumar A, Deed JS, Bhasin B, et al. Comparison of the effect of diclofenac with hyoscine-N-butylbromide in the symptomatic treatment of acute biliary colic. ANZ J Surg 2004;74(7):573–6.
63. Al-Waili N, Saloom KY. The analgesic effect of intravenous tenoxicam in symptomatic treatment of biliary colic: a comparison with hyoscine N-butylbromide. Eur J Med Res 1998;3(10):475–9.

64. Akriviadis EA, Hatzigavriel M, Kapnias D, et al. Treatment of biliary colic with diclofenac: a randomized, double-blind, placebo-controlled study. Gastroenterology 1997;113(1):225–31.

65. Goldman G, Kahn PJ, Alon R, et al. Biliary colic treatment and acute cholecystitis prevention by prostaglandin inhibitor. Dig Dis Sci 1989;34(6):809–11.

66. Gurusamy KS, Samraj K. Early versus delayed laparoscopic cholecystectomy for acute cholecystitis. Cochrane Database Syst Rev 2006;(4):CD005440.

67. Gracie WA, Ransohoff DF. The natural history of silent gallstones: the "innocent gallstone" is not a myth. N Engl J Med 1982;307:798–800.

68. Friedman GD. Natural history of asymptomatic and symptomatic gallstones. Am J Surg 1993;165(4):399–404.

69. Tint GS, Salen G, Colalillo A, et al. Ursodeoxycholic acid: a safe and effective agent for dissolving cholesterol gallstones. Ann Intern Med 1982;97(3):351–6.

70. Meredith TJ, Williams GV, Maton PN, et al. Retrospective comparison of 'Cheno' and 'Urso' in the medical treatment of gallstones. Gut 1982;23(5):382–9.

71. Tomida S, Abei M, Yamaguchi T, et al. Long-term ursodeoxycholic acid therapy is associated with reduced risk of biliary pain and acute cholecystitis in patients with gallbladder stones: a cohort analysis. Hepatology 1999;30:6–13.

72. Venneman NG, Besselink MG, Keulemans YC, et al. Ursodeoxycholic acid exerts no beneficial effect in patients with symptomatic gallstones awaiting cholecystectomy. Hepatology 2006;43(6):1276–83.

73. Paumgartner G, Pauletzki J, Sackmann M. Ursodeoxycholic acid treatment of cholesterol gallstone disease. Scand J Gastroenterol Suppl 1994;204:27–31.

74. Rewbridge AG. The disappearance of gallstone shadows following the prolonged administration of bile acids. Surgery 1937;1:395–400.

75. Schiff M. Il coleinato di soda nella cura dei calcoli biliari. L'imparziale 1873;13: 97–8 [in Italian].

76. Dabney WC. The use of choleate of soda to prevent the formation of gallstones. Am J Med Sci 1876;71:410.

77. Danzinger RG, Hofmann AF, Schoenfield LJ. Dissolution of cholesterol gallstones by chenodeoxycholic acid. N Engl J Med 1972;286:1–8.

78. Makino I, Shinozaki K, Yoshino K, et al. [Dissolution of cholesterol gallstones by long-term administration of ursodeoxycholic acid]. Nippon Shokakibyo Gakkai Zasshi 1975;72:690–702 [in Japanese].

79. Kupfer RM, Maudgal DP, Northfield TC. Gallstone dissolution rate during chenic acid therapy. Effect of bedtime administration plus low cholesterol diet. Dig Dis Sci 1982;27(11):1025–9.

80. Lanzini A, Facchinetti D, Northfield TC. Maintenance of hepatic bile acid secretion rate during overnight fasting by bedtime bile acid administration. Gastroenterology 1988;95(4):1029–35.

81. van Erpecum KJ, Portincasa P, Stolk MF, et al. Effects of bile salt and phospholipid hydrophobicity on lithogenicity of human gallbladder bile. Eur J Clin Invest 1994;24:744–50.

82. van Erpecum KJ, Portincasa P, Gadellaa M, et al. Effects of bile salt hydrophobicity on nucleation behaviour of cholesterol crystals in model bile. Eur J Clin Invest 1996;26:602–8.

83. Portincasa P, van Erpecum KJ, Jansen A, et al. Behavior of various cholesterol crystals in bile from gallstone patients. Hepatology 1996;23:738–48.

84. Moschetta A, vanBerge-Henegouwen GP, Portincasa P, et al. Cholesterol crystallization in model biles. Effects of bile salt and phospholipid species composition. J Lipid Res 2001;42(8):1273–81.

85. Hardison WG, Grundy SM. Effect of ursodeoxycholate and its taurine conjugate on bile acid synthesis and cholesterol absorption. Gastroenterology 1984;87(1): 130–5.

86. Uchida K, Akiyoshi T, Igimi H, et al. Differential effects of ursodeoxycholic acid and ursocholic acid on the formation of biliary cholesterol crystals in mice. Lipids 1991;26:526–30.

87. Wang DQ, Tazuma S, Cohen DE, et al. Feeding natural hydrophilic bile acids inhibits intestinal cholesterol absorption: studies in the gallstone-susceptible mouse. Am J Physiol Gastrointest Liver Physiol 2003;285(3):G494–502.

88. van de Heijning BJ, van de Meeberg P, Portincasa P, et al. Effects of ursodeoxycholic acid therapy on in vitro gallbladder contractility in patients with cholesterol gallstones. Dig Dis Sci 1999;44:190–6.

89. Guarino MP, Cong P, Cicala M, et al. Ursodeoxycholic acid improves muscle contractility and inflammation in symptomatic gallbladders with cholesterol gallstones. Gut 2007;56(6):815–20.

90. Portincasa P, Di Ciaula A, vanBerge-Henegouwen GP. Smooth muscle function and dysfunction in gallbladder disease. Curr Gastroenterol Rep 2004;6(2): 151–62.

91. Xiao ZL, Rho AK, Biancani P, et al. Effects of bile acids on the muscle functions of guinea pig gallbladder. Am J Physiol Gastrointest Liver Physiol 2002;283(1): G87–94.

92. Stolk MF, van de Heijning BJ, van Erpecum KJ, et al. Effect of bile salts on in vitro gallbladder motility: preliminary study. Ital J Gastroenterol Hepatol 1996;28: 105–10.

93. Xiao ZL, Biancani P, Carey MC, et al. Hydrophilic but not hydrophobic bile acids prevent gallbladder muscle dysfunction in acute cholecystitis. Hepatology 2003;37(6):1442–50.

94. Maurer KJ, Rao VP, Ge Z, et al. T-cell function is critical for murine cholesterol gallstone formation. Gastroenterology 2007;133(4):1304–15.

95. Pauletzki JG, Althaus R, Holl J, et al. Gallbladder emptying and gallstone formation: a prospective study on gallstone recurrence. Gastroenterology 1996;111: 765–71.

96. Portincasa P, van Erpecum KJ, van de Meeberg PC, et al. Apolipoprotein (Apo) E4 genotype and galbladder motility influence speed of gallstone clearance and risk of recurrence after extracorporeal shock-wave lithotripsy. Hepatology 1996;24:580–7.

97. Venneman NG, vanBerge-Henegouwen GP, Portincasa P, et al. Absence of apolipoprotein E4 genotype, good gallbladder motility and presence of solitary stones delay rather than prevent gallstone recurrence after extracorporeal shock wave lithotripsy. J Hepatol 2001;35(1):10–6.

98. Festi D, Frabboni R, Bazzoli F, et al. Gallbladder motility in cholesterol gallstone disease. Effect of ursodeoxycholic acid administration and gallstone dissolution. Gastroenterology 1990;99:1779–85.

99. Sackmann M, Eder H, Spengler U, et al. Gallbladder emptying is an important factor in fragment disappearance after shock wave lithotripsy. J Hepatol 1993; 17:62–6.

100. Leopold GR, Amberg J, Gosink BB, et al. Gray scale ultrasonic cholecystography: a comparison with conventional radiographic techniques. Radiology 1976; 121(2):445–8.

101. Portincasa P, Di Ciaula A, Palmieri VO, et al. Sonographic evaluation of gallstone burden in humans. Ital J Gastroenterol Hepatol 1994;26(3):141–4.

102. Everson GT, Braverman DZ, Johnson ML, et al. A critical evaluation of real-time ultrasonography for the study of gallbladder volume and contraction. Gastroenterology 1980;79:40–6.

103. Portincasa P, Moschetta A, Colecchia A, et al. Measurement of gallbladder motor function by ultrasonography: towards for standardization. (già Ital J Gastroenterol Hepatol). Dig Liver Dis 2003;35(Suppl 3):S56–61.

104. Portincasa P, Di Ciaula A, Baldassarre G, et al. Gallbladder motor function in gallstone patients: sonographic and *in vitro* studies on the role of gallstones, smooth muscle function and gallbladder wall inflammation. J Hepatol 1994;21: 430–40.

105. Portincasa P, Moschetta A, Di Ciaula A, et al. Pathophysiology of cholesterol gallstone disease. In: Borzellino G, Cordiano C, editors. Biliary lithiasis. Basic science, current diagnosis and management. Milano (Italy): Springer Italia S.r.l; 2008. p. 19–49.

106. Pereira SP, Veysey MJ, Kennedy C, et al. Gallstone dissolution with oral bile acid therapy. Importance of pretreatment CT scanning and reasons for nonresponse. Dig Dis Sci 1997;42(8):1775–82.

107. Pereira SP, Hussaini SH, Kennedy C, et al. Gallbladder stone recurrence after medical treatment. Do gallstones recur true to type? Dig Dis Sci 1995;40: 2568–75.

108. Senior JR, Johnson MF, DeTurck DM, et al. In vivo kinetics of radiolucent gallstone dissolution by oral dihydroxy bile acids. Gastroenterology 1990;99(1): 243–51.

109. Jazrawi RP, Pigozzi MG, Galatola G, et al. Optimum bile acid treatment for rapid gall stone dissolution. Gut 1992;33:381–6.

110. Paumgartner G. Therapeutic options and choice of appropriate treatment. Bile acids-cholestasis-gallstones. Advances in basic and clinical bile acid research. Dordrecht (The Netherlands): Kluwer Academic Publishers; 1996. p. 205–10.

111. Bateson MC, Bouchier IA, Trash DB, et al. Calcification of radiolucent gall stone during treatment with ursodeoxycholic acid. Br Med J (Clin Res Ed) 1981; 283(6292):645–6.

112. Bazzoli F, Festi D, Mazzella G, et al. Acquired gallstone opacification during cholelitholytic treatment with chenodeoxyholic, ursodeoxycholic, and tauroursodeoxycholic acids. Am J Gastroenterol 1995;90(6):978–81.

113. Lanzini A, Jazrawi RP, Kupfer RM, et al. Gallstone recurrence after medical dissolution. An overestimated threat? J Hepatol 1986;3:241–6.

114. Rabenstein T, Radespiel-Troger M, Hopfner L, et al. Ten years experience with piezoelectric extracorporeal shockwave lithotripsy of gallbladder stones. Eur J Gastroenterol Hepatol 2005;17(6):629–39.

115. Sackmann M, Ippisch E, Sauerbruch T, et al. Early gallstone recurrence rate after successful shock-wave therapy. Gastroenterology 1990;98:392–6.

116. Villanova N, Bazzoli F, Taroni F, et al. Gallstone recurrence after successful oral bile acid treatment: a 12 year follow-up study and evaluation of long term post-dissolution treatment. Gastroenterology 1989;97:726–31.

117. Petroni ML, Jazrawi RP, Pazzi P, et al. Risk factors for the development of gallstone recurrence following medical dissolution. The British-Italian Gallstone Study Group. Eur J Gastroenterol Hepatol 2000;12(6):695–700.

118. Petroni ML, Jazrawi RP, Lanzini A, et al. Repeated bile acid therapy for the long-term management of cholesterol gallstones. J Hepatol 1996;25:719–24.

119. O'Leary DP, Johnson AG. Future directions for conservative treatment of gallbladder calculi. Br J Surg 1993;80(2):143–7.

120. Gilat T, Konikoff F. Pregnancy and the biliary tract. Can J Gastroenterol 2000; 14(Suppl D):55D–9D.
121. Sugerman HJ, Brewer WH, Shiffman ML, et al. A multicenter, placebo-controlled, randomized, double-blind, prospective trial of prophylactic ursodiol for the prevention of gallstone formation following gastric-bypass-induced rapid weight loss. Am J Surg 1995;169(1):91–6.
122. Lammert F, Neubrand MW, Bittner R, et al. [S3-guidelines for diagnosis and treatment of gallstones. German Society for Digestive and Metabolic Diseases and German Society for Surgery of the Alimentary Tract]. Z Gastroenterol 2007;45(9):971–1001 [in German].
123. Portincasa P, Di Ciaula A, Wang HH, et al. Medicinal treatments of cholesterol gallstones: old, current and new perspectives. Curr Med Chem 2009;16(12):1531–42.
124. Istvan ES, Deisenhofer J. Structural mechanism for statin inhibition of HMG-CoA reductase. Science 2001;292(5519):1160–4.
125. Kallien G, Lange K, Stange EF, et al. The pravastatin-induced decrease of biliary cholesterol secretion is not directly related to an inhibition of cholesterol synthesis in humans. Hepatology 1999;30(1):14–20.
126. Duane WC, Hunninghake DB, Freeman ML, et al. Simvastatin, a competitive inhibitor of HMG-CoA reductase, lowers cholesterol saturation index of gallbladder bile. Hepatology 1988;8:1147–50.
127. Loria P, Bertolotti M, Cassinadri MT, et al. Short-term effects of simvastatin on bile acid synthesis and bile lipid secretion in human subjects. Hepatology 1994;19:882–8.
128. Hanson DS, Duane WC. Effects of lovastatin and chenodiol on bile acid synthesis, bile lipid composition, and biliary lipid secretion in healthy human subjects. J Lipid Res 1994;35(8):1462–8.
129. Saunders KD, Cates JA, Abedin MZ, et al. Lovastatin and gallstone dissolution: a preliminary study. Surgery 1993;113:28–35.
130. Smit JW, van Erpecum KJ, Renooij W, et al. The effects of the 3-hydroxy, 3-methylglutaryl coenzyme A reductase inhibitor pravastatin on bile composition and nucleation of cholesterol crystals in cholesterol gallstone disease. Hepatology 1995;21(6):1523–9.
131. Tazuma S, Hatsushika S, Aihara N, et al. Inhibitory effects of pravastatin, a competitive inhibitor of hydroxymethylglutaryl coenzyme A reductase, on cholesterol gallstone formation in prairie dogs. Digestion 1992;51:179–84.
132. Abedin MZ, Narins SC, Park EH, et al. Lovastatin alters biliary lipid composition and dissolves gallstones: a long-term study in prairie dogs. Dig Dis Sci 2002; 47(10):2192–210.
133. Davis KG, Wertin TM, Schriver JP. The use of simvastatin for the prevention of gallstones in the lithogenic prairie dog model. Obes Surg 2003;13(6):865–8.
134. Chapman BA, Burt MJ, Chisholm RJ, et al. Dissolution of gallstones with simvastatin, an HMG CoA reductase inhibitor. Dig Dis Sci 1998;43(2):349–53.
135. Porsch-Ozcurumez M, Hardt PD, Schnell-Kretschmer H, et al. Effects of fluvastatin on biliary lipids in subjects with an elevated cholesterol saturation index. Eur J Clin Pharmacol 2001;56(12):873–9.
136. Smith JL, Roach PD, Wittenberg LN, et al. Effects of simvastatin on hepatic cholesterol metabolism, bile lithogenicity and bile acid hydrophobicity in patients with gallstones. J Gastroenterol Hepatol 2000;15(8):871–9.
137. Wilson IR, Hurrell MA, Pattinson NR, et al. The effect of simvastatin and bezafibrate on bile composition and gall-bladder emptying in female non-insulin-dependent diabetics. J Gastroenterol Hepatol 1994;9(5):447–51.

138. Miettinen TE, Kiviluoto T, Taavitsainen M, et al. Cholesterol metabolism and serum and biliary noncholesterol sterols in gallstone patients during simvastatin and ursodeoxycholic acid treatments. Hepatology 1998;27(3):649–55.

139. Sharma BC, Agarwal DK, Baijal SS, et al. Pravastatin has no effect on bile lipid composition, nucleation time, and gallbladder motility in persons with normal levels of cholesterol. J Clin Gastroenterol 1997;25(2):433–6.

140. Caroli-Bosc FX, Le GP, Pugliese P, et al. Role of fibrates and HMG-CoA reductase inhibitors in gallstone formation: epidemiological study in an unselected population. Dig Dis Sci 2001;46(3):540–4.

141. Gonzalez-Perez A, Garcia-Rodriguez LA. Gallbladder disease in the general population: association with cardiovascular morbidity and therapy. Pharmacoepidemiol Drug Saf 2007;16(5):524–31.

142. Tsai CJ, Leitzmann MF, Willett WC, et al. Statin use and the risk of cholecystectomy in women. Gastroenterology 2009;136(5):1593–600.

143. Bodmer M, Brauchli YB, Krahenbuhl S, et al. Statin use and risk of gallstone disease followed by cholecystectomy. JAMA 2009;302(18):2001–7.

144. Wang DQ. Regulation of intestinal cholesterol absorption. Annu Rev Physiol 2007;69:221–48.

145. Davis HR Jr, Zhu LJ, Hoos LM, et al. Niemann-Pick C1 Like 1 (NPC1L1) is the intestinal phytosterol and cholesterol transporter and a key modulator of whole-body cholesterol homeostasis. J Biol Chem 2004;279(32):33586–92.

146. Altmann SW, Davis HR Jr, Zhu L, et al. Niemann-Pick C1 Like 1 protein is critical for intestinal cholesterol absorption. Science 2004;303:1201–4.

147. Davies JP, Scott C, Oishi K, et al. Inactivation of NPC1L1 causes multiple lipid transport defects and protects against diet-induced hypercholesterolemia. J Biol Chem 2005;280(13):12710–20.

148. Ge L, Wang J, Qi W, et al. The cholesterol absorption inhibitor ezetimibe acts by blocking the sterol-induced internalization of NPC1L1. Cell Metab 2008;7(6):508–19.

149. Valasek MA, Repa JJ, Quan G, et al. Inhibiting intestinal NPC1L1 activity prevents diet-induced increase in biliary cholesterol in Golden Syrian hamsters. Am J Physiol Gastrointest Liver Physiol 2008;(4):G813–22.

150. Davis HR, Veltri EP. Zetia: inhibition of Niemann-Pick C1 Like 1 (NPC1L1) to reduce intestinal cholesterol absorption and treat hyperlipidemia. J Atheroscler Thromb 2007;14(3):99–108.

151. Zuniga S, Molina H, Azocar L, et al. Ezetimibe prevents cholesterol gallstone formation in mice. Liver Int 2008;28(7):935–47.

152. Wang DQ, Tazuma S. Effect of beta-muricholic acid on the prevention and dissolution of cholesterol gallstones in C57L/J mice. J Lipid Res 2002;43(11):1960–8.

153. Mathur A, Walker JJ, Al-Azzawi HH, et al. Ezetimibe ameliorates cholecystosteatosis. Surgery 2007;142(2):228–33.

154. Mangelsdorf DJ, Thummel C, Beato M, et al. The nuclear receptor superfamily: the second decade. Cell 1995;83(6):835–9.

155. Janowski BA, Willy PJ, Devi TR, et al. An oxysterol signalling pathway mediated by the nuclear receptor LXR alpha. Nature 1996;383(6602):728–31.

156. Parks DJ, Blanchard SG, Bledsoe RK, et al. Bile acids: natural ligands for an orphan nuclear receptor. Science 1999;284(5418):1365–8.

157. Makishima M, Okamoto AY, Repa JJ, et al. Identification of a nuclear receptor for bile acids. Science 1999;284(5418):1362–5.

158. Repa JJ, Mangelsdorf DJ. The liver X receptor gene team: potential new players in atherosclerosis. Nat Med 2002;8(11):1243–8.

159. Kalaany NY, Mangelsdorf DJ. LXRS and FXR: the yin and yang of cholesterol and fat metabolism. Annu Rev Physiol 2006;68:159–91.
160. Modica S, Moschetta A. Nuclear bile acid receptor FXR as pharmacological target: are we there yet? FEBS Lett 2006;580(23):5492–9.
161. Moschetta A, Bookout AL, Mangelsdorf DJ. Prevention of cholesterol gallstone disease by FXR agonists in a mouse model. Nat Med 2004;10(12):1352–8.
162. Liu Y, Binz J, Numerick MJ, et al. Hepatoprotection by the farnesoid X receptor agonist GW4064 in rat models of intra- and extrahepatic cholestasis. J Clin Invest 2003;112(11):1678–87.
163. Uppal H, Zhai Y, Gangopadhyay A, et al. Activation of liver X receptor sensitizes mice to gallbladder cholesterol crystallization. Hepatology 2008;47(4):1331–42.
164. Keus F, de Jong JA, Gooszen HG, et al. Small-incision versus open cholecystectomy for patients with symptomatic cholecystolithiasis. Cochrane Database Syst Rev 2006;(4):CD004788.
165. Keus F, de Jong JA, Gooszen HG, et al. Laparoscopic versus open cholecystectomy for patients with symptomatic cholecystolithiasis. Cochrane Database Syst Rev 2006;(4):CD006231.
166. Keus F, de Jong JA, Gooszen HG, et al. Laparoscopic versus small-incision cholecystectomy for patients with symptomatic cholecystolithiasis. Cochrane Database Syst Rev 2006;(4):CD006229.
167. Pokorny WJ, Saleem M, O'Gorman RB, et al. Cholelithiasis and cholecystitis in childhood. Am J Surg 1984;148(6):742–4.
168. Amaral JF, Thompson WR. Gallbladder disease in the morbidly obese. Am J Surg 1985;149(4):551–7.
169. Sleisenger MH, Fordtran JS. Gastrointestinal disease: pathophysiology, diagnosis, management. 8th edition. Philadelphia: WB Saunders; 2006.
170. Lowenfels AB, Walker AM, Althaus DP, et al. Gallstone growth, size, and risk of gallbladder cancer: an interracial study. Int J Epidemiol 1989;18:50–4.
171. Randi G, Franceschi S, La Vecchia C. Gallbladder cancer worldwide: geographical distribution and risk factors. Int J Cancer 2006;118(7):1591–602.
172. Ashur H, Siegal B, Oland Y, et al. Calcified ballbladder (porcelain gallbladder). Arch Surg 1978;113(5):594–6.
173. Lowenfels AB, Lindstrom CG, Conway MJ, et al. Gallstones and risk of gallbladder cancer. J Natl Cancer Inst 1985;75(1):77–80.
174. Bonatsos G, Birbas K, Toutouzas K, et al. Laparoscopic cholecystectomy in adults with sickle cell disease. Surg Endosc 2001;15(8):816–9.
175. Wang DQH, Carey MC. Complete mapping of crystallization pathways during cholesterol precipitation from model bile: influence of physical-chemical variables of pathophysiologic relevance and identification of a stable liquid crystalline state in cold, dilute and hydrophilic bile salt-containing system. J Lipid Res 1996;37:606–30.

# Gallbladder Imaging

Richard M. Gore, MD[a,b,*], Kiran H. Thakrar, MD[a,b],
Geraldine M. Newmark, MD[a,b], Uday K. Mehta, MD[a,b],
Jonathan W. Berlin, MD[a,b]

**KEYWORDS**

- Computed tomography - Gallbladder - Ultrasonography
- Magnetic resonance imaging

Recent technical advances in ultrasonography, multidetector computed tomography (CT), magnetic resonance imaging (MRI), and scintigraphy have significantly improved the accuracy of the noninvasive imaging of benign and malignant gallbladder pathology.[1–4] Because of high diagnostic accuracy, wide availability, and ease of performance, ultrasonography and CT are the primary imaging tests for patients with suspected gallbladder and biliary tract pathology. MRI with magnetic resonance cholangiopancreatography (MRCP) is assuming an increasingly important role in the imaging armamentarium and has largely replaced diagnostic endoscopic retrograde cholangiopancreatography (ERCP).[5] Evaluation of acute cholecystitis using hepatobiliary scintigraphy has diminished over the past decade.[1] Positron emission tomographic (PET) imaging is being used with increased frequency to stage gallbladder neoplasms.[6] This article presents the imaging findings of common gallbladder diseases, and the role of each of the imaging modalities is placed in perspective for optimizing patient management.

## CHOLELITHIASIS

The nature and size of a gallstone affects its imaging characteristics. Gallstones are comprised mainly of cholesterol, bilirubin, and calcium salts, with smaller amounts of protein and other materials including bile acids, fatty acids, and inorganic salts. In Western countries, cholesterol is the principal constituent of more than 75% of gallstones, with smaller amounts of calcium bilirubinate.[7–9] Pure cholesterol stones contain more than 90% cholesterol and account for less than 10% of biliary calculi.[7–9] The more cholesterol and less calcium a stone contains, the less likely will it be seen on CT scan, which best depicts predominantly calcified stones. Black or brown pigment stones consist of calcium salts of bilirubin and contain less than 25% cholesterol. These stones compose only 10% to 25% of gallstones in North

[a] Department of Radiology, NorthShore University Health System, 2650 Ridge Avenue, Evanston, IL 60201, USA
[b] Department of Radiology, University of Chicago Pritzker School of Medicine, Evanston, IL, USA
* Corresponding author. Department of Radiology, NorthShore University Health System, 2650 Ridge Avenue, Evanston, IL 60201.
E-mail address: rgore@uchicago.edu

Gastroenterol Clin N Am 39 (2010) 265–287
doi:10.1016/j.gtc.2010.02.009
0889-8553/10/$ – see front matter © 2010 Elsevier Inc. All rights reserved.

gastro.theclinics.com

America. These stones show a less-dramatic duct shadow than cholesterol or more calcified stones, particularly when present in the bile duct.

## Plain Radiographic Findings

The abdominal plain radiograph is insensitive in depicting gallstones because only 15% to 20% are sufficiently calcified to be visualized.[10] Oral cholecystography was the mainstay of gallstone detection for more than 50 years but was replaced in the late 1970s by ultrasonography.

## Sonographic Findings

Ultrasonography is now the gold standard for the noninvasive diagnosis of cholelithasis.[11] This imaging test is highly accurate (>96%), can be performed at the patient's bedside, and does not require the use of ionizing radiation. Gallstones must fulfill 3 major sonographic criteria. They must (1) show an echogenic focus, (2) cast an acoustic shadow, and (3) seek gravitational dependence.[1–4] Gallstones are accurately diagnosed when a 5 mm or larger defect meets all 3 major criteria. Stones smaller than 2 to 3 mm may be difficult to visualize. Small stones, however, are usually multiple in occurrence, assisting their detection.[12–14]

Gallstones produce 3 patterns of shadowing. The first is a discrete shadow (**Fig. 1**A) emanating from a solitary stone. The second pattern is confluent shadowing because of multiple stones (see **Fig. 1**B) or gravel that abut each other in the gallbladder. The third pattern, the wall-echo-shadow (WES) complex (see **Fig. 1**C) occurs when a contracted gallbladder is completely filled with gallstones. These stones give an echogenic double arc appearance, which consists of 2 parallel arcuate hyperechoic lines separated by a thin hypoechoic space and distal acoustic shadowing. The more superficial hyperechoic arc represents reflections from gallstones, and the hypoechoic space in between represents either a small sliver of bile between the wall and the stones or a hypoechoic portion of the gallbladder wall. The WES sign must be differentiated from a partially collapsed duodenal bulb, porcelain gallbladder, emphysematous cholecystitis, xanthogranulomatous cholecystitis, and a calcified hepatic artery aneurysm.[15]

Gallstones characteristically produce "clean" shadowing without reverberation because most of the sound is absorbed by the stone. Bowel gas reflects 99% of the incident sound energy producing reverberations and backscatter echoes (dirty shadowing).[11] Reverberation artifacts may be seen posterior to calcified stones that contain gas within fissures.

## CT Findings

The CT appearance of gallstones is variable (**Fig. 2**), depending on their composition; pattern of calcification; and the presence of lamellation, fissuring, or gas.[15–17] Stones with high cholesterol content are difficult to visualize because they are isodense with the surrounding bile. Well-calcified stones are readily detected on CT scan. Stones that are denser than bile may be seen because of a rim or nidus of calcification. The CT attenuation of gallstones correlates more closely with the cholesterol content of the stones than with the calcium content. On CT scan, gallstones can be simulated by the enhancing mucosa of a contracted gallbladder wall or neck, which often folds on itself.[13]

## MRI Findings

On MRI, most gallstones (**Fig. 3**) produce little or no signal because of the restricted motion of water and cholesterol molecules in the crystalline lattice of the stone.

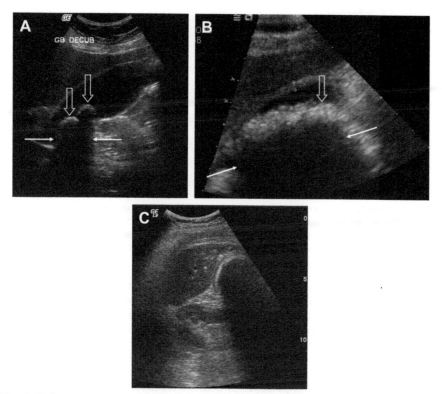

**Fig. 1.** Gallstones: sonographic findings. (*A*) Longitudinal sonogram shows 2 echogenic shadowing foci (*open arrows*) in the gallbladder, which cast clean acoustic shadows (*solid arrows*) distal to the stones. (*B*) Multiple small stones and gravel abut each other (*open arrow*) and cast a confluent acoustic shadow (*arrows*) on this longitudinal sonogram. There is mural thickening of the gallbladder (*calipers*) as well. (*C*) The wall-echo-shadow sign caused by shadowing emanating from a contracted gallbladder filled with stones.

Gallstones and bile duct stones are best seen on T2-weighted imaging sequences that produce bright bile. MRI is superior to CT in detecting small calculi because of the inherent contrast between low signal intensity stones and high signal intensity bile.[18–20]

## CHOLEDOCHOLITHIASIS

Choledocholithiasis is found in 7% to 20% of patients undergoing cholecystectomy and 2% to 4% of patients after cholecystectomy.[21–23] These stones are usually silent unless they obstruct the common bile duct (CBD). Small calculi may intermittently cause colicky pain as they obstruct at the ampulla of Vater but generally pass into the duodenum. Larger stones between 5 and 10 mm in size are difficult to pass and can result in intermittent long-term symptoms and sequelae such as cholangitis and sepsis.

The detection of bile duct stones is easiest in the setting of biliary dilatation. But biliary dilatation is present in only 66% to 75% of patients with bile duct stones, and depiction of the stones may be difficult.[21]

### Sonographic Findings

Bile duct stones appear as echogenic foci within the fluid-filled duct that may cast an acoustic shadow in a sonograph.[24] The stone may appear as an echogenic curved

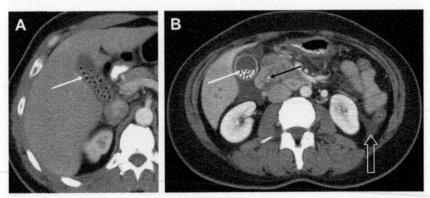

**Fig. 2.** Gallstones: CT findings. (*A*) Multiple gas-containing stones (*arrow*) with peripheral calcification are present within the gallbladder. (*B*) Multiple calcified stones (*white arrow*) are present within the gallbladder. There is a distal common bile duct stone (*black arrow*) causing pancreatitis and upper abdominal fluid collections (*open arrow*).

line; therefore, only the anterior margin is visualized. Stones may also appear with homogeneous echogenicity throughout the stone, with or without acoustic shadowing. Adjacent duodenal and colonic gas can make it difficult to image the distal CBD; therefore, sonography only has a sensitivity of 18% to 45% in the detection of CBD stones.[25,26]

### CT Findings

As with gallstones, the CT appearance of CBD stones is variable, depending on their composition and pattern of calcification.[27] High-attenuation stones can be easily seen with the duct lumen even in the absence of biliary dilatation. Only 20% of common bile stones have a homogeneously high density.[28] Other findings include a rim of high

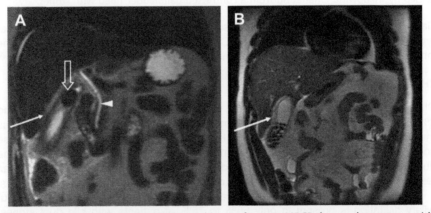

**Fig. 3.** Gallstones: MRI findings. (*A*) Coronal image from an MRCP shows a large stone with very low signal intensity (*open arrow*) lodged in the gallbladder neck causing acute cholecystitis associated with mural thickening of the gallbladder and high signal intensity pericholecystic fluid (*solid arrow*). Note the normal common bile duct (*arrowhead*). (*B*) Coronal T2-weighted, fat-suppressed image shows multiple small stones within the gallbladder and high signal intensity pericholecystic fluid (*arrow*) related to acute cholecystitis.

attenuation (which may be difficult to detect when impacted against the duct wall), soft tissue attenuation, and homogeneous near-water attenuation. Stones may rarely have sufficient pure cholesterol to appear in lower attenuation than surrounding bile. Multi-detector CT with coronal reformatted images has a sensitivity of 76% to 80% in the depiction of bile duct stones.[1]

### MRI Findings

On MRI, CBD stones appear as foci of low signal intensity surrounded by bright bile on T2-weighted sequences (**Fig. 4**). Stones as small as 2 mm can be depicted by this technique, which has an excellent sensitivity (81%–100%) and specificity (85%–99%).[18,21,29,30] MRCP is superior to CT and ultrasonography in selecting patients who may benefit from preoperative ERCP. MRCP is recommended in patients with gallstones and a moderate-to-high suspicion of CBD stones based on clinical, sonographic, and laboratory data.[31] MRCP can rule out CBD stones in up to 48% of patients with high preoperative probability of CBD stones.[32]

## GALLBLADDER SLUDGE

Gallbladder sludge is thick viscous bile that consists of cholesterol monohydrate crystals and calcium bilirubinate granules embedded in a gel matrix of mucus glycoproteins. It often develops in patients with prolonged fasting in intensive care units, trauma patients receiving total parenteral nutrition, and within 5 to 7 days of fasting in patients who have undergone gastrointestinal surgery. Sludge typically has a fluctuating course and may disappear and reappear over several months or years. Sludge may be an intermediate step in the formation of gallstones. Some 8% of patients with sludge will develop asymptomatic gallstones.[11,33]

Sludge produces low-amplitude, nonshadowing echoes that tend to layer in the most dependent portion of the gallbladder and moves slowly when the patient changes positions (**Fig. 5**). Aggregated sludge may appear as a mobile nonshadowing, echogenic, intraluminal mass (sludge ball) or as a nonshadowing polypoid mass (tumefactive sludge) in the dependent portion of the gallbladder. A gallbladder

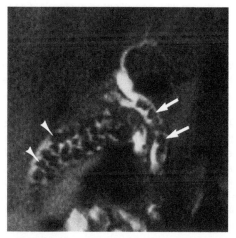

**Fig. 4.** Choledocholithiasis: MRI findings. Multiple common bile duct (*arrows*) and gallbladder (*arrowheads*) stones are seen on this coronal image from an MRCP examination. There is only mild biliary dilatation.

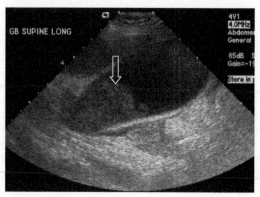

**Fig. 5.** Biliary sludge: sonographic findings. Sludge produces low-amplitude, nonshadowing echoes (*arrow*) that layer in the most dependent portion of the gallbladder.

completely filled with sludge may be isoechoic with the adjacent liver and difficult to identify, hence called hepatization of the gallbladder. Sludge is also different in appearance from gravel and multiple small stones in that sludge is echogenic but does not cast an acoustic shadow. In addition, sludge is more viscous and does not seek gravitational dependence as rapidly as gravel.[1,11]

## ACUTE CHOLECYSTITIS

Acute cholecystitis results from obstruction of the gallbladder neck or cystic duct by a gallstone in 80% to 95% of patients.[34] Acute acalculous cholecystitis (AAC) composes 5% to 15% of cases of acute cholecystitis and is typically caused by diminished gallbladder emptying (eg, in patients with severe trauma/surgery, burns, shock, anesthesia, diabetes); by decreased blood flow in the cystic artery because of obstruction, hypotension, or embolization; or by bacterial infection.[35,36] Although most patients present with typical right upper quadrant symptoms, this diagnosis may be challenging in patients with complicated systemic disease and sepsis.

Patients with suspected cholecystitis should be imaged for 2 major reasons. First, most patients (60%–85%) referred to exclude cholecystitis have other causes of right upper quadrant pain, including peptic ulcer disease, pancreatitis, hepatitis, appendicitis, hepatic congestion from right-sided heart failure, perihepatitis from pelvic inflammatory disease (Fitz-Hugh-Curtis syndrome), right lower lobe pneumonia, right-sided pyelonephritis, or nephroureterolithiasis. If the patient does not have acute cholecystitis, the clinical workup can be redirected before the patient's clinical condition deteriorates. Secondly, imaging can diagnose severe complications such as emphysematous cholecystitis and perforation, which require immediate surgery.[37]

Patients with suspected acute cholecystitis should be evaluated with ultrasonography as the initial imaging procedure. If the diagnosis is in doubt, it can be confirmed with hepatobiliary scintigraphy or CT. Multidetector CT is often initially performed in many cases because the diagnosis is unclear. CT is also helpful in suspected complications of acute cholecystitis, such as emphysematous cholecystitis or gallbladder perforation. MRI is usually used to exclude obstructing and nonobstructing biliary tract stones.

The morphologic changes that occur in acute cholecystitis are well depicted in imaging studies and result from the presence of stones, increased mural blood flow, and capillary leakage caused by inflammatory changes, mural thickening of the gall-bladder, and pericholecystic fluid.

### Sonographic Findings

The sonographic findings of acute uncomplicated cholecystitis include gallstones often impacted in the cystic duct or gallbladder neck (**Fig. 6**), mural thickening (>3 mm), a 3-layered appearance of the gallbladder wall, hazy delineation of the gall-bladder, localized pain with maximal tenderness elicited over the gallbladder (sono-graphic Murphy's sign), pericholecystic fluid, and gallbladder distension.[38,39] Gallstones and the sonographic Murphy's sign are the most specific indicators of acute cholecystitis with a positive predictive value of 92%.[38,39] The sonographic Murphy's sign may be difficult to elicit in obtunded patients and those who have received pain medication. The sign may be absent in patients with gangrenous chole-cystitis. Finding an impacted stone in the cystic duct or gallbladder neck also increases the likelihood of acute cholecystitis.[38–42]

### Multidetector CT Findings

The CT findings (**Fig. 7**) of acute cholecystitis have been well described and include gallstones, mural thickening of the gallbladder, mural edema, pericholecystic fluid and inflammation, and transient increased enhancement of the liver parenchyma adja-cent to the gallbladder caused by hyperemia.[1,2,4,17] CT is less sensitive (75%) than ultrasonography in the depiction of gallstones. Stones with significant calcification or the presence of gas in a noncalcified stone (the Mercedes-Benz sign) are best seen with CT.[17] The CT findings of acute cholecystitis have been divided into major and minor criteria. Major findings include calculi, mural thickening of the gallbladder, pericholecystic fluid, and subserosal edema. Minor findings are gallbladder distension and sludge. The overall sensitivity, specificity, and accuracy of CT for the diagnosis of acute cholecystitis are 91.7%, 99.1%, and 94.3%, respectively.[41–45]

### MRI Findings

MRI (**Fig. 8**) rivals ultrasonography and CT in the depiction of acute cholecystitis. On postgadolinium T1-weighted images, acute cholecystitis manifests as increased mural enhancement, mural thickening, and transient increased enhancement of the adjacent liver parenchyma. Findings on T2-weighted images include the presence of gallstones, the presence of an intramural abscess appearing as a hyperintense

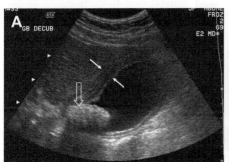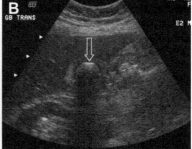

**Fig. 6.** Acute cholecystitis: sonographic findings. Longitudinal (*A*) and transverse (*B*) sono-grams show a large obstructing stone (*open arrow*) within the gallbladder neck associated with a thick, hypoechoic gallbladder wall (*arrows*). The patient also had a sonographic Murphy sign.

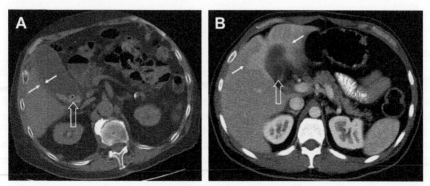

**Fig. 7.** Acute cholecystitis: CT findings. (*A*) Multiple calcified stones (*open arrow*) are seen in the dependent portion of the gallbladder. Mural thickening (*solid arrows*) of the gall-bladder is also present. (*B*) In a different patient, the inflamed gallbladder (*open arrow*) is causing hyperenhancement of the adjacent liver (*solid arrows*).

focus in the gallbladder wall, and increased wall thickness. Periportal edema depicted as periportal high signal intensity may be observed but is a nonspecific finding.[46–48]

### Hepatobiliary Scintigraphy

Radionuclide cholescintigraphy with technetium Tc 99m-labelled iminodiacetic acid analogs (hepatobiliary iminodiacetic acid scan) was first introduced in the late 1970s. In this study, hepatic parenchymal uptake is observed within 1 minute, with peak activity occurring at 10 to 15 minutes. The bile ducts are usually visualized within 10 minutes, and the gallbladder should fill with isotope within 1 hour if the cystic duct is patent. If the gallbladder is not identified, delayed imaging up to 4 hours should be performed.[1–3] Prompt biliary excretion of the isotope without visualization of the gall-bladder is the hallmark of acute cholecystitis (**Fig. 9**).

False-positive results may occur in patients with abnormal bile flow because of hepatic parenchymal disease or a prolonged fast with a distended, sludge-filled gall-bladder. Delayed gallbladder filling can be seen in the setting of chronic cholecystitis.[1]

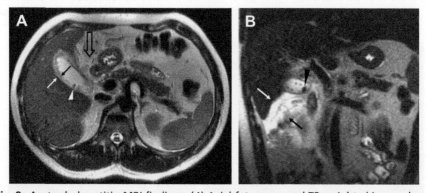

**Fig. 8.** Acute cholecystitis: MRI findings. (*A*) Axial fat-suppressed T2-weighted image shows a gallstone (*arrowhead*), mural thickening (*solid arrows*) of the gallbladder and high signal intensity pericholecystic fluid (*open arrow*). (*B*) Coronal MRCP image shows gallstones (*arrowhead*) and a large amount of subhepatic, pericholecystic fluid (*open arrows*) in a more severe case of acute cholecystitis.

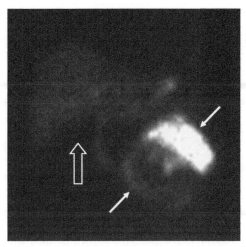

**Fig. 9.** Acute cholecystitis: hepatobiliary scintigraphy findings. A 60-minute image from a heptobiliary scintiscan shows isotope in the duodenum and small bowel (*solid arrows*) but none in the gallbladder (*open arrow*).

## ACUTE ACALCULOUS CHOLECYSTITIS

Acute gallbladder inflammation in the absence of stones, AAC, is seen in 2% to 15% of patients undergoing cholecystectomy and accounts for 47% of cases of postoperative cholecystitis and 50% of children with acute cholecystitis. It is difficult to make the diagnosis of AAC clinically and on imaging.[49]

AAC has a mortality rate approaching 60% and should be considered in every postoperative, posttraumatic, or coronary care patient with sepsis.[50] AAC typically results from a gradual increase of bile viscosity because of prolonged stasis that leads to functional obstruction of the cystic duct. Mural necrosis occurs in 60% of cases, and gangrene and perforation are common.[1,51]

Sonographic findings of AAC include gallbladder distention and sludge, with more specific signs of mural thickening, hypoechoic regions within the wall (**Fig. 10**A), pericholecystic fluid, diffuse increased echogenicity within the gallbladder resulting from hemorrhage, pus, intraluminal membranes, and a positive sonographic Murphy's sign.[11]

CT demonstrates inhomogeneous mural thickening (see **Fig. 10**B), perihepatitis, pericholecystic inflammation, and increased attenuation within the gallbladder lumen.

Diagnostic percutaneous aspiration of intraluminal bile under sonographic guidance confirms the diagnosis. Percutaneous cholecystectomy can help temporize the critically ill patient with AAC.[52]

## COMPLICATIONS OF ACUTE CHOLECYSTITIS
### Empyema

Suppurative cholecystitis (empyema) develops when pus fills the distended and inflamed gallbladder. The complication usually develops in diabetic patients and may behave like an intraabdominal abscess with rapid progression of symptoms. On ultrasonography, pus within the gallbladder resembles sludge. On CT scan, the attenuation of the intraluminal pus is high (>30 HU). The diagnosis can be established by sonographically guided percutaneous needle aspiration of the gallbladder.[2–4]

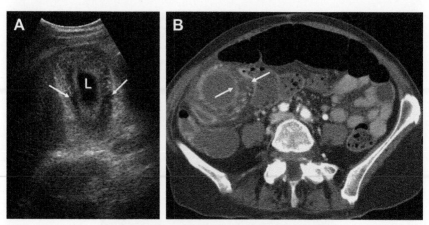

**Fig. 10.** Acute acalculous cholecystitis: imaging features. (*A*) Sonogram shows marked mural thickening of the gallbladder with hypoechoic regions (*arrows*) within the wall. L, gallbladder lumen. (*B*) CT in a different patient shows marked mural thickening (*arrows*) of the gallbladder with hypo- and hyperenhancing areas. Both patients were in the intensive care unit.

### Gangrenous Cholecystitis

Gangrenous cholecystitis is associated with significantly increased morbidity and mortality and usually requires emergent surgery. This complication is characterized by intramural hemorrhage, mucosal ulcers, and intraluminal purulent debris, hemorrhage, and strands of fibrinous exudates.[2–4]

There are several sonographic findings that suggest the diagnosis of gangrenous cholecystitis in the appropriate clinical setting: intraluminal membranes (**Fig. 11**A) relating to strands of fibrinous exudates and desquamated mucosa causing coarse, nonlayering intraluminal echoes. In addition, there may be marked asymmetry of the thickened gallbladder wall because of the presence of intramural hemorrhage or microabscess formation. Complex pericholecystic fluid collections containing debris are usually the result of microperforations of the gallbladder.[53,54]

CT scan may demonstrate intraluminal membranes, mural necrosis, intramural or intraluminal hemorrhage or gas, pericholecystic abscess (see **Fig. 11**B), and irregular or absent gallbladder wall enhancement during contrast-enhanced CT.[55–60]

### Emphysematous Cholecystitis

Emphysematous cholecystitis develops in fewer than 1% of cases of acute cholecystitis and is more common in men and in patients with diabetes and splanchnic ischemia.[61] This rapidly progressive and often fatal disease is characterized by the presence of gas within the wall or lumen of the gallbladder. *Clostridium perfringens*, *Clostridium welchii*, *Escherichia coli*, and *Klebsiella* are the most common gas-forming bacteria that cause this disease. Patients with emphysematous cholecystitis have a fivefold increased risk of perforation.[61]

The CT (**Fig. 12**A) and MRI diagnosis of emphysematous cholecystitis is fairly straightforward if intraluminal or intramural air is present. The diagnosis may be more difficult to establish sonographically. Intraluminal gas produces hyperechoic reflectors in the nondependent portion of the gallbladder (see **Fig. 12**B), with "dirty" acoustic shadowing that contains "comet tail" or "ring-down" artifacts. These

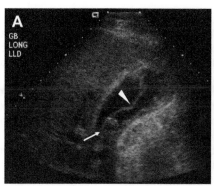
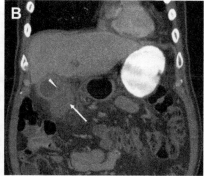

**Fig. 11.** Gangrenous cholecystitis: imaging features. (*A*) Longitudinal sonogram shows membranes (*arrowhead*) and a shadowing stone (*arrow*) within the gallbladder lumen. (*B*) Coronal reformatted CT image shows marked mural thickening of the gallbladder, an intraluminal membrane (*arrowhead*), and pericholecystic inflammatory change extending to the hepatic flexure of the colon (*arrow*).

artifacts must be differentiated from the WES sign of a contracted gallbladder filled with stones. Intramural gas manifests as a hyperechoic ring around the fluid-filled gallbladder. These features must be differentiated from shadowing that is secondary to a porcelain gallbladder or comet-tail artifacts that are due to cholesterol deposits within Rokitansky-Aschoff sinuses (RASs).[62–66]

### Gallbladder Perforation

Some 5% to 10% of patients with acute cholecystitis develop gallbladder perforation.[67] It occurs most commonly in the setting of gangrenous cholecystitis with other risk factors including gallstones, impaired vascular supply, infection, malignancy, and steroid use. The fundus of the gallbladder is the most common site of perforation because it has the most tenuous blood supply.[68,69]

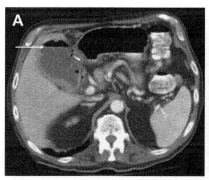
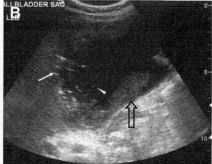

**Fig. 12.** Emphysematous cholecystitis: imaging features. (*A*) Longitudinal sonogram shows intramural (*solid arrows*) and intraluminal (*arrowhead*) gas bubbles as well as debris (*open arrow*) within this necrotic gallbladder. (*B*) CT scan in the same patient shows intraluminal (*solid arrow*) and intramural (*arrowhead*) gas, as well as mural thickening of the gallbladder.

### Hemorrhagic Cholecystitis

This rare complication of acute cholecystitis results from hemorrhage secondary to mucosal ulceration and necrosis and has been reported in the presence and absence of gallstones. Atherosclerosis of the gallbladder wall is a major predisposing factor. Classically the patient presents with biliary colic, jaundice, and melena.[2–4]

On sonography, intraluminal blood appears as echogenic material with a higher echogenicity than sludge, which may form a dependent layer; however, blood clots may appear as clumps or masses adherent to the gallbladder wall. With evolving hemorrhage this may have a cystic appearance.[70–73]

On CT scan there is hyperdensity of the bile in addition to the other findings of acute cholecystitis. A fluid-fluid level may develop and if perforation occurs, hemoperitoneum may result. Prompt diagnosis is essential because hemorrhagic cholecystitis is associated with a high mortality rate.[70,74–76]

## CHRONIC CHOLECYSTITIS

Gallbladders that are subjected to repeated bouts of acute cholecystitis are at risk for developing chronic cholecystitis. Chronic cholecystitis is several times more common pathologically in cholecystectomy specimens than in acute cholecystitis, and both conditions are often present simultaneously. Many cases that are pathologically diagnosed as "chronic cholecystitis" have the imaging diagnosis of "acute cholecystitis" because the findings on cross-sectional imaging may be identical. Also, from a clinical standpoint it may be difficult at times to distinguish the pain caused by physiologic contraction of a chronically inflamed gallbladder from that associated with an attack of acute cholecystitis. This distinction is made easier if the patient presents with fever, leukocytosis, and imaging findings suggesting acute inflammation and cystic duct obstruction.[71,72]

Chronic acalculous cholecystitis represents fewer than 5% of all cases of chronic cholecystitis. It may be caused by biliary stasis, bile duct abnormalities, recent stone passage, or chronic diseases such as diabetes and connective tissue and collagen vascular disease. Patients present with symptoms of intermittent biliary colic but without stones. The diagnosis is often one of exclusion.

CT, ultrasonography, and MRI typically show nonspecific mural thickening of the gallbladder.[3,73] There is increasing evidence to suggest that cholecystokinin (CCK)-enhanced hepatobiliary scintigraphy can predict which patients with chronic acalculous cholecystitis or biliary dyskinesia will obtain symptomatic relief from surgery. After the gallbladder fills with the isotope, CCK is administered and the gallbladder ejection fraction is calculated. A post-CCK ejection fraction of less than 30% to 40% may indicate chronic cholecystitis. Although CCK-enhanced cholescintigraphy is an improvement on historically difficult, ambiguous, and suboptimal imaging diagnosis, many surgeons, are unwilling to perform cholecystectomy based solely on a reduced ejection fraction.[73,77,78]

### Milk of Calcium Bile

Milk of calcium bile or limey bile is an uncommon disorder characterized by puttylike, thickened bile composed of calcium carbonate. It is usually associated with cystic duct obstruction and chronic cholecystitis.[10]

Sonographically, milk of calcium bile demonstrates echogenic layering material with a flat or convex meniscus usually associated with acoustic shadowing. Occasionally a weak reverberation artifact may be produced. CT and plain radiographs show high-attenuation material layering within the gallbladder lumen.

### Porcelain Gallbladder

In this uncommon disorder, chronic cholecystitis produces mural calcification of the gallbladder. The term derives from the brittle consistency of the gallbladder. Porcelain gallbladder, seen in 0.06% to 0.8% of cholecystectomy specimens, presents with 2 types of histologic calcification: (1) a broad continuous band of calcification of the muscularis and (2) multiple punctuate calcifications scattered through the mucosa and submucosa.[2,3,11] The entire wall or only part of the wall of the gallbladder may be calcified. Porcelain gallbladder is 5 times more frequent in men than in women, with a mean age of 54 years at presentation. Patients often have few symptoms, and the diagnosis is often made by detecting a palpable right upper quadrant mass or finding typical calcifications on plain radiographs. Prophylactic cholecystectomy is advocated in these patients, even in the paucity of symptoms, because of the strikingly high incidence (11%–33%) of carcinoma of the gallbladder.[2,3,11]

Sonographically, porcelain gallbladder presents with 3 patterns of mural calcification: (1) a hyperechoic linear or semilunar structure with acoustic shadowing; (2) an irregular clump of echoes with acoustic shadowing; or (3) a biconvex, curvilinear hyperechoic structure with variable acoustic shadowing.[11]

CT depicts the mural calcification and may directly visualize an associated carcinoma. The CT appearance of porcelain gallbladder can be simulated by a contracted gallbladder containing a large stone with a calcified rim and a bile attenuation center or by lipoidal deposition caused by transarterial chemoembolization of hepatic tumors.[2,3]

### Gallstone Ileus

Gallstone ileus occurs in the setting of chronic cholecystitis and results from erosion of a gallstone into the gastrointestinal tract, with subsequent development of bowel obstruction. The patient usually has symptoms of only chronic colic without evidence of acute cholecystitis before the obstruction. The stone, which needs to be larger than 2 cm to cause obstruction, typically erodes into the duodenum and may get lodged at narrow portions of the gut, such as the duodenum, ligament of Treitz, ileocecal valve, sigmoid colon, or any area of stricture.[2,3]

Radiographically, gallstone ileus manifests as gas in the biliary tract, intestinal obstruction, and the presence of a radiopaque gallstone (**Fig. 13**) surrounded by fluid or gas in the obstructed bowel.[11]

## GALLBLADDER ADENOMYOMATOSIS

Adenomyomatosis is a relatively common acquired, hyperplastic lesion of the gallbladder characterized by excessive proliferation of surface epithelium, with invaginations into the thickened, hypertrophied muscularis propria. The intramural diverticula formed by these invaginations are referred to as RASs and are a prominent feature of this disorder. This disorder, which is found in up to 8% of patients undergoing cholecystectomy, has been postulated to result from mechanical obstruction of the gallbladder (from stones, cystic duct kinking, or congenital septum), chronic inflammation, and anomalous pancreaticobiliary ductal union.[79–82]

The association of this disorder with clinical findings is controversial. More than 90% of cases are associated with gallstones, which may be responsible for biliary symptoms. There is also a higher frequency of gallbladder carcinoma in gallbladders with segmental adenomyomatosis than in those without segmental adenomyomatosis.[81]

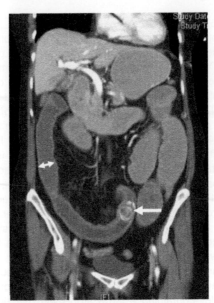

**Fig. 13.** Gallstone ileus: CT findings. Coronal reformatted CT image shows a calcified gallstone (*arrow*) within the lumen of the distal ileum causing obstruction and fluid-filled dilatation (*double headed arrow*) of the proximal small bowel.

Adenomyomatosis may be generalized, segmental, or focal, the last being most common. Diffuse adenomyomatosis causes thickening and irregularity of the musosal and muscular layers with associated RASs. In the segmental or annular form, a circumferential stricture divides the gallbladder lumen into separate chambers. The focal form causes a focal mass or nodule, usually in the fundus, which is called an adenomyoma.[79–82]

### Sonographic Findings

The sonographic findings in adenomyomatosis include diffuse or segmental thickening of the gallbladder wall and anechoic intramural diverticula. A V-shaped reverberation or comet-tail artifact (**Fig. 14**A) may emanate from small cholesterol crystals or stones that are lodged in the RASs. This artifact occurs as a result of sound reverberating in or between cholesterol crystals and is useful in differentiating mural thickening related to adenomyomatosis from other abnormalities. If the diverticula and their associated artifacts are not present, nonspecific mural thickening indistinguishable from acute or chronic cholecystitis and gallbladder carcinoma may be present.[83]

The segmental form of adenomyomatosis results in annular narrowing, usually of the gallbladder body, with segmentation of the gallbladder lumen. Stones are often trapped in the fundal compartment. If stones and reverberation artifact are not seen, this focal mural thickening can simulate carcinoma.[79–82]

The focal form of adenomyomatosis most commonly presents as a sessile, polypoid mass in the fundus, protruding into the gallbladder lumen.[79–82]

### CT Findings

On CT, adenomyomatosis may be difficult to diagnose because the RASs are often small and can be overlooked. The segmental and focal forms can be particularly

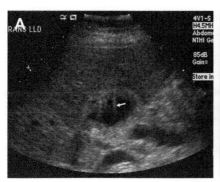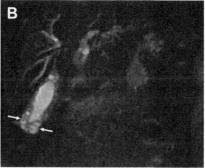

**Fig. 14.** Adenomyomatosis of the gallbladder: imaging features. (*A*) Transverse right upper quadrant sonogram shows a thick gallbladder wall and echogenic intramural foci that produce "ring-down" reverberation artifacts (*arrow*). These foci are caused by the cholesterol crystals within RASs. (*B*) Coronal MRCP image shows multiple high signal intensity structures (*arrows*) within the gallbladder wall, which represent the RASs. This produces a so-called string of pearls appearance.

difficult to differentiate from carcinoma because they appear as focal mural thickening or as a fundal mass. Ultrasonography has the advantage of being able to show the ring-down artifact related to the RASs.[2,3]

### MRI Findings

Because MRI offers more complete visualization of the gallbladder and more definitive identification of RASs, MRI has become the primary imaging examination in patients with known or suspected gallbladder adenomyomatosis. The RASs appear as small intramural foci of low signal intensity on T1-weighted images and of high signal intensity on T2-weighted images. The RASs imaged longitudinally can produce a so-called string of pearls appearance (see **Fig 14**B), a sign that is 92% specific for adenomyomatosis. In one study, MRI was more accurate than CT or ultrasonography (93%, 75%, 66%, respectively) in establishing this diagnosis.[72]

### GALLBLADDER CARCINOMA

Cross-sectional imaging is needed to expedite the diagnosis and appropriate treatment of patients with gallbladder malignancies, who often present with nonspecific symptoms of right upper quadrant pain, jaundice, and weight loss.[2,3,84–86]

Initial assessment of patients with right upper quadrant pain should include examination by ultrasonography. The diagnostic accuracy of ultrasonography is more than 80%, but it has limitations in the diagnosis of involved lymph nodes and the staging of disease.[72,86] Endoscopic ultrasonography demonstrates a diagnostic value for predicting the depth of tumor involvement and for differential diagnosis of polypoid lesions.

CT is superior to ultrasonography in assessing lymphadenopathy and spread of the disease into liver, porta hepatis, or adjacent structures, and is valuable in being able to predict which patients may benefit from surgical therapy.[72,84–86] Although MRI is not typically used as a primary imaging modality for the gallbladder, it may be useful in cases of focal or diffuse mural thickening to distinguish gallbladder cancer from adenomyomatosis and chronic cholecystitis. In addition, MRCP can provide more detailed information regarding biliary involvement of the tumor than ultrasonography or CT.[2,72,86,87]

Although direct cholangiography, such as ERCP or percutaneous transhepatic cholangiography, is of little value in detecting the presence of gallbladder carcinoma, it is helpful in planning the surgical approach because they can show tumor growth in adjacent intrahepatic ducts or in the CBD. The cholangiographic differential diagnosis includes cholangiocarcinoma, metastases, Mirizzi syndrome, and pancreatic carcinoma.

Gallbladder carcinomas have 3 major patterns of presentation histologically and on cross-sectional imaging: (1) focal or diffuse thickening and/or irregularity of the gallbladder wall, (2) polypoid mass originating in the gallbladder wall and projecting into the lumen, and (3) most commonly, a mass obscuring or replacing the gallbladder, often invading adjacent liver.[2,86]

### Carcinoma Manifesting as Mural Thickening

Focal or diffuse thickening of the gallbladder wall is the least common presentation of gallbladder carcinoma and is the most difficult to diagnose, particularly in the early stages. Gallbladder carcinoma may cause mild to marked mural thickening in a focal or diffuse pattern. This thickening is best appreciated on sonography, in which the gallbladder wall is normally 3 mm or less in thickness. Carcinomas confined to the gallbladder mucosa may present as flat or slightly raised lesions with mucosal irregularity that are difficult to appreciate sonographically. In one sonographic series, half the patients with these early carcinomas had no protruding lesions, and fewer than one-third were identified preoperatively.[88] More advanced gallbladder carcinomas can cause marked mural thickening, often with irregular and mixed echogenicity (**Fig. 15**A, B). The gallbladder may be contracted, normal sized, or distended, and gallstones are usually present.[2,3,86]

Two factors interfere with the sonographic recognition of carcinoma as the cause of gallbladder wall thickening: (1) Changes of early gallbladder carcinoma may be only subtle mucosal irregularity or mural thickening. (2) Gallbladder wall thickening is a nonspecific finding that can also be caused by acute or chronic cholecystitis; hyperalimentation; portal hypertension; adenomyomatosis; inadequate gallbladder distention; hypoalbuminemia; hepatitis; or hepatic, cardiac, or renal failure. Sometimes the echo architecture of the wall can help narrow the differential diagnosis.[2,3,11,86] Although CT is inferior to ultrasonography in evaluating the gallbladder wall for mucosal irregularity, mural thickening, and cholelithiasis, it is superior in evaluating the thickness of portions of the gallbladder wall that are obscured by interposed gallstones or mural calcifications on ultrasonograph. On CT scans, focal malignant wall thickening (**Fig. 16**C) usually enhances after administration of intravenous contrast material. When focal or irregular thickening of the gallbladder wall is encountered on CT scans, the images should be carefully inspected for bile duct dilatation, local invasion, metastasis, or adenopathy.[87,89]

### Carcinoma Manifesting as a Polypoid Mass

About one-fourth of gallbladder carcinomas manifest as a polypoid mass projecting into the gallbladder lumen.[3] Identification of these neoplasms is particularly important because they are well differentiated and are more likely to be confined to the gallbladder mucosa or muscularis when discovered.

On sonography, polypoid carcinomas usually have a homogeneous tissue texture, are fixed to the gallbladder wall at their base, and do not cast an acoustic shadow. Most carcinomas are broad based with smooth borders, although occasional tumors have a narrow stalk or villous fronds. The polyp may be hyperechoic, hypoechoic, or

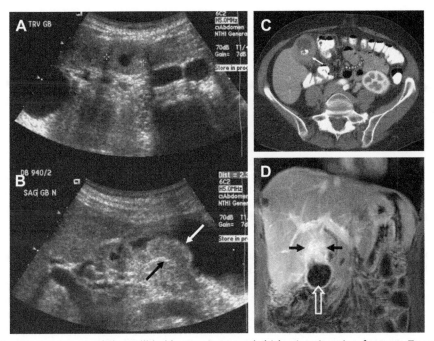

**Fig. 15.** Carcinoma of the gallbladder causing mural thickening: imaging features. Transverse (*A*) and longitudinal (*B*) sonograms show marked mural thickening of the neck of the gallbladder (*calipers and arrow*). (*C*) CT shows irregular mural thickening (*arrows*) of the gallbladder associated with multiple calcified stones. (*D*) Coronal contrast-enhanced MRI shows mural thickening and hyperenhancement (*solid arrows*) caused by cancer of the neck of the gallbladder. Open arrow indicates a large gallstone in the gallbladder fundus producing virtually no MR signal.

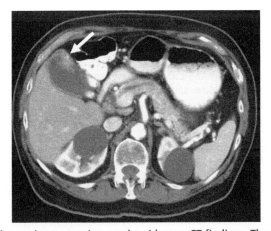

**Fig. 16.** Gallbladder carcinoma causing a polypoid mass: CT findings. There is an enhancing mass (*arrow*) present along the anterior aspect of the gallbladder lumen.

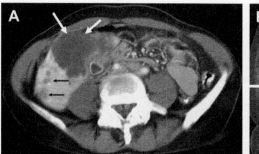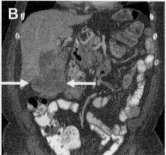

**Fig. 17.** Gallbladder carcinoma presenting as a gallbladder fossa mass: CT findings. (*A*) Axial CT scan shows a carcinoma of the gallbladder directly invading the liver (*white arrows*) and causing hematogenous metastases (*black arrows*). (*B*) Coronal reformatted CT scan in a different patient shows a mass occupying the gallbladder fossa (*arrows*).

isoechoic relative to the liver. Gallstones are usually present, and the gallbladder is either normal sized or expanded by the mass.[2,3,11]

A small polypoid carcinoma can be indistinguishable from a cholesterol polyp, adenoma, or adherent stone. Most benign polyps are small, measuring less than 1 cm. If a gallbladder polyp is larger than 1 cm in diameter and is not clearly benign, cholecystectomy should be considered. Tumefactive sludge or blood clot can simulate a polypoid carcinoma. Positional maneuvers usually differentiate these entities; clots and sludge move, albeit slowly, whereas cancers do not.[2,3,11]

When polypoid carcinomas are sufficiently large, they manifest as soft tissue masses that are denser than surrounding bile on CT scans (see **Fig. 16**). The polypoid cancer usually enhances homogeneously after administration of contrast medium, and the adjacent gallbladder wall may be thickened. Necrosis or calcification is uncommon.[90,91]

### Carcinoma Manifesting as a Gallbladder Fossa Mass

A large mass obscuring or replacing the gallbladder is the most common (42%–70%) presentation of gallbladder carcinoma. Sonographically the mass is often complex, with regions of necrosis, and small amounts of pericholecystic fluid are often present. Gallstones are commonly seen within the ill-defined mass, which typically invades hepatic parenchyma.[92,93]

On CT scans, infiltrating carcinomas that replace the gallbladder often show irregular contrast enhancement with scattered regions of internal necrosis (**Fig. 17**). Unless the associated gallstones are densely calcified, they may be difficult to identify. Invasion of the liver or hepatoduodenal ligament, satellite lesions, hepatic or nodal metastases, and bile duct dilatation are also common.

MRI findings in gallbladder carcinoma are similar to those reported with CT. MRI demonstrates prolongation of the T1 and T2 relaxation time in gallbladder carcinoma and is therefore heterogeneously hyperintense on T2-weighted images and hypointense on T1-weighted images compared with liver parenchyma. Ill-defined early enhancement is a typical appearance of gallbladder carcinoma in dynamic gadolinium-enhanced MRI. Combining MRI and MRCP offers the potential of evaluating parenchymal, vascular, biliary, and nodal involvement with a single noninvasive examination. Based on MRI alone, however, it may be difficult to distinguish carcinoma of the gallbladder from inflammatory and metastatic disease.[88,94]

## REFERENCES

1. Turner MA, Fulcher AC. Gallbladder and biliary tract: normal anatomy and examination techniques. In: Gore RM, Levine MS, editors. Textbook of gastrointestinal radiology. 3rd edition. Philadelphia (PA): W.B. Saunders; 2008. p. 1333–56.
2. Gore RM, Yaghmai V, Newmark GM, et al. Imaging benign and malignant disease of the gallbladder. Radiol Clin North Am 2002;40:1307–27.
3. Bennett GL. Cholelithiasis, cholecystitis, choledocholithiasis, and hyperplastic cholecystoses. In: Gore RM, Levine MS, editors. Textbook of gastrointestinal radiology. 3rd edition. Philadelphia (PA): W.B. Saunders; 2008. p. 1411–57.
4. Bennett GL, Balthazar EJ. Ultrasound and CT evaluation of emergent gallbladder pathology. Radiol Clin North Am 2003;41:1203–16.
5. Shanmugam V, Beattie GC, Yule SR, et al. Is magnetic resonance cholangio-pancreatography the new gold standard in biliary imaging? Br J Radiol 2005;78:888–93.
6. Ramos-Font C, Santiago Chinchilla A, Rodríguez-Fernández A, et al. Gallbladder cancer staging with 18F-FDG PET-CT. Rev Esp Med Nucl 2009;28:74–7.
7. Chan WC, Joe BN, Coakley FV, et al. Gallstone detection at CT in vitro: effect of peak voltage setting. Radiology 2006;241:546–53.
8. Stewart L, Griffiss JM, Way LW. Spectrum of gallstone disease in the veterans population. Am J Surg 2005;190:746–51.
9. Brackel K, LaMerris JS, Nijs HGT, et al. Predicting gallstone composition with CT: in vivo and in vitro analysis. Radiology 1990;174:337–41.
10. Baker SR. Abdominal calcifications. In: Gore RM, Levine MS, editors. Textbook of gastrointestinal radiology. 3rd edition. Philadelphia (PA): W.B. Saunders; 2008. p. 225–34.
11. Laing FC. The gallbladder and bile ducts. In: Rumack CM, Wilson SR, Charboneau JW, editors. Diagnostic ultrasound. 3rd edition. St Louis (MO): Elsevier Mosby; 2004. p. 247–315.
12. Hough DM, Glazebrook KN, Paulson EK, et al. Value of prone position in ultrasonographic diagnosis of gallstones. J Ultrasound Med 2000;19:633–8.
13. Bortoff GA, Chen MY, Ott DJ, et al. Gallstones: imaging and intervention. Radiographics 2000;20:751–66.
14. Cooperberg PC. Imaging the gallbladder. Radiology 1987;163:605–14.
15. Rybick FJ. The WES sign. Radiology 2000;214:581–2.
16. Brakos JA, Ralls PW, Lapin SA, et al. Cholelithiasis: evaluation with CT. Radiology 1987;162:415–8.
17. Grand D, Horton KM, Fishman EK. CT of the gallbladder: spectrum of disease. AJR Am J Roentgenol 2004;183:163–70.
18. Kim JH, Kim MJ, Park SI, et al. MR cholangiography in symptomatic gallstones: diagnostic accuracy according to clinical risk group. Radiology 2002;224:410–6.
19. Tsai HM, Lin XZ, Chen CY, et al. MRI of gallstones with different compositions. AJR Am J Roentgenol 2004;182:1513–9.
20. Catalano OA, Sahani DV, Kalva SP, et al. MR imaging of the gallbladder: a pictorial essay. Radiographics 2008;28:135–55.
21. Millat B, Decker G, Fingerhut A. Imaging of choledocholithiasis: what does the surgeon need? Abdom Imaging 2001;26:3–6.
22. Kim YJ, Kim MJ, Kim KW, et al. Preoperative evaluation of common bile duct stones in patients with gallstone disease. AJR Am J Roentgenol 2005;184:1854–9.
23. Coelho JC, Buffara M, Possobon CE, et al. Incidence of common bile duct stones in patients with acute and chronic cholecystitis. Surg Gynecol Obstet 1984;158:76–80.

24. Cronan JJ. Prospective diagnosis of choledocholithiasis. Radiology 1983;146: 467–9.
25. Gross BH, Harter LP, Gore RM, et al. Ultrasonographic evaluation of common bile duct stones: prospective comparison with endoscopic retrograde cholangiopancreatography. Radiology 1983;146:471–4.
26. Mitchell SE, Clark RA. A comparison of computed tomography and sonography in choledocholithiasis. AJR Am J Roentgenol 1984;142:729–33.
27. Baron RL, Tublin ME, Peterson MS. Imaging the spectrum of biliary tract disease. Radiol Clin North Am 2002;40:1325–54.
28. Baron RL. Diagnosing choledocholithiasis: how far can we push helical CT? Radiology 1997;204:753–7.
29. Samaraee AA, Khan U, Almashta Z, et al. Preoperative diagnosis of choledocholithiasis: the role of MRCP. Br J Hosp Med 2009;70:339–43.
30. Norero E, Norero B, Huete A, et al. Accuracy of magnetic resonance cholangiopancreatography for the diagnosis of common bile duct stones. Rev Med Chil 2008;136:600–5.
31. Bilgin M, Shaikh F, Semelka RC, et al. Magnetic resonance imaging of gallbladder and biliary system. Top Magn Reson Imaging 2009;20:31–42.
32. Sakai Y, Tsuyuguchi T, Tsuchiya S, et al. Diagnostic value of MRCP and indications for ERCP. Hepatogastroenterology 2007;54:2212–5.
33. Dill JE. Biliary sludge. Ann Intern Med 1999;131:630–1.
34. Chang TC, Lin MT, Wu MH, et al. Evaluation of early versus delayed laparoscopic cholecystectomy in the treatment of acute cholecystitis. Hepatogastroenterology 2009;56:26–8.
35. Elwood DR. Cholecystitis. Surg Clin North Am 2008;88:1241–52.
36. Dehni N, Schielke A. Acute cholecystitis. Rev Prat 2007;57:2134–8.
37. Smith EA, Dillman JR, Elsayes KM, et al. Cross-sectional imaging of acute and chronic gallbladder inflammatory disease. AJR Am J Roentgenol 2009;192:188–96.
38. Spence SC, Teichgraeber D, Chandrasekhar C. Emergent right upper quadrant sonography. J Ultrasound Med 2009;28(4):479–96.
39. Teefey SA, Baron RL, Bigler SA. Sonography of the gallbladder: significance of striated (layered) thickening of the gallbladder wall. AJR Am J Roentgenol 1991;156:945–7.
40. Harvey RT, Miller WJ Jr. Acute biliary disease: initial CT and follow-up US versus initial US and follow-up CT. Radiology 1999;213:831–6.
41. Bree RL. Further observations on the usefulness of the sonographic Murphy sign in the evaluation of suspected acute cholecystitis. J Clin Ultrasound 1995;23: 169–72.
42. Uggowitzer M, Kugler C, Schramayer G, et al. Sonography of acute cholecystitis: comparison of color and power Doppler sonography in detecting a hypervascular gallbladder wall. AJR Am J Roentgenol 1997;203:93–7.
43. Paulson EK. Acute cholecystitis: CT findings. Semin Ultrasound CT MR 2000;21: 56–63.
44. Fidler J, Paulson EK, Layfield L. CT evaluation of acute cholecystits: findings useful in diagnosis. AJR Am J Roentgenol 1996;166:1085–8.
45. Stoker J, van Randen A, Laméris W, et al. Imaging patients with acute abdominal pain. Radiology 2009;253:31–46.
46. Bader TR, Semelka RC. Gallbladder and biliary system. In: Semelka RC, editor. Abdominal-pelvic MRI. 2nd edition. Hoboken (NJ): Wiley; 2006. p. 447–507.
47. Loud PA, Semelka RC, Kettritz U, et al. MRI of acute cholecystitis: comparison with normal gallbladder and other entities. Magn Reson Imaging 1996;14:349–55.

48. Kim KW, Park MS, Yu JS, et al. Acute cholecystitis at T2-weighted and manganese-enhanced T1-weighted MR cholangiography: preliminary study. Radiology 2003;227:580–4.
49. Strasberg SM. Acute calculous cholecystitis. N Engl J Med 2008;26(358): 2804–11.
50. Mirvis SE, Vainright JR, Nelson AW, et al. The diagnosis of acute acalculous cholecystitis: comparison of sonography, scintigraphy, and CT. AJR Am J Roentgenol 1986;147:1171–5.
51. Boland GW, Slater G, Lu DS, et al. Prevalence and significance of gallbladder abnormalities seen on sonography in intensive care unit patients. AJR Am J Roentgenol 2000;174:973–7.
52. Amaral J, Xiao ZL, Chen Q, et al. Gallbladder muscle dysfunction in patients with acalculous disease. Gastroenterology 2001;120:506–11.
53. Teefey SA, Baron RL, Radke HM, et al. Gangrenous cholecystitis: new observations on sonography. J Ultrasound Med 1991;134:191–4.
54. Jeffrey RB, Laing FC, Wong W, et al. Gangrenous cholecystitis: diagnosis by ultrasound. Radiology 1983;148:219–21.
55. Bridges MD, Jones BC, Morgan DE, et al. Acute cholecystitis and gallbladder necrosis: value of contrast enhanced helical CT. AJR Am J Roentgenol 1999;172:34–5.
56. Chopra S, Dodd GD, Mumbower AL, et al. Treatment of acute cholecystitis in non-critically ill patients at high surgical risk: comparison of clinical outcomes after gallbladder aspiration and after percutaneous cholecystostomy. AJR Am J Roentgenol 2001;176:1025–31.
57. Bennett GL, Rusienk H, Lisi V, et al. CT findings in acute gangrenous cholecystitis. AJR Am J Roentgenol 2002;178:275–81.
58. Singh AK, Sagar P. Gangrenous cholecystitis: prediction with CT imaging. Abdom Imaging 2005;30:218–21.
59. Hunt DR, Chu FC. Gangrenous cholecystitis in the laparoscopic era. Aust N Z J Surg 2000;70:428–30.
60. Varma DG, Faust JM. Computed tomography of gangrenous acute postoperative acalculous cholecystitis. J Comput Tomogr 1988;12:29–31.
61. Gill KS, Chapman AJ, Weston MJ. The changing face of emphysematous cholecystitis. Br J Radiol 1997;70:986–91.
62. Konno K, Ishida H, Naganuma H, et al. Emphysematous cholecystitis: sonographic findings. Abdom Imaging 2002;27:191–5.
63. Altun E, Semelka RC, Elias J Jr, et al. Acute cholecystitis: MR findings and differentiation from chronic cholecystitis. Radiology 2007;244:174–83.
64. Chiu HH, Chen CM, Mo LR. Emphysematous cholecystitis. Am J Surg 2004;188: 325–6.
65. Grayson DE, Abbott RM, Levy AD, et al. Emphysematous infections of the abdomen and pelvis: a pictorial review. Radiographics 2002;22:543–61.
66. Koenig T, Tamm EP, Kawashima A. Magnetic resonance imaging findings in emphysematous cholecystitis. Clin Radiol 2004;59:455–8.
67. Morris BS, Balpande PR, Morani AC, et al. The CT appearances of gallbladder perforation. Br J Radiol 2007;80:898–901.
68. Kim PN, Lee KS, Kim IY, et al. Gallbladder perforation: comparison of US findings with CT. Abdom Imaging 1994;19:239–42.
69. Konno K, Ishida H, Sato M, et al. Gallbladder perforation: color Doppler findings. Abdom Imaging 2002;27:47–50.
70. Moskos MM, Eschelman DJ. Hemorrhagic cholecystitis. AJR Am J Roentgenol 1991;156:1304–5.

71. Tsimmerman IS. Chronic cholecystitis and its clinical masks: diagnosis and differential diagnosis. Klin Med 2006;84:4–12.

72. Kim SJ, Lee JM, Lee JY, et al. Analysis of enhancement pattern of flat gallbladder wall thickening on MDCT to differentiate gallbladder cancer from cholecystitis. AJR Am J Roentgenol 2008;191:765–71.

73. Ziessman HA. Functional hepatobiliary disease: chronic acalculous gallbladder and chronic acalculous biliary disease. Semin Nucl Med 2006;36:119–32.

74. Yiu-Chiu VS, Chiu LC, Wedel VJ. Acalculous hemorrhagic cholecystitis. J Comput Tomogr 1980;4:201–6.

75. Pandya R, O'Malley C. Hemorrhagic cholecystitis as a complication of anticoagulant therapy: role of CT in its diagnosis. Abdom Imaging 2008;33:652–3.

76. Jenkins M, Golding RH, Cooperberg PL. Sonography and computed tomography of hemorrhagic cholecystitis. AJR Am J Roentgenol 1983;140:1197–9.

77. Ziessman HA. Interventions used with cholescintigraphy for the diagnosis of hepatobiliary disease. Semin Nucl Med 2009;39(3):174–85.

78. Jung SE, Lee JM, Lee K, et al. Gallbladder wall thickening: MR imaging and pathologic correlation with emphasis on layered pattern. Eur Radiol 2005;15:694–701.

79. Yoon JH, Cha SS, Han SS, et al. Gallbladder adenomyomatosis: imaging findings. Abdom Imaging 2006;31:555–63.

80. Boscak AR, Al-Hawary M, Ramsburgh SR. Adenomyomatosis of the gallbladder. Radiographics 2006;26:941–6.

81. Hwang JI, Chou YH, Tsay SH, et al. Radiologic and pathologic correlation of adenomyomatosis of the gallbladder. Abdom Imaging 1998;23:73–7.

82. Lichtenstein JE. Adenomyomatosis and cholestrolosis. In: Gore RM, Levine MS, editors. Textbook of gastrointestinal radiology. 2nd edition. Philadelphia: WB Saunders; 2000. p. 1353–9.

83. LaFortune M, Gariepy G, Dumont A, et al. The V-shaped artifact of the gallbladder wall. AJR Am J Roentgenol 1986;147:505–8.

84. Kiran RP, Pokala N, Dudrick SJ. Incidence pattern and survival for gallbladder cancer over three decades—an analysis of 10301 patients. Ann Surg Oncol 2007;14:827–32.

85. Furlan A, Ferris JV, Hosseinzadeh K, et al. Gallbladder carcinoma update: multimodality imaging evaluation, staging, and treatment options. AJR Am J Roentgenol 2008;191:1440–7.

86. Gore RM, Shelhamer RP. Biliary tract neoplasms: diagnosis and staging. Cancer Imaging 2007;7:S15–23.

87. Kim SJ, Lee JM, Lee JY, et al. Accuracy of preoperative T-staging of gallbladder carcinoma using MDCT. AJR Am J Roentgenol 2008;190:74–80.

88. Yoshimitsu K, Irie H, Aibe H, et al. Well-differentiated adenocarcinoma of the gallbladder with intratumoral cystic components due to abundant mucin production: a mimicker of adenomyomatosis. Eur Radiol 2005;15:229–33.

89. Soyer P, Gouhiri M, Boudiaf M, et al. Carcinoma of the gallbladder: imaging features with surgical correlation. AJR Am J Roentgenol 1997;169:781–4.

90. Wilbur AC, Sagireddy PB, Aizenstein RI. Carcinoma of the gallbladder: color Doppler ultrasound and CT findings. Abdom Imaging 1997;22:187–90.

91. Levy AD, Murakata LA, Rohrmann CA Jr. Gallbladder carcinoma: radiologic-pathologic correlation. Radiographics 2001;21:295–314.

92. Onoyama H. Diagnostic imaging of early gallbladder cancer: retrospective study of 53 cases. World J Surg 1999;23:708–12.

93. Yoshimitsu K, Honda H, Jimi M, et al. MR diagnosis of adenomyomatosis of the gallbladder and differentiation from gallbladder carcinoma: importance of showing Rokitansky-Aschoff sinuses. AJR Am J Roentgenol 1999;172: 1535–40.
94. Schwartz LH, Black J, Fong Y, et al. Gallbladder carcinoma: findings at MR imaging with MR cholangiopancreatography. J Comput Assist Tomogr 2002;26: 405–10.

# Endoscopic Ultrasonography in Diseases of the Gallbladder

Darby E. Robinson O'Neill, MD, Michael D. Saunders, MD*

**KEYWORDS**

- Endoscopic ultrasonography • Gallbladder • Cholelithiasis
- Choledocholithiasis • Microlithiasis • Gallbladder polyp
- Gallbladder mass • Gallbladder cancer

Endoscopic ultrasonography (EUS) was introduced in 1980 and has developed considerably in the past 30 years. Primarily useful for the detection and staging of gastrointestinal cancers, EUS is now established as an important diagnostic modality that is necessary for the optimal management of gastrointestinal disease. EUS and magnetic resonance cholangiopancreatography (MRCP) have been largely responsible for the diminishing role of diagnostic endoscopic retrograde cholangiopancreatography (ERCP). EUS has become an essential tool for the complete pancreaticobiliary endoscopist.

EUS is an accurate modality for imaging gallbladder structures because of the close proximity of the duodenum to the gallbladder and extrahepatic biliary tree (**Fig. 1**). EUS is considered superior to transabdominal ultrasonography (US) for imaging the biliary system, using higher ultrasound frequencies (5–12 MHz vs 2–5 MHz).[1] EUS can differentiate the double-layered structure of the gallbladder wall and provide higher resolution for imaging small polypoid lesions. Both types of echoendoscopes, radial and linear (transverse and longitudinal imaging, respectively), can be used to image the biliary tree. In addition to imaging, EUS-guided needle puncture using the linear instrument enables transluminal aspiration of tissue for diagnosis and provides direct access to the biliary tree for therapeutic interventions. The development of intraductal ultrasonography (IDUS) miniprobes has further advanced the study of pancreaticobiliary tree disorders.

Clinical situations in which EUS can be used for evaluation of gallbladder disease include investigation of suspected cholelithiasis or biliary sludge, evaluation of

Division of Gastroenterology, University of Washington Medical Center, 1959 NE Pacific Street, PO Box 356424, Seattle, WA 98195, USA
* Corresponding author.
*E-mail address:* michaels@medicine.washington.edu

Gastroenterol Clin N Am 39 (2010) 289–305
doi:10.1016/j.gtc.2010.03.001
0889-8553/10/$ – see front matter. Published by Elsevier Inc.

gastro.theclinics.com

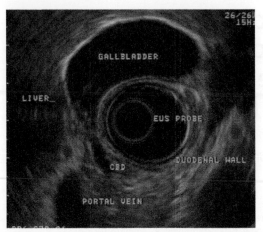

**Fig. 1.** Endosonographic image obtained from the duodenal bulb showing the close proximity of the gallbladder and common bile duct to the duodenal wall.

suspected choledocholithiasis, imaging of polypoid lesions of the gallbladder, and diagnosis and staging of gallbladder cancer. This article reviews the use of EUS in these settings.

## EUS INSTRUMENTS

The currently available instruments for biliary imaging with EUS include radial and linear echoendoscopes and catheter-based IDUS probes. There are 2 types of echoendoscopes, denoted radial or linear based on the piezoelectric crystals that generate the EUS image.[2] In EUS, ultrasound pulses are generated by a transducer containing a piezoelectric crystal that converts an electronic pulse into an acoustic wave that propagates into the tissue. The same transducer then detects returning acoustic waves that contain information about the tissue through which the waves have propagated.[3] In a radial echoendoscope, the crystals are arranged in a band around the shaft of the endoscope, perpendicular to the long axis of the instrument, generating a cross-sectional image (**Fig. 2**). Radial scanning instruments provide detailed circumferential images, making them useful for orientation, and electronic radial instruments with Doppler capabilities help distinguish small vessels from ducts and improve vascular staging. In a linear echoendoscope, the crystals are arranged along one side of the endoscope's tip, generating a longitudinal image parallel to

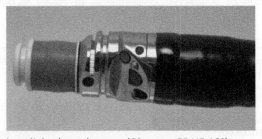

**Fig. 2.** The electronic radial echoendoscope (Olympus GF-UE 160).

the long axis of the instrument. Only the linear echoendoscope can be used to guide fine-needle puncture. The ability of the linear echoendoscope to provide scanning in the same plane as the instrument's shaft allows the endoscopist to trace the path of a needle as it is inserted out of the working channel of the echoendoscope (**Fig. 3**). Hence, a linear echoendoscope can be used for diagnostic evaluation and to facilitate interventional EUS, such as EUS-guided fine-needle aspiration, EUS-guided injection therapies, and EUS-guided drainage procedures. The availability of high-frequency catheter ultrasound probes allows imaging from within the biliary tree. IDUS probes are placed during ERCP, most often over a guide wire, and can be advanced into the common bile duct, hilar region, intrahepatic ducts, gallbladder, and across biliary strictures.

## EUS TECHNIQUE

Endoscopic expertise using a duodenoscope (radial and linear echoendoscopes are primarily oblique viewing) and a detailed understanding of the regional cross-sectional anatomy are essential to obtain and interpret EUS images of the biliary tree. The optimal position for imaging the gallbladder is variable. The gallbladder is most commonly and easily imaged from the duodenal bulb but may also be imaged from the antrum or descending duodenum. EUS imaging is usually commenced in the duodenal bulb with the echoendoscope in the long position, with the endoscope advanced to the superior angle of the duodenal bulb and the tip deflected downward. To image the body, fundus, and neck of the gallbladder, the transducer is moved slowly along the course of the gallbladder using torque and tip deflection as needed.[1] The normal gallbladder appears as a large fluid-filled (anechoic) structure with a thin, layered wall (**Fig. 4**). With the echoendoscope in the same position, the common bile duct and common hepatic duct are seen in their long axis alongside and superficial to the portal vein (**Fig. 5**). When it is dilated, the bile duct is often readily recognized. If Doppler is available, it can be used to confirm bile duct identification and distinguish

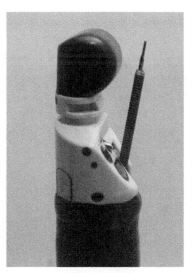

**Fig. 3.** The linear array echoendoscope (Olympus GF-UC-140P AL5) with needle in accessory channel.

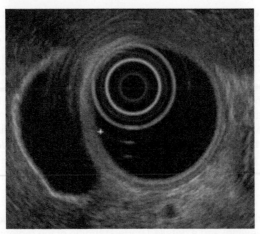

**Fig. 4.** Endosonographic image of a normal gallbladder from the duodenal bulb. The gallbladder appears as an anechoic (fluid-filled) structure with a thin layered wall.

the duct from vessels such as the portal vein or gastroduodenal artery. Imaging is then continued with the echoendoscope in the short position at the level of the papilla, similar to the endoscope position when performing ERCP. In this position, the bile duct is identified at the periampullary portion of the pancreas and followed proximally to the level of the bifurcation and gallbladder.

## EUS AND OCCULT CHOLECYSTOLITHIASIS OR MICROLITHIASIS

Gallstone disease is common in the United States, with a prevalence of approximately 10% to 15% among adults.[4] The gold standard for evaluation for gallbladder stones is transabdominal US, which has been shown to have a sensitivity of 98% for the detection of cholecystolithiasis.[5] However, US may miss gallstones in some patients, particularly those with small gallstones, and a high clinical suspicion for cholelithiasis may

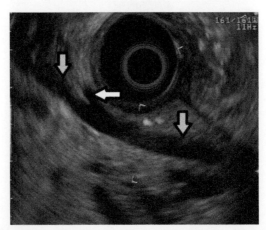

**Fig. 5.** Transluminal view from the duodenal bulb of the common bile and common hepatic ducts (*vertical arrows*). The cystic duct takeoff is visualized (*horizontal arrow*).

make additional studies warranted. Given its higher-frequency resolution and the closer proximity of the echoendoscope to the biliary system compared with US, EUS can be used to evaluate for occult cholecystolithiasis among patients in whom gallbladder stones are suspected but cannot be confirmed after US (**Fig. 6**).

The performance of EUS in the diagnosis of occult cholelithiasis was evaluated by Dahan and colleagues.[6] They prospectively studied 45 patients with acute idiopathic pancreatitis (n = 25) or transient biliary-type pain associated with fever, jaundice, and increased liver enzymes (n = 20). All patients previously had at least 2 normal trans-abdominal US scans. EUS showed gallbladder stones or sludge in 26 of the 45 patients, with the diagnosis of macrolithiasis or microlithiasis confirmed at cholecystectomy in 23 of the 26. Among the 19 patients in whom EUS did not suggest cholelithiasis, 7 underwent cholecystectomy for other reasons, and the others were followed clinically; only 1 patient was subsequently diagnosed with cholelithiasis. EUS therefore had a sensitivity of 96% for detection of occult cholelithiasis (94% for

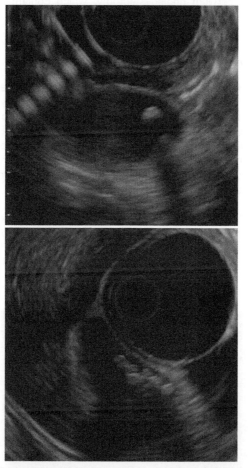

**Fig. 6.** EUS images of a patient with suspected biliary colic but negative transabdominal US. (*Top*) The gallbladder containing a single mobile echogenic structure with posterior shadowing. (*Bottom*) Numerous small echogenic shadowing foci consistent with stones.

macroscopically visible stones) and a specificity of 86%. This result compared with a sensitivity of 67% for the microscopic examination of duodenal bile from the same patients (P<.03).

Liu and colleagues[7] performed EUS in 18 patients with acute pancreatitis in whom no cause was identified after history, laboratory evaluation, and conventional abdominal imaging. Of these patients, all had undergone at least 1 US, 9 had multiple US, and 6 had also been evaluated with computed tomography (CT); each of these imaging studies had failed to detect biliary calculi. EUS revealed small gallstones in 14 of the 18 patients (78%); 10 of these 14 also had gallbladder sludge (**Fig. 7**), and 3 had concomitant choledocholithiasis. The diagnosis of cholelithiasis was confirmed at cholecystectomy in all 14 patients. The 4 patients without cholelithiasis by EUS remained free of gallstone disease as determined by laboratory, clinical, and US follow-up for a median of 22 months. Similar results were obtained by Thorbøll and colleagues,[8] who evaluated 35 consecutive patients with biliary colic who had undergone at least 1 (mean = 2.1) normal US. EUS showed cholecystolithiasis in 18 of the 35 (52%). Seventeen of these patients underwent cholecystectomy, which confirmed the presence of stones in the gallbladder in 15 of 17 (88%).

## EUS AND CHOLEDOCHOLITHIASIS

Choledocholithiasis is a frequent complication of gallstone disease, occurring in 15% to 20% of patients with symptomatic cholelithiasis.[9] Historically, ERCP has been considered the gold standard for the diagnosis of common bile duct stones. However, ERCP is an invasive procedure that is associated with a small, but not insignificant, risk of serious complications such as pancreatitis, cholangitis, perforation, and hemorrhage,[10] and thus should ideally be reserved for patients with proven common bile duct stones who require endoscopic therapy. It is therefore important to use initial safe, noninvasive diagnostic modalities for choledocholithiasis to select appropriate patients for ERCP.

In recent years, EUS has emerged as a minimally invasive procedure that is useful for the diagnosis of common bile duct stones (**Fig. 8**). Several studies have been performed to compare the performance of EUS with those of conventional imaging techniques such as US and CT, as well as a newer modality, MRCP. The performance of EUS has also been compared with ERCP. In addition, several groups have recently

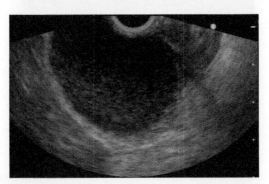

**Fig. 7.** Linear EUS image of gallbladder sludge, seen as minute, echogenic, nonshadowing particles layering in the dependent part of the gallbladder.

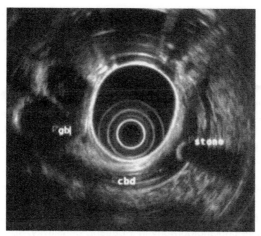

**Fig. 8.** Transluminal view of the common bile duct with a stone, seen as an echogenic focus with posterior shadowing. The gallbladder is visualized adjacent and superior to the bile duct.

proposed and studied an EUS-guided ERCP approach for diagnosis of choledocholithiasis among patients with intermediate probability of common duct stones.

Transabdominal US is routinely used for the diagnosis of cholelithiasis, but it is not sensitive in the detection of common bile duct stones. In a prospective series of 155 patients with suspected choledocholithiasis, 51 of whom had common duct stones at ERCP that were later confirmed by sphincterotomy or surgery, Sugiyama and Atomi[11] found that EUS had a higher sensitivity (96%) than US (63%) for detection of choledocholithiasis (P<.001). The specificity and accuracy of EUS (100% and 99%, respectively) for common duct stones were also significantly higher than those of US (95% and 83%). The extrahepatic bile duct was wholly displayed in 96% of patients by EUS but in only 60% by US (P<.0001). Amouyal and colleagues[12] obtained similar results when they evaluated 62 consecutive patients with suspected common bile duct stones. They found that EUS was more sensitive (97%) than US (25%, P<.0001) and had a significantly higher negative predictive value (97% vs 56%; P<.0001). Specificity and positive predictive value of the 2 modalities were not significantly different.

The sensitivity of CT for common duct stones, although higher than that of US, is lower than the sensitivity of EUS. Earlier studies[11,12] performed before helical CT scanning was widely available, found that CT had a sensitivity for detection of common bile duct stones ranging from 71% to 75%. More recent investigations have found improved test performance using helical CT, albeit not equal to that of EUS. In a prospective study of 52 inpatients referred for ERCP for suspected choledocholithiasis, Polkowski and colleagues[13] compared the performance of EUS with helical CT. Thirty-four of the 50 patients (68%) who underwent successful ERCP (which was considered the gold standard) were shown to have bile duct stones. The sensitivity, specificity, and accuracy of EUS (91%, 100%, and 94%, respectively) were higher than those of CT (85%, 88%, and 86%), but these differences were not statistically significant. Likewise, Kondo and colleagues[14] evaluated the performance of EUS versus helical CT in 28 patients considered likely to have common bile duct stones. Twenty-four of the 28 patients (85.7%) were found to have choledocholithiasis using a combination of ERCP and intraductal US, which was considered the gold standard. The sensitivity of EUS (100%) was higher than that of helical CT (88%). Among patients with small (1–4 mm) common duct stones, sensitivity of EUS remained 100%, whereas sensitivity of CT fell to 67%. The investigators concluded that, when immediate diagnosis and treatment are required, EUS should be the first-choice study because of its improved sensitivity for small stones.

MRCP, as a noninvasive and increasingly available study, has been advocated as an alternative to EUS for the evaluation of choledocholithiasis, particularly among patients with low to intermediate probability of common bile duct stones. Schmidt and colleagues[15] prospectively evaluated 57 patients with suspected choledocholithiasis using MRCP and EUS. If either study detected choledocholithiasis or unexplained common bile duct dilation, ERCP or intraoperative cholangiography was considered the gold standard for final diagnosis. Among patients with negative EUS and MRCP, the gold standard was clinical follow-up. Common bile duct stones were found in 18 of the 57 patients (31.6%) and confirmed by ERCP in 17 patients and by intraoperative cholangiography in 1 patient. Sensitivity, specificity, and accuracy for MRCP were 94.8%, 94.4%, and 94.7%, respectively. Corresponding values for EUS, which were not statistically different, were 97.4%, 94.4%, and 96.5%. A systematic review[16] of 5 prospective studies comparing EUS and MRCP, with a pooled data set of 301 patients, yielded similar results. The aggregated sensitivities of EUS and MRCP for the detection of choledocholithiasis were 93% and 85%, respectively, and their aggregated specificities were 96% and 93%. The aggregated positive predictive values were 93% and 87%, with negative predictive values of 96% and 92%. The systematic review showed no statistically significant differences between EUS and MRCP for the detection of choledocholithiasis.

Several studies[17–21] have compared the performance of EUS with ERCP in the detection of common duct stones, and most have failed to find a significant difference in test performance between the 2 procedures. Palazzo and colleagues[17] retrospectively evaluated 219 patients who had undergone EUS and ERCP for evaluation of suspected choledocholithiasis. Common bile duct stones were detected by ERCP in 77 patients, and, in all of these cases, stones were also diagnosed by EUS. In 19 patients, choledocholithiasis was diagnosed by EUS but not confirmed by ERCP, and EUS and ERCP failed to diagnose common duct stones in 1 patient later found to have choledocholithiasis during surgical exploration. EUS and ERCP findings were therefore concordant in 91.3% of cases. In a prospective study, Prat and colleagues[18] evaluated 119 patients strongly suspected of choledocholithiasis, and performed EUS and ERCP. Endoscopic sphincterotomy with basket and balloon exploration of the common bile duct was considered the gold standard for diagnosis of choledocholithiasis and was performed in all but 1 case; 78 (66%) of the patients were found to have common bile duct stones at sphincterotomy. The findings at ERCP and EUS were concordant in 95% of cases. The sensitivity, specificity, positive predictive value, and negative predictive value of EUS were 93%, 97%, 98%, and 88%, respectively. These values were not significantly different than those for ERCP (89%, 100%, 100%, and 83%).

Given the comparable test performances of EUS and ERCP, and the risk of morbidity associated with ERCP, a strategy has been proposed in which EUS is used as the initial diagnostic test before ERCP, particularly for patients with intermediate or lower probability of common bile duct stones. Several recent randomized controlled trials[22–25] have evaluated this approach. Karakan and colleagues[22] randomized 120 patients with an intermediate risk for choledocholithiasis (baseline probability of bile duct stones no more than 67%) in a 1:1 fashion to EUS or ERCP as their initial study. Those who underwent EUS first (the EUS-guided ERCP group) proceeded to ERCP only if choledocholithiasis was detected on EUS, and sphincter-otomy and stone extraction were performed if either procedure showed common duct stones. Among patients in the ERCP group, sphincterotomy and stone extraction were performed if the cholangiogram revealed choledocholithiasis. There was a trend for an increased number of endoscopic procedures in the ERCP group (mean 1.63 proce-dures per patient) compared with the EUS-guided ERCP group (mean 1.38 proce-dures per patient), although this difference was not statistically significant. There was also a trend for an increased rate of complications in the ERCP group (10%) compared with the EUS-guided ERCP group (1.7%; $P = .06$), and Kaplan-Meier anal-ysis showed a significantly higher rate of negative outcomes in the ERCP group ($P = .049$). Polkowski and colleagues,[23] in a study of similar design, randomized 100 patients with intermediate probability of common bile duct stones to EUS or ERCP first. They found no significant difference in the number of procedures performed in the EUS-guided ERCP versus ERCP groups (1.42 and 1.31 procedures per patient, respectively), but more patients in the ERCP group (40%) than the EUS-guided ERCP group (10%; $P<.001$) experienced a negative outcome. A recent systematic review[26] that included 423 patients from the Polkowski and Karakan studies as well as 2 other randomized controlled trials, showed that the EUS-guided ERCP approach avoided ERCP in 67% of patients when EUS did not show choledocholithiasis. The risk of undergoing an additional endoscopic procedure was higher in the EUS-guided ERCP group (risk ratio [RR] 2.46, $P = .004$). The EUS-guided ERCP approach was also associated with a significantly lower risk of overall complications (complication rate 6.6% vs 19%; RR 0.35; $P<.001$) and post-ERCP pancreatitis (RR 0.21, $P = .03$).

## EUS AND POLYPOID LESIONS OF THE GALLBLADDER

Polypoid lesions of the gallbladder are common, being found in 3% to 7% of healthy subjects undergoing US.[27,28] On US, these masses have echogenicity similar to the gallbladder wall, project into the lumen, are fixed, and lack an acoustic shadow (**Fig. 9**).[29] Most polypoid gallbladder lesions are cholesterol polyps, which appear

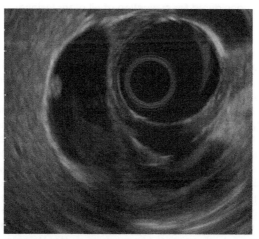

**Fig. 9.** EUS image of a gallbladder polyp, seen as a small echogenic, nonshadowing, nonmo-bile structure adherent to the gallbladder wall. The findings are consistent with a small cholesterol polyp.

as pedunculated lesions with a granular surface and an internal echo pattern of a tiny echogenic spot or spots, sometimes with echopenic areas. In 1 large series,[30] cholesterol polyps accounted for 62.8% of gallbladder polyps. Other polypoid lesions include adenomyomatosis, adenoma, and adenocarcinoma. Adenomyomatoses are sessile echogenic masses containing multiple microcysts or with a comet tail artifact. Adenocarcinomas, which account for 3% to 8% of polypoid gallbladder lesions,[29] and adenomas are sessile or pedunculated masses with a hypoechoic to isoechoic internal echo and without echogenic spots, microcysts, or comet tail artifact. Risk factors for malignant polypoid lesions include older patient age, solitary lesions, coexistent gallstones, and presence of symptoms.[29]

Current recommendations for the management of gallbladder polyps are based largely on polyp size. The risk of adenocarcinoma is higher in polyps larger than 1 cm, particularly among patients more than 50 years of age, so these patients should undergo cholecystectomy, as should those with symptomatic gallbladder polyps.[29] Smaller, asymptomatic lesions can be followed with serial US. EUS can be helpful to further distinguish benign from malignant or potentially malignant gallbladder polyps, and is superior to transabdominal US for this purpose. Sugiyama and colleagues[31] performed a retrospective analysis of 65 patients who underwent cholecystectomy for small (≤20 mm) polypoid lesions of the gallbladder, comparing preoperative EUS and US findings with the eventual pathologic diagnoses. Lesions were classified as cholesterol polyps, adenomyomatoses, or adenoma/adenocarcinoma. EUS correctly identified the polypoid lesions in 97% of patients, versus 71% for US (P<.0001). A second retrospective study by Azuma and colleagues,[32] which reviewed 89 patients with gallbladder polyps less than 20 mm in size who underwent EUS and US before surgery, found that EUS precisely diagnosed the lesions in 86.5% of cases, compared with 51.7% for US. In determining whether or not the polyp was carcinoma, the sensitivity, specificity, positive predictive value, and negative predictive value of EUS were 91.7%, 87.7%, 75.9%, and 96.6%, respectively. US had a specificity of 54.2%, sensitivity of 53.8%, and positive and negative predictive values of 54.2% and 94.6%; all of these values were lower than those for EUS. The investigators suggested that US diagnosis and continued ultrasonographic surveillance are likely sufficient for polyps less than 10 mm in size that are diagnosed as cholesterol polyps, but EUS should be considered for evaluation of all other lesions.

To further aid in differential diagnosis and management decisions, 2 groups have devised EUS scoring systems for evaluation of polypoid gallbladder lesions. Choi and colleagues[33] used preoperative EUS data from a reference group of 79 patients with gallbladder polyps 5 to 15 mm in diameter to construct an EUS scoring system to predict risk of neoplasia (adenoma or adenocarcinoma). Their scoring system (Table 1) uses 5 variables: the layer structure of the gallbladder wall, the echo pattern of the polyp, the nature of the polyp margin, the presence or absence of a stalk, and the number of polyps. The areas under the receiver operating characteristic curves were 0.91 for an EUS score of more than 6, versus 0.63 for polyp size more than 10 mm (P<.01). Sensitivity, specificity, and accuracy for the risk of neoplastic polyp using a cutoff EUS score of 6 were 81%, 86%, and 83.7%, respectively, compared with 60%, 64%, and 62.7% using polyp size alone and a 10-mm cutoff diameter. Evaluation of the scoring system in a validation group of 26 patients yielded comparable results. A second group, Sadamoto and colleagues,[34] created a similar EUS scoring system (Table 2) using only 3 variables: maximum polyp diameter, internal echo pattern, and presence or absence of hyperechoic spots. Using a cutoff EUS score of 12, the sensitivity, specificity, and accuracy for the risk of neoplasia were 77.8%, 82.7%, and 82.9%, respectively. If size alone was considered, the sensitivity,

**Table 1**
**EUS scoring system to predict neoplastic gallbladder polyps**

| Variable | Score |
|---|---|
| Layer structure of gallbladder wall | |
| Preserved | 0 |
| Lost | 6 |
| Echo pattern of polyp | |
| Hyperechoic spots | 0 |
| Hyperechoic homogeneous | 1 |
| Isoechoic homogeneous | 2 |
| Isoechoic heterogeneous | 5 |
| Margin of polyp | |
| Not lobulated | 0 |
| Lobulated | 4 |
| Stalk | |
| Pedunculated | 0 |
| Sessile | 3 |
| Number of polyps | |
| Multiple | 0 |
| Single | 2 |

*Data from* Choi WB, Lee SK, Kim MH, et al. A new strategy to predict the neoplastic polyps of the gallbladder based on a scoring system using EUS. Gastrointest Endosc 2000;52(3):376; with permission.

specificity, and accuracy for the risk of a neoplastic polyp 11 mm or more in diameter were 83.3%, 65.3%, and 70.0%, respectively.

Once a gallbladder polyp or mass has been identified, EUS can also be used to perform fine-needle aspiration (FNA) to obtain a histologic diagnosis. Historically, the diagnosis of gallbladder carcinoma has been established by percutaneous

**Table 2**
**EUS scoring system to predict neoplastic gallbladder polyps**

| Variable | Score |
|---|---|
| Maximum polyp diameter, mm | |
| X | X |
| Internal echo pattern | |
| Heterogeneous | 4 |
| Homogeneous | 0 |
| Hyperechoic spot(s) | |
| Presence | −5 |
| Absence | 0 |

Total score = maximum polyp size + internal echo pattern (heterogeneous 4, homogeneous 0) + hyperechoic spots (present −5, absent 0).

*Data from* Sadamoto Y, Oda S, Tanaka M, et al. A useful approach to the differential diagnosis of small polypoid lesions of the gallbladder, using an endoscopic ultrasound scoring system. Endoscopy 2002;34(12):963; with permission.

US-guided or CT-guided biopsy. However, percutaneous FNA is associated with minor abdominal pain in 4.5% of cases[35] and bile peritonitis in 1% to 6%.[35,36] Two small case series suggest that EUS-guided FNA of gallbladder masses is safe and can provide a definitive diagnosis (**Fig. 10**). Jacobson and colleagues[37] reported on 6 cases in which EUS-FNA was performed for suspected gallbladder masses initially found by CT and ranging from less than 2 to more than 10 cm in size. FNA of the mass was performed in all 6 cases, and regional lymph nodes were also sampled in 5. The final diagnosis was gallbladder carcinoma in 5 cases and xanthogranulomatous cholecystitis in 1. Of the 5 confirmed cases of gallbladder carcinoma, FNA of the gallbladder mass yielded a specimen positive for malignancy in 3 and suspicious for carcinoma in 1. In the latter case, FNA of a regional lymph node established the diagnosis of carcinoma. FNA was negative for malignancy in 1 case of proven carcinoma. No immediate or delayed complications were noted, and operative findings in the 4 patients who underwent surgery suggested no bleeding, perforation, bile leakage, or other complications related to the FNA. In a second series[38] of 6 patients who underwent EUS-FNA of gallbladder masses ranging in size from 1.8 to 7.4 cm, all 5 patients with adenocarcinoma had FNA positive for malignancy. In 4 cases, FNA of the mass itself was positive; in the other case, aspiration of the mass was not possible but FNA of a hilar lymph node revealed adenocarcinoma. There were no immediate or late complications.

## EUS AND GALLBLADDER CARCINOMA

Gallbladder carcinoma is an uncommon disease. It is estimated that approximately 9760 cases of gallbladder and other biliary tract cancers were diagnosed in the United States in 2009 and that these were responsible for 3370 deaths.[39] Because the signs and symptoms of gallbladder carcinoma (including abdominal pain, nausea, vomiting, weight loss, and anorexia) are nonspecific, the disease is often diagnosed at an advanced stage and is associated with a high mortality.[40] Accurate preoperative staging (**Box 1**) of gallbladder carcinoma is crucial, because staging determines the operative approach,[41] and depth of invasion (T stage) closely correlates with prognosis.[42] Because EUS allows detailed visualization of the layers of the gallbladder wall, there has been interest in using EUS for preoperative staging of gallbladder carcinoma.

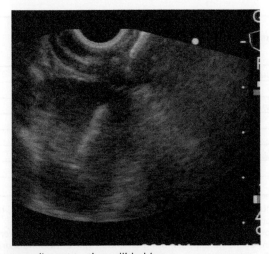

**Fig. 10.** FNA of a mass adjacent to the gallbladder.

---

**Box 1**
**TNM staging of gallbladder carcinoma**

Primary tumor (T)

    TX, Primary tumor cannot be assessed

    T0, No evidence of primary tumor

    Tis, Carcinoma in situ

    T1, Tumor invades lamina propria or muscle layer

    T1a, Tumor invades lamina propria

    T1b, Tumor invades muscle layer

    T2, Tumor invades perimuscular connective tissue; no extension beyond serosa or into liver

    T3, Tumor perforates the serosa (visceral peritoneum) and/or directly invades the liver and/or one other adjacent organ or structure, such as the stomach, duodenum, colon, pancreas, omentum, or extrahepatic bile ducts

    T4, Tumor invades main portal vein or hepatic artery or invades two or more extrahepatic organs or structures

Regional lymph nodes (N)

    NX, Regional lymph nodes cannot be assessed

    N0, No regional lymph node metastasis

    N1, Metastases to nodes along the cystic duct, common bile duct, hepatic artery, and/or portal vein

    N2, Metastases to periaortic, pericaval, superior mesenteric artery, and/or celiac artery lymph nodes

Distant metastasis (M)

    M0, No distant metastasis

    M1, Distant metastasis

*From* American Joint Committee on Cancer. AJCC Cancer Staging Manual. 7th ed. New York: Springer; 2010; with permission.

---

Fujita and colleagues[43] proposed EUS criteria for T staging of gallbladder cancer (**Table 3**). They retrospectively reviewed the records of 39 patients who had undergone EUS and surgical resection for gallbladder cancer and divided their EUS images into 4 types. Type A tumors are pedunculated, with a fine nodular surface, and the gallbladder wall has preserved outer hyperechoic and inner hypoechoic layers. Type B tumors are broad-based masses or areas of wall thickening, again associated with a normal gallbladder wall structure. Type C tumors are broad-based lesions that cause irregularity of the outer hyperechoic layer of the gallbladder wall, whereas type D tumors disrupt the entire layer structure of the gallbladder wall. After classifying the EUS images into these categories, they then correlated the endosonographic types with histologic depth of invasion. All type A tumors were confined to the mucosa (pTis), and type B lesions invaded varying depths between the mucosa and subserosa (pT1–2). Type C tumors invaded the subserosa or beyond (mainly pT2), and type D tumors invaded beyond the serosa (pT3–4).

To assess the accuracy of these EUS T staging criteria, Sadamoto and colleagues[44] retrospectively analyzed EUS and histopathologic findings in 41 patients with

| Table 3<br>EUS classification of gallbladder cancer | | | |
|---|---|---|---|
| Type | Shape | Surface | Outer Hyperechoic Layer |
| A | Pedunculated | Nodular | Intact |
| B | Broad-based protrusion or wall thickening | Irregular | Intact |
| C | Broad-based protrusion or wall thickening | Irregular | Irregular |
| D | Broad-based protrusion or wall thickening | Irregular | Disrupted |

*Data from* Fujita N, Noda Y, Kobayashi G, et al. Diagnosis of the depth of invasion of gallbladder carcinoma by EUS. Gastrointest Endosc 1999;50(5):660; with permission.

surgically resected gallbladder cancer who had undergone preoperative EUS. They found that all type A tumors were confined to the mucosa, 84.6% of the type C tumors invaded the subserosa, and 85.7% of the type D lesions invaded the serosa or beyond. Similar to the findings of Fujita and colleagues,[43] the type B tumors exhibited varying depths of invasion. When type A tumors were considered to correspond to pTis, type B to pT1, type C to pT2, and type D to pT3-4, the accuracies of the EUS criteria for T staging were 100%, 75.6%, 85.3%, and 92.7%, respectively.

These findings should be confirmed with prospective studies, but the performance of EUS seems to be similar to that of multidetector CT (MDCT), which has been shown to have an accuracy of 83.9% for determining the local extent of gallbladder carcinoma.[45] The performance of EUS for T staging of gallbladder cancer is also similar to that of high resolution transabdominal ultrasonography (HRUS). A recent prospective study by Jang and colleagues[46] evaluated 144 patients with polypoid gallbladder lesions greater than 1 cm in size but without definite local invasion into an adjacent organ. Twenty-seven of these patients were ultimately found to have adenocarcinoma of the gallbladder. All underwent preoperative HRUS, MDCT, and EUS, and these findings were compared with operative and histopathologic findings. There was no significant difference between the diagnostic accuracy of EUS (55.5%) and those of MDCT and HRUS (44.4% and 62.9%, respectively).

## SUMMARY

EUS is an important addition to our armamentarium of endoscopic tools for the evaluation of gallbladder disease. EUS can effectively identify patients with occult cholelithiasis and gallbladder sludge, and is sensitive for the evaluation of choledocholithiasis; it is particularly helpful in determining which patients with intermediate probability of common duct stones should go on to ERCP. Polypoid lesions of the gallbladder can be accurately classified by EUS, which can also be safely used to perform FNA to provide a histologic diagnosis. EUS staging of gallbladder carcinoma can help guide therapy and predict prognosis. With the recent introduction of technologies such as intraductal US and interventional EUS, the future will likely bring further expansion of the role of EUS in the evaluation and management of diseases of the gallbladder and biliary tract.

## REFERENCES

1. Stevens P, Eswaran S. Endoscopic ultrasound for biliary disease. In: Gress F, Savides T, editors. Endoscopic ultrasonography. 2nd edition. Chichester, West Sussex (UK): Wiley-Blackwell; 2009. p. 151–9.

2. Jacobson BC. EUS instruments, room setup, and assistants. In: Gress F, Savides T, editors. Endoscopic ultrasonography. 2nd edition. Wiley-Blackwell; 2009. p. 15–22.
3. Hwang JH, Kimmey MB. Basic principles and fundamentals of EUS imaging. In: Gress F, Savides T, editors. Endoscopic ultrasonography. 2nd edition. Wiley-Blackwell; 2009. p. 5–14.
4. Shaffer EA. Gallstone disease: epidemiology of gallbladder stone disease. Best Pract Res Clin Gastroenterol 2006;20(6):981–96.
5. Cooperberg PL, Burhenne HJ. Real-time ultrasonography. Diagnostic technique of choice in calculous gallbladder disease. N Engl J Med 1980; 302(23):1277–9.
6. Dahan P, Andant C, Levy P, et al. Prospective evaluation of endoscopic ultrasonography and microscopic examination of duodenal bile in the diagnosis of cholecystolithiasis in 45 patients with normal conventional ultrasonography. Gut 1996;38(2):277–81.
7. Liu CL, Lo CM, Chan JK, et al. EUS for detection of occult cholelithiasis in patients with idiopathic pancreatitis. Gastrointest Endosc 2000;51(1):28–32.
8. Thorbøll J, Vilmann P, Jacobsen B, et al. Endoscopic ultrasonography in detection of cholelithiasis in patients with biliary pain and negative transabdominal ultrasonography. Scand J Gastroenterol 2004;39(3):267–9.
9. Hermann RE. The spectrum of biliary stone disease. Am J Surg 1989;158(3): 171–3.
10. Andriulli A, Loperfido S, Napolitano G, et al. Incidence rates of post-ERCP complications: a systematic survey of prospective studies. Am J Gastroenterol 2007;102(8):1781–8.
11. Sugiyama M, Atomi Y. Endoscopic ultrasonography for diagnosing choledocholithiasis: a prospective comparative study with ultrasonography and computed tomography. Gastrointest Endosc 1997;45(2):143–6.
12. Amouyal P, Amouyal G, Levy P, et al. Diagnosis of choledocholithiasis by endoscopic ultrasonography. Gastroenterology 1994;106(4):1062–7.
13. Polkowski M, Palucki J, Regula J, et al. Helical computed tomographic cholangiography versus endosonography for suspected bile duct stones: a prospective blinded study in non-jaundiced patients. Gut 1999;45(5):744–9.
14. Kondo S, Isayama H, Akahane M, et al. Detection of common bile duct stones: comparison between endoscopic ultrasonography, magnetic resonance cholangiography, and helical-computed-tomographic cholangiography. Eur J Radiol 2005;54(2):271–5.
15. Schmidt S, Chevallier P, Novellas S, et al. Choledocholithiasis: repetitive thickslab single-shot projection magnetic resonance cholangiopancreatography versus endoscopic ultrasonography. Eur Radiol 2007;17(1):241–50.
16. Verma D, Kapadia A, Eisen GM, et al. EUS vs MRCP for detection of choledocholithiasis. Gastrointest Endosc 2006;64(2):248–54.
17. Palazzo L, Girollet P, Salmeron M, et al. Value of endoscopic ultrasonography in the diagnosis of common bile duct stones: comparison with surgical exploration and ERCP. Gastrointest Endosc 1995;42(3):225–31.
18. Prat F, Amouyal G, Amouyal P, et al. Prospective controlled study of endoscopic ultrasonography and endoscopic retrograde cholangiography in patients with suspected common bile duct lithiasis. Lancet 1996;347(8994):75–9.
19. Canto MI, Chak A, Stellato T, et al. Endoscopic ultrasonography versus cholangiography for the diagnosis of choledocholithiasis. Gastrointest Endosc 1998; 47(6):439–48.

20. Ney MV, Maluf-Filho F, Sakai P, et al. Echo-endoscopy versus endoscopic retrograde cholangiography for the diagnosis of choledocholithiasis: the influence of the size of the stone and diameter of the common bile duct. Arq Gastroenterol 2005;42(4):239–43.

21. Chak A, Hawes HR, Cooper GS, et al. Prospective assessment of the utility of EUS in the evaluation of gallstone pancreatitis. Gastrointest Endosc 1999;49(5): 599–604.

22. Karakan T, Cindoruk M, Alagozlu H, et al. EUS versus endoscopic retrograde cholangiopancreatography for patients with intermediate probability of bile duct stones: a prospective randomized trial. Gastrointest Endosc 2009;69(2): 244–52.

23. Polkowski M, Regula J, Tilszer A, et al. Endoscopic ultrasound versus endoscopic retrograde cholangiography for patients with intermediate probability of bile duct stones: a randomized trial comparing two management strategies. Endoscopy 2007;39(4):296–303.

24. Lee YT, Chan FK, Leung WK, et al. Comparison of EUS and ERCP in the investigation with suspected biliary obstruction caused by choledocholithiasis: a randomized study. Gastrointest Endosc 2008;67(4):660–8.

25. Liu CL, Fan ST, Lo CM, et al. Comparison of early endoscopic ultrasonography and endoscopic retrograde cholangiopancreatography in the management of acute biliary pancreatitis: a prospective randomized study. Clin Gastroenterol Hepatol 2005;3(12):1238–44.

26. Petrov MS, Savides TJ. Systematic review of endoscopic ultrasonography versus endoscopic retrograde cholangiopancreatography for suspected choledocholithiasis. Br J Surg 2009;96(9):967–74.

27. Segawa K, Arisawa T, Niwa Y, et al. Prevalence of gallbladder polyps among apparently healthy Japanese: ultrasonographic study. Am J Gastroenterol 1992;87(5):630–3.

28. Chen CY, Lu CL, Chang FY, et al. Risk factors for gallbladder polyps in the Chinese population. Am J Gastroenterol 1997;91(11):2066–8.

29. Lee KF, Wong J, Li JC, et al. Polypoid lesions of the gallbladder. Am J Surg 2004; 188(2):186–90.

30. Yang HL, Sun YG, Wang Z. Polypoid lesions of the gallbladder: diagnosis and indications for surgery. Br J Surg 1992;79(3):227–9.

31. Sugiyama M, Xie XY, Atomi Y, et al. Differential diagnosis of small polypoid lesions of the gallbladder: the value of endoscopic ultrasonography. Ann Surg 1999; 229(4):498–504.

32. Azuma T, Yoshikawa T, Araida T, et al. Differential diagnosis of polypoid lesions of the gallbladder by endoscopic ultrasonography. Am J Surg 2001;181(1): 65–70.

33. Choi WB, Lee SK, Kim MH, et al. A new strategy to predict the neoplastic polyps of the gallbladder based on a scoring system using EUS. Gastrointest Endosc 2000;52(3):372–9.

34. Sadamoto Y, Oda S, Tanaka M, et al. A useful approach to the differential diagnosis of small polypoid lesions of the gallbladder, utilizing an endoscopic ultrasound scoring system. Endoscopy 2002;34(12):959–65.

35. Zargar SA, Khuroo MS, Mahajan R, et al. US-guided fine-needle aspiration biopsy of gallbladder masses. Radiology 1991;179(1):275–8.

36. Wu SS, Lin KC, Soon MS, et al. Ultrasound-guided percutaneous transhepatic fine needle aspiration cytology study of gallbladder polypoid lesions. Am J Gastroenterol 1996;91(8):1591–4.

37. Jacobson BC, Pitman MB, Brugge WR. EUS-guided FNA for the diagnosis of gall-bladder masses. Gastrointest Endosc 2003;57(2):251–4.
38. Varadarajulu S, Eloubeidi MA. Endoscopic ultrasound-guided fine-needle aspiration in the evaluation of gallbladder masses. Endoscopy 2005;37(8):751–4.
39. Jemal A, Siegel R, Ward E, et al. Cancer statistics, 2009. CA Cancer J Clin 2009; 59(4):225–49.
40. Reid KM, Ramos-De la Medina A, Donohue JH. Diagnosis and surgical management of gallbladder cancer: a review. J Gastrointest Surg 2007;11(5):671–81.
41. Shih SP, Schulick RD, Cameron JL, et al. Gallbladder cancer: the role of laparoscopy and radical resection. Ann Surg 2007;245(6):893–901.
42. Yamaguchi K, Chijiiwa K, Saiki S, et al. Retrospective analysis of 70 operations for gallbladder carcinoma. Br J Surg 1997;84(2):200–4.
43. Fujita N, Noda Y, Kobayashi G, et al. Diagnosis of the depth of invasion of gallbladder carcinoma by EUS. Gastrointest Endosc 1999;50(5):659–63.
44. Sadamoto Y, Kubo H, Harada N, et al. Preoperative diagnosis and staging of gallbladder carcinoma by EUS. Gastrointest Endosc 2003;58(4):536–41.
45. Kim SJ, Lee JM, Lee JY, et al. Accuracy of preoperative T-staging of gallbladder carcinoma using MDCT. AJR Am J Roentgenol 2008;190(1):74–80.
46. Jang JY, Kim SW, Lee SE, et al. Differential diagnostic and staging accuracies of high resolution ultrasonography, endoscopic ultrasonography, and multidetector computed tomography for gallbladder polypoid lesions and gallbladder cancer. Ann Surg 2009;250(6):943–9.

# Epidemiology of Gallbladder Cancer

Guy D. Eslick, PhD, MMedSc(Clin Epi), MMedStat[a,b,c,*]

---

**KEYWORDS**

- Gallbladder cancer • Gallstones • Obesity • Incidence
- Mortality • Female gender

---

Gallbladder cancer is a rare cancer that was first described more than 2 centuries ago.[1] Individuals with gallbladder cancer usually have no symptoms or signs[2] and deteriorate quickly with the development of metastatic disease. Unfortunately, this gastrointestinal cancer continues to have a poor prognosis because of late diagnosis and few effective treatment options. Gallbladder cancer is an unusual gastrointestinal cancer in that it is much more common among older women than men. The incidence of gallbladder cancer also shows wide geographic and ethnic variations.[3] Understanding the epidemiology of gallbladder cancer has and will continue to provide valuable insights into determining causes and risk factors for gallbladder cancer.

## DESCRIPTIVE EPIDEMIOLOGY
### Incidence

In describing the incidence of gallbladder cancer, two sources of data have been used. First, the *Cancer Incidence in Five Continents, Volume IX* (CI5) presents incidence data from populations worldwide.[4] The reference period for this volume was defined as 1998 to 2002. In addition, data was obtained from the Surveillance, Epidemiology, and End Results (SEER) Program of the National Cancer Institute (NCI), which is a leading source of information on cancer incidence and survival in the United States.[5] SEER currently collects and publishes cancer incidence and survival data from population-based cancer registries covering approximately 26% of the United States population. SEER coverage includes 23% of African Americans, 40% of Hispanics, 42% of American Indians and Alaska Natives, 53% of Asians, and 70% of Hawaiian/Pacific Islanders.

---

[a] Discipline of Surgery, The University of Sydney, Sydney Medical School, Nepean, Penrith, Australia
[b] School of Public Health, The University of Sydney, Sydney, New South Wales, Australia
[c] Department of Nutrition, Harvard School of Public Health, Boston, MA, USA
* Corresponding author. Department of Surgery, Nepean Hospital, Level 5, South Block, P.O. Box 63, Penrith, New South Wales, Australia.
*E-mail address:* eslickg@med.usyd.edu.au

Gastroenterol Clin N Am 39 (2010) 307–330
doi:10.1016/j.gtc.2010.02.011
0889-8553/10/$ – see front matter Crown Copyright © 2010 Published by Elsevier Inc. All rights reserved.

**gastro.theclinics.com**

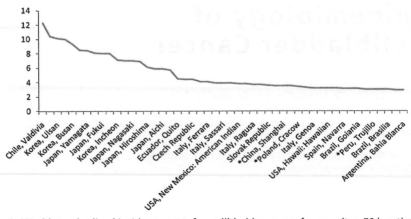

**Fig. 1.** World standardized incidence rates for gallbladder cancer for men (top 50 locations).

### World

Using data from the CI5 database, the world standardized incidence rates for gall-bladder cancer for men (**Fig. 1**) and women (**Fig. 2**) was determined. Chile (Valdivia) was found to have the highest incidence of gall bladder cancer among men and women: 12.3 and 27.3 per 100,000 population, respectively (ASW, age-standardized to the world population). Among the top 10 locations around the world, men seem to have very little geographic variation, with regions in Korea and Japan making up most of these. Most of the top 50 locations for gallbladder cancer have an incidence of approximately 3.0 to 4.0 per 100,000. Geographic locations for women however, shows more variation for gallbladder cancer, with regions in India, Peru, Korea, Japan, Columbia, and the United States among the top 10 locations. Among women, incidences of gallbladder cancer among the top 50 locations around the world are higher than those for men, with most between 4.0 and 6.0. The highest incidence rates among women are twice those of men, but incidence rates decline sharply for women and show a steady decline among men.

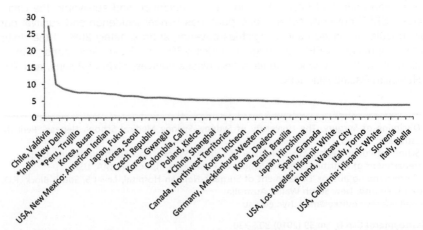

**Fig. 2.** World standardized incidence rates for gallbladder cancer for women (top 50 locations).

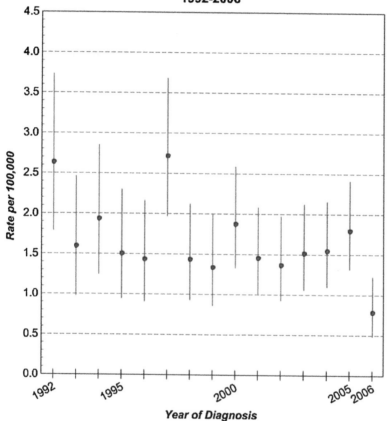

**Age-Adjusted SEER Incidence Rates and 95% Confidence Intervals
Cancer Site: Gallbladder
All Ages, Asian/Pacific Islander, Female
1992-2006**

Cancer sites include invasive cases only unless otherwise noted.
Incidence source: SEER 13 areas (San Francisco, Connecticut, Detroit, Hawaii, Iowa, New
Mexico, Seattle, Utah, Atlanta, San Jose-Monterey, Los Angeles, Alaska Native Registry and
Rural Georgia).
Rates are per 100,000 and are age-adjusted to the 2000 US Std Population (19 age groups -
Census P25-1130).

**Fig. 3.** SEER incidence data for Asian/Pacific Islander women between 1992 and 2006 in the
United States. (*From* National Cancer Institute. Surveillance, Epidemiology, and End Results
(SEER) Program. Available at: http://seer.cancer.gov/.)

## United States

According to the CI5 data, the highest incidence of gallbladder cancer in the United
States occurs among Korean men in Los Angeles and American Indian women in
New Mexico (ASW, 5.9 and 7.1, respectively). Among men, American Indians are
next in terms of incidence (3.8), with Hawaiians (3.2) in Hawaii, Japanese (2.6) in
Los Angeles, and African Americans (2.5) in Connecticut constituting the top five
United States locations.

Among the top five United States locations with the highest incidence of gallbladder
cancer for women, Hispanic Whites (3.9) from Los Angeles were second, followed by

Koreans (3.6) in Los Angeles, Hispanic Whites (3.5) from California, and Hispanic Whites from San Francisco (3.3) . The high incidence of gallbladder cancer among non-White ethnic groups suggests that either genetic or environment factors are responsible for these high rates.

Data from the United States (**Figs. 3–6**) show changes in incidence over time for women (1992–2006), with Asian/Pacific Islanders showing a gradual decline in gallbladder cancer incidence from 2.7 in 1992 to 0.7 in 2006 (see **Fig. 3**). Hispanics also showed a decreased incidence from 4.5 in 1992 to 2.5 in 2006 (see **Fig. 4**). African Americans showed no real change in incidence over this 15-year period (see **Fig. 5**),

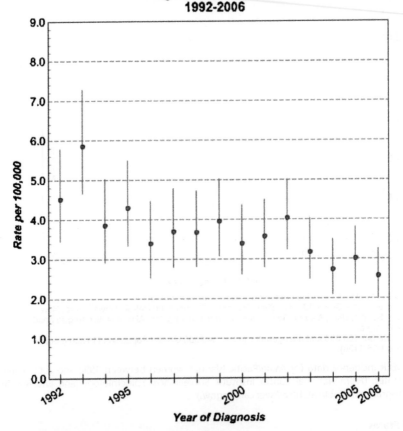

**Age-Adjusted SEER Incidence Rates and 95% Confidence Intervals
Cancer Site: Gallbladder
All Ages, Hispanic, Female
1992-2006**

Cancer sites include invasive cases only unless otherwise noted.
Incidence source: SEER 13 areas (San Francisco, Connecticut, Detroit, Hawaii, Iowa, New Mexico, Seattle, Utah, Atlanta, San Jose-Monterey, Los Angeles, Alaska Native Registry and Rural Georgia).
Rates are per 100,000 and are age-adjusted to the 2000 US Std Population (19 age groups - Census P25-1130).
Hispanics and Non-Hispanics are not mutually exclusive from whites, blacks, Asian/Pacific Islanders, and American Indians/Alaska Natives.
Incidence data for Hispanics and Non-Hispanics are based on NHIA and exclude cases from the Alaska Native Registry.

**Fig. 4.** SEER incidence data for Hispanic women between 1992 and 2006 in the United States. (*From* National Cancer Institute. Surveillance, Epidemiology, and End Results (SEER) Program. Available at: http://seer.cancer.gov/.)

which is similar to non-Hispanic White women, who show a very slight decrease during this timeframe (see **Fig. 6**).

### Mortality

Worldwide data suggest that Mapuche Indians in Chile and Hispanics have the highest mortality, with North American Indians and Mexican Americans following closely behind. This finding is believed to be caused partly by the lack of medical care available in certain geographic locations.[6]

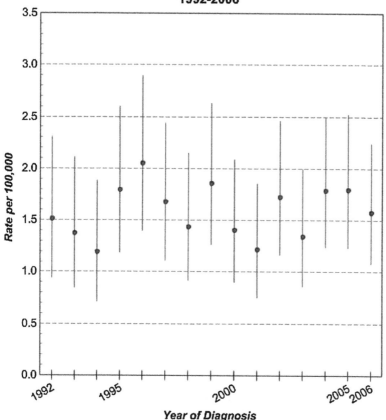

**Age-Adjusted SEER Incidence Rates and 95% Confidence Intervals
Cancer Site: Gallbladder
All Ages, Black, Female
1992-2006**

*Year of Diagnosis*

Cancer sites include invasive cases only unless otherwise noted.
Incidence source: SEER 13 areas (San Francisco, Connecticut, Detroit, Hawaii, Iowa, New Mexico, Seattle, Utah, Atlanta, San Jose-Monterey, Los Angeles, Alaska Native Registry and Rural Georgia).
Rates are per 100,000 and are age-adjusted to the 2000 US Std Population (19 age groups - Census P25-1130).

**Fig. 5.** SEER incidence data for African American women between 1992 and 2006 in the United States. (*From* National Cancer Institute. Surveillance, Epidemiology, and End Results (SEER) Program. Available at: http://seer.cancer.gov/.)

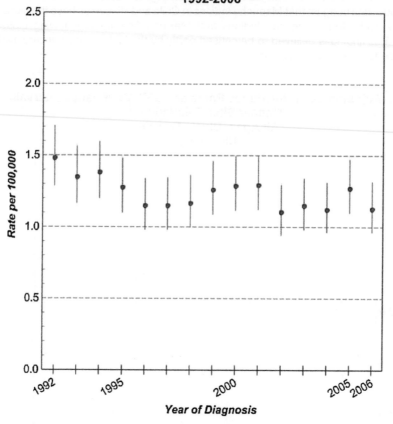

**Fig. 6.** SEER incidence data for non-Hispanic White women between 1992 and 2006 in the United States. (*From* National Cancer Institute. Surveillance, Epidemiology, and End Results (SEER) Program. Available at: http://seer.cancer.gov/.)

In the United States, SEER mortality data between 1992 and 2006 suggest that the mortality rates for gallbladder cancer are decreasing for some ethnic groups. This decline can be seen among Hispanics (**Fig. 7**) and Asian/Pacific Islanders (**Fig. 8**), whereas no change has occurred for African Americans or non-Hispanic Whites (**Figs. 9** and **10**).

### Geographic Variation

Currently, the geographic distribution of gallbladder cancer is not well described.[7] A study on the descriptive epidemiologic trends of gallbladder cancer among 25

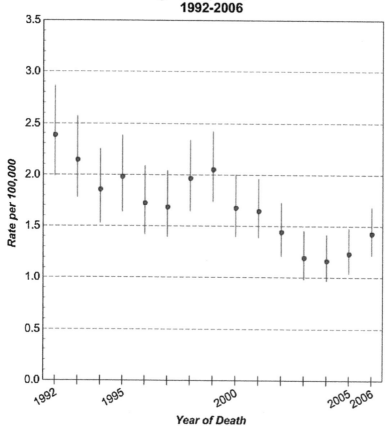

**Age-Adjusted U.S. Mortality Rates and 95% Confidence Intervals**
**Cancer Site: Gallbladder**
**All Ages, Hispanic, Female**
**1992-2006**

Cancer sites include invasive cases only unless otherwise noted.
Mortality source: US Mortality Files, National Center for Health Statistics, CDC.
Rates are per 100,000 and are age-adjusted to the 2000 US Std Population (19 age groups - Census P25-1130).
Hispanics and Non-Hispanics are not mutually exclusive from whites, blacks, Asian/Pacific Islanders, and
American Indians/Alaska Natives.
Mortality data for Hispanics and Non-Hispanics do not include cases from Connecticut, Maine, Maryland,
Minnesota, New Hampshire, New York, North Dakota, Oklahoma, Vermont.

**Fig. 7.** SEER mortality data for Hispanic women between 1992 and 2006 in the United States. (*From* National Cancer Institute. Surveillance, Epidemiology, and End Results (SEER) Program. Available at: http://seer.cancer.gov/.)

European countries between 1965 to 1989[7] reported the highest mortality rates in Hungary (3.9/100,000 men; 7.4/100,000 women), with high rates also in Germany, Austria, Czechoslovakia, Hungary, and Poland. During the 25-year period assessed, mortality rates were found to have increased in Czechoslovakia and Hungary but were stable in Poland and declined in Austria and Germany. The lowest mortality rates were reported in Belgium, France, Britain, Ireland, Norway, Bulgaria, and Mediterranean countries. Trends among this group found that over the 25-year period, mortality rates declined in Bulgaria and Great Britain but increased in all other countries.

In terms of geographic location in the United States, data from the National Cancer Institute (NCI) between 1970 and 1994 highlight states with high mortality for

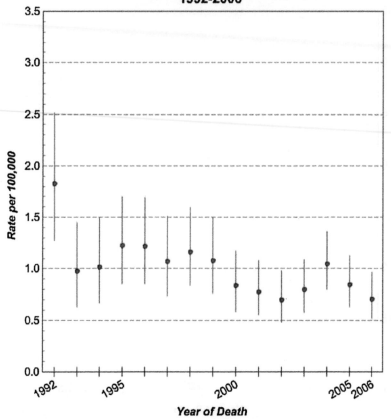

Age-Adjusted U.S. Mortality Rates and 95% Confidence Intervals
Cancer Site: Gallbladder
All Ages, Asian/Pacific Islander, Female
1992-2006

Cancer sites include invasive cases only unless otherwise noted.
Mortality source: US Mortality Files, National Center for Health Statistics, CDC.
Rates are per 100,000 and are age-adjusted to the 2000 US Std Population (19 age groups -
Census P25-1130).

**Fig. 8.** SEER mortality data for Asian/Pacific Islander women between 1992 and 2006 in the United States. (*From* National Cancer Institute. Surveillance, Epidemiology, and End Results (SEER) Program. Available at: http://seer.cancer.gov/.)

gallbladder cancer. Among White men, the highest mortality rates occurred in New Mexico, Arizona, Minnesota, North Dakota, Ohio, West Virginia, Maine, and Rhode Island (**Figs. 11** and **12**). African American had very few high mortality states in during this period, with these only consisting of Oklahoma, Missouri, Massachusetts, and New Jersey (**Fig. 13**). The highest mortality rates for African American women were seen in Oklahoma, Kansas, Wisconsin, Kentucky, South Carolina, and West Virginia. (**Fig. 14**).

Another recent study reported that most countries in Europe, Canada, the United States, and the United Kingdom show a decline in gallbladder cancer–associated mortality for both genders. However, increases in mortality among men were found for Iceland, Costa Rica, and Korea.[8] The variation seen in Europe and the United

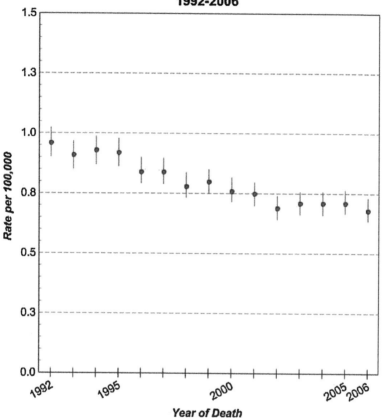

**Age-Adjusted U.S. Mortality Rates and 95% Confidence Intervals**
**Cancer Site: Gallbladder**
**All Ages, Non-Hispanic White, Female**
**1992-2006**

Cancer sites include invasive cases only unless otherwise noted.
Mortality source: US Mortality Files, National Center for Health Statistics, CDC.
Rates are per 100,000 and are age-adjusted to the 2000 US Std Population (19 age groups - Census P25-1130).
Hispanics and Non-Hispanics are not mutually exclusive from whites, blacks, Asian/Pacific Islanders, and American Indians/Alaska Natives.
Mortality data for Hispanics and Non-Hispanics do not include cases from Connecticut, Maine, Maryland, Minnesota, New Hampshire, New York, North Dakota, Oklahoma, Vermont.

**Fig. 9.** SEER mortality data for non-Hispanic White women between 1992 and 2006 in the United States. (*From* National Cancer Institute. Surveillance, Epidemiology, and End Results (SEER) Program. Available at: http://seer.cancer.gov/.)

States could reflect the movement of certain populations, International Classification of Diseases coding for gallbladder cancer, changes in diet, or increases in rates of obesity, or that these locations do not offer sufficient diagnostic modalities for individuals with gallbladder cancer or screen high-risk populations within these states.

## RISK FACTORS

Traditionally, risk factors for the development of gallbladder cancer have essentially been chronic cholelithiasis and female gender. However, other factors also promote

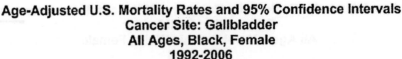

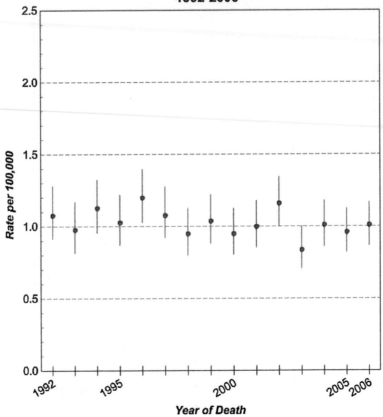

Cancer sites include invasive cases only unless otherwise noted.
Mortality source: US Mortality Files, National Center for Health Statistics, CDC.
Rates are per 100,000 and are age-adjusted to the 2000 US Std Population (19 age groups -
Census P25-1130).

**Fig. 10.** SEER mortality data for African American women between 1992 and 2006 in the United States. (*From* National Cancer Institute. Surveillance, Epidemiology, and End Results (SEER) Program. Available at: http://seer.cancer.gov/.)

the development of gallbladder cancer. An important risk factor seems to be infection, with studies supporting the relationship with *Salmonella typhi*.[9] The continual discovery of new organisms presents new possibilities for elucidating important and potentially treatable risk factors.[10]

### Age

The incidence of gallbladder cancer increases with age, with the highest incidence usually found in individuals older than 65 years.[2] However, a recent analysis of the SEER database between 1973 to 2002 found a substantial decrease has occurred

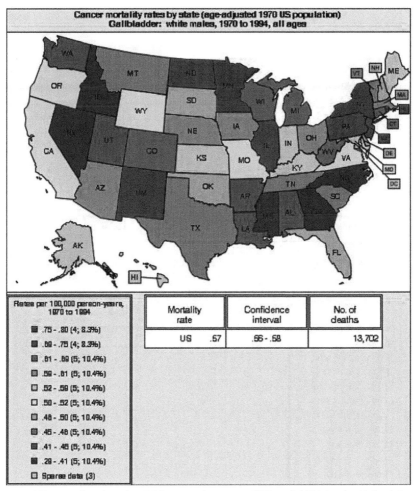

Fig. 11. NCI mortality data for White men between 1970 and 1994 in the United States. (*From* National Cancer Institute. Available at: http://www.cancer.gov/.)

in the incidence of gallbladder cancer among individuals older than 50 years, and actually reported an increased incidence of gallbladder cancer in younger age groups (<50 years).[11]

### Gender

It has long been known that women are more likely to develop gallbladder cancer, with odds ratios suggesting an increased risk ranging between 2 and 8 times that of men.[11] Gallbladder disease has always been associated with the four Fs: (1) fat (overweight); (2) age older than 40 years; (3) female gender; and (4) fertile. These risk factors certainly increase a woman's chance of developing gallbladder disease, but other factors also contribute to the development of gallbladder cancer.

### Gallbladder Disease

Gallstone disease is an important risk factor for the development of gallbladder cancer; however, not all individuals with gallstones will develop gallbladder cancer.

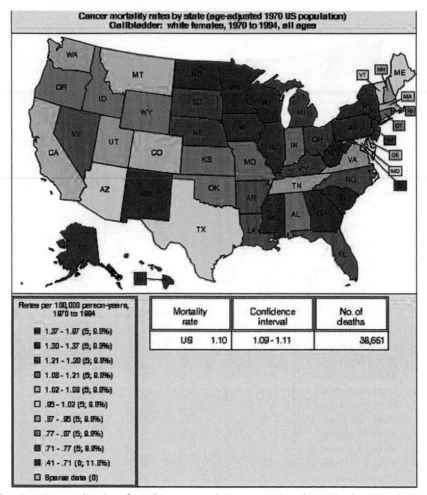

**Fig. 12.** NCI mortality data for White women between 1970 and 1994 in the United States. (*From* National Cancer Institute. Available at: http://www.cancer.gov/.)

Moreover, having a history of benign gallbladder diseases increases the risk for developing gallbladder cancer, although some studies do not support this statement (**Table 1**). Most case-control studies strongly suggest a relationship, whereas cohort studies also support a link but with less strength.

A family history of gallbladder disease also increases the risk for developing gallbladder cancer, with case-control and cohort studies supporting this hypothesis. Studies have also shown that individuals who develop gallstones are four times (95% CI, 1.5–11) more likely to develop gallbladder cancer at a younger age. These patients are likely to present with gallbladder cancer an average of 6 years earlier than those with no gallstones.[12]

### Obesity

Clearly, increasing body mass index (BMI), particularly in the overweight (BMI, 25.0–29.9) and obese (BMI, >30) range, increases risk for developing gallstones.[3] Studies

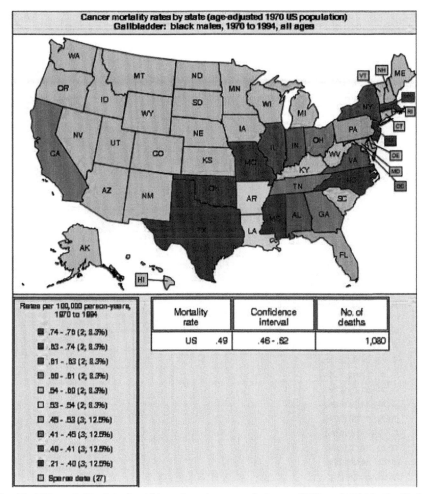

**Fig. 13.** NCI mortality data for African American men between 1970 and 1994 in the United States. (*From* National Cancer Institute. Available at: http://www.cancer.gov/.)

assessing increasing BMI as a risk factor for gallbladder cancer have reported conflicting findings (**Table 2**). A recent meta-analysis focusing on the potential relationship between excess body weight and risk for gallbladder cancer[13] included three case-control and eight cohort studies in the final random-effects analysis, which had a total of 3288 cases of gallbladder cancer. No heterogeneity was reported among the studies. Compared with normal-weight subjects, individuals who were overweight or obese had a relative risk (RR) for developing gallbladder cancer of 1.15 (95% CI, 1.01–1.30) or 1.66 (95% CI, 1.47–1.88), respectively. Moreover, obese women (RR, 1.88; 95% CI, 1.66–2.13) were at greater risk than obese men (RR, 1.35; 95% CI, 1.09–1.68). In the United States, correlations between increasing rates of gallbladder disease and obesity have been made among Hispanics, who are more likely to be obese or overweight than non-Hispanic whites.[14] This finding suggests that the effect of obesity may be mediated by other factors, such as ethnicity. Further research is needed to elucidate the mechanisms responsible.

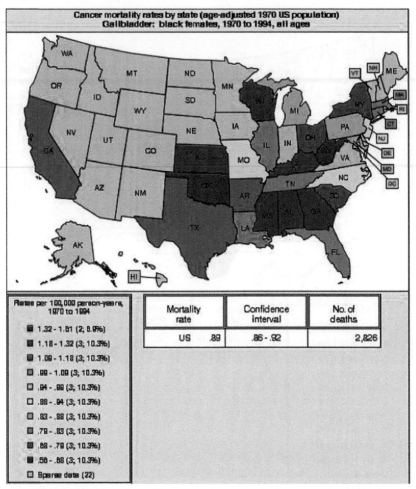

**Fig. 14.** NCI mortality data for African American women between 1970 and 1994 in the United States. (*From* National Cancer Institute. Available at: http://www.cancer.gov/.)

### Reproductive Factors

Studies linking reproductive factors, such as increased parity and gravidity, to gallbladder cancer have provided conflicting results (**Table 3**). Previous research suggests an association between these reproductive factors and the development of gallstones. Other factors, such as oral contraceptives, have not been shown to increase the risk for gallbladder cancer. Furthermore, conflicting studies provide no clear picture of the potential link between menopause and hormone replacement therapy in relation to gallbladder cancer.

A prospective case-control study from India assessed lifestyle and reproductive factors in 78 incident cases of gallbladder cancer and 78 age- and gender-matched controls with gallstones.[14] Almost two thirds of the cases and controls were women (68%), and the mean ages were 50 years for cases and 43 years for controls. Tobacco use (odds ratio [OR], 2.71; 95% CI, 1.22–6.02) and chewing tobacco (OR, 2.50; 95%

**Table 1**

**Relative risks for gallbladder cancer among patients with a history of selected gallbladder diseases**

| Study | Participants | Relative Risk (95% CI) | Adjustment |
|---|---|---|---|
| History of benign gallbladder diseases[a] | | | |
| Cohort studies[b] | | | |
| Maringhini et al, 1987 (USA)[15] | | 2.8 (0.9–6.6) | Age and sex |
| | Men | 8.3 (1.0–30.0)[c] | Age and sex |
| | Women | 2.0 (0.4–5.7)[c] | Age and sex |
| Chow et al,[16] 1999 (Denmark) | | 3.6 (2.6–4.9) | Age and sex |
| Yagyu et al,[17] 2004 (Japan) | Men | 1.2 (0.3–4.7) | Age |
| | Women | 1.1 (0.4–2.9) | Age |
| Case-control studies[d] | | | |
| Lowenfels et al,[18] 1985 (USA) | Non-Indians | 4.4 (2.6–7.3) | Age, sex, center, alcohol, smoking, education, and response status |
| | Indians | 20.9 (8.1–54.0) | Age, sex, center, alcohol, smoking, education, and response status |
| Nervi et al,[19] 1988 (Chile) | | 7.0 (5.9–8.3) | Age, sex, country |
| WHO,[20] 1989[e] | | 2.3 (1.2–4.4) | None reported |
| Kato et al,[21] 1989 (Japan) | | 34.4 (4.51–266.0) | None reported |
| Zatonski et al,[22] 1997[f] | | 4.4 (2.6–7.5) | Age and sex |
| Okamoto et al,[23] 1999 (Japan) | | 10.8 (4.1–28.4)[g] | Sex, age, ethnicity, smoking, and socioeconomic status |
| Khan et al,[24] 1999 (USA) | Women | 26.6 (7.0–101.4) | Age, ethnicity, socioeconomic status, hysterectomy, menopause, parity, diabetes, and smoking |
| | | 28.9 (4.7–173.0)[c] | |
| Family history of benign gallbladder diseases | | | |
| Case-control studies[h] | | | |
| Kato et al,[21] 1989 (Japan) | | 3.0 (1.3–6.5) | None reported |

(continued on next page)

**Table 1**
*(continued)*

| Study | Participants | Relative Risk (95% CI) | Adjustment |
|---|---|---|---|
| Strom et al,[25] 1995 (Bolivia, Mexico) | | 3.6 (1.3–11.4) | Age, sex, and hospital |
| Family history of gallbladder cancer[i] | | | |
| Cohort studies[j] | | | |
| Goldgar et al,[26] 1994 (USA) | First-degree relatives | 2.1 (0.2–6.1) | Age at diagnosis |
| Hemminki et al,[27] 2003 (Sweden) | Parents | 5.1 (2.4–9.3) | Age, sex, region, period, and socioeconomic status |
| | Offspring | 4.1 (2.0–7.6)[c] | Age, sex, region, period, and socioeconomic status |
| Case-control studies | | | |
| Fernandez et al,[28] 1994 (Italy) | First degree relatives | 13.9 (1.2–163.9) | Age, sex, residence, and education |

[a] Summary relative risk for all studies was 4.9 (95% CI, 3.3–7.4) and heterogeneity test between studies was $\chi^2_6 = 57.361$; $P<.001$.

[b] Summary relative risk for cohort studies was 2.2 (95% CI, 1.2–4.2) and heterogeneity test between studies was $\chi^2_3 = 6.918$; $P = .075$.

[c] Not included in the summary estimates.

[d] Summary relative risk for case-control studies was 7.1 (95% CI, 4.5–11.2) and heterogeneity test between studies was $\chi^2_7 = 28.540$; $P<.001$.

[e] Chile, China, Colombia, Israel, Kenya, Mexico.

[f] Australia, Canada, Netherlands, Poland.

[g] Estimated from available data.

[h] Summary relative risk for case-control studies was 3.2 (95% CI, 1.7–6.1) and heterogeneity test between studies was $\chi^2_1 = 0.007$; $P = .791$.

[i] Summary relative risk for all studies was 4.8 (95% CI, 2.6–8.9) and heterogeneity test between studies was $\chi^2_2 = 1.647$; $P = .439$.

[j] Summary relative risk for cohort studies was 4.5 (95% CI, 2.4–8.5) and heterogeneity test between studies was $\chi^2_2 = 0.895$; $P = .344$.

*From* Randi G, Franceschi S, La Vecchia C. Gallbladder cancer worldwide: Geographical distribution and risk factors. Int J Cancer 2006;118:1591–602; with permission.

**Table 2**
Relative risks for gallbladder cancer for highest versus lowest category of body mass index

| Study | Reference Category | Highest Category | Participants | Relative Risk (95% CI) | Adjustment |
|---|---|---|---|---|---|
| Cohort studies | | | | | |
| Moller et al,[29] 1994 (Denmark) | Non obese | Obese | Men | 0.5 (0.1–1.8) | None reported |
| | Non obese | Obese | Women | 1.4 (0.9–2.1) | None reported |
| Calle et al,[30] 2003 (USA) | 18.5–24.9 | 30.0–34.9 | Men | 1.8 (1.1–2.9) | Age, race, education, and many (8) lifestyle variables |
| | 18.5–24.9 | 30.0–34.9 | Women | 2.1 (1.6–2.9) | Age, race, education, and many (8) lifestyle variables |
| Samanic et al,[31] 2004 (USA) | Non obese | Obese | White men | 1.7 (1.1–2.6) | Age and calendar year |
| | Non obese | Obese | Black men | 0.9 (0.2–3.9) | Age and calendar year |
| Kuriyama et al,[32] 2005 (Japan) | 18.5–24.9 | 25.0–27.4 | Men | 0.5 (0.1–3.9) | Age and many (11) lifestyle and reproductive variables |
| | 18.5–24.9 | ≥30 | Women | 4.5 (1.4–14.2) | Age and many (11) lifestyle and reproductive variables |
| Case-control studies | | | | | |
| Moerman et al,[33] 1994 (Netherlands) | <27 | ≥27 | Women | 1.4 (0.7–2.6)[a] | Subjects frequently matched for age and sex |
| Strom et al,[25] 1995 (Bolivia, Mexico) | <24 | >28 | Body mass index average | 1.6 (0.4–6.1) | Age and sex |
| | <25 | >29 | Body mass index maximum | 2.6 (0.5–18.6) | Age and sex |
| Zatonski et al,[22] 1997[b] | I quartile | IV quartile | Men | 1.0 (0.3–2.8) | Age, center, alcohol, smoking, education, and response status |
| | I quartile | IV quartile | Women | 2.1 (1.2–3.8) | Age, center, alcohol, smoking, education, and response status |
| Serra et al,[34] 2002 (Chile) | <24.9 | >30 | | 0.9 (0.4–1.8) | Age, sex, gallstone disease |

a Estimated from available data.
b Australia, Canada, Netherlands, Poland.
*Data from* Randi G, Franceschi S, La Vecchia C. Gallbladder cancer worldwide: Geographical distribution and risk factors. Int J Cancer 2006;118:1591–602.

**Table 3**
Relative risks for gallbladder cancer for highest versus lowest category of the selected reproductive and lifestyle factors

| Study | Reference Category | Highest Category | Relative Risk (95% CI) | Adjustment |
|---|---|---|---|---|
| Parity: number of births | | | | |
| Lambe et al,[35] 1993 (Sweden) | 0 | ≥6 | 3.0 (1.1–8.0) | Age |
| | 1 | ≥6 | 1.7 (0.6–4.7) | Age and age at first birth |
| De Aretxabala et al,[36] 1995 (Chile) | <5 | ≥5 | 4.2 (1.5–12.8) | Subjects matched for age |
| Tavani et al,[37] 1996 (Italy) | 0 | ≥1 | 1.3 (0.5–3.4) | Age and cholelithiasis |
| | 0 | ≥4 | 2.9 (0.9–9.6) | Age and cholelithiasis |
| Pandey et al,[38] 2003 (India) | ≤3 | >3 | 3.9 (1.4–10.3) | None reported |
| Number of pregnancies | | | | |
| Moerman et al,[33] 1994 (Netherlands) | 0 | ≥1 | 2.2 (0.7–6.7) | Age |
| | 1–2 | ≥5 | 1.7 (0.7–4.1) | Age |
| | 1–2 | ≥5 | 1.5 (0.6–3.7) | Age and age at first pregnancy |
| De Aretxabala et al,[36] 1995 (Chile) | <5 | ≥5 | 3.4 (1.2–9.9) | Subjects matched for age |
| Zatonski et al,[22] 1997[a] | 1 | ≥3 | 2.2 (0.9–5.4) | Age, sex, center, alcohol, smoking, education, and response status |
| Khan et al,[24] 1999 (USA) | 0 | ≥1 | 1.0 (0.6–1.6) | Age, ethnicity, socioeconomic status, cholelithiasis, hysterectomy, and postmenopause |
| Serra et al,[34] 2002 (Chile) | ≤5 | >5 | 1.5 (0.8–2.7) | Age, sex, gallstone disease |
| Pandey et al,[38] 2003 (India) | ≤3 | >3 | 6.7 (1.8–23.4) | None reported |
| Age at first childbirth | | | | |
| Lambe et al,[35] 1993 (Sweden) | <20 | ≥35 | 0.5 (0.2–1.4) | Age and number of births |
| Tavani et al,[37] 1996 (Italy) | <20 | >30 | 0.9 (0.2–4.0) | Age and cholelithiasis |

| Study | | | RR (95% CI) | Adjustments |
|---|---|---|---|---|
| Zatonski et al,[22] 1997[a] | <20 | ≥20 | 0.5 (0.3–1.0) | Age, center, alcohol, smoking, schooling, parity, and response status |
| Pandey et al,[38] 2003 (India) | ≤20 | >20 | 0.8 (0.4–1.6) | None reported |
| **Oral contraceptive use[b]** | | | | |
| WHO,[20] 1989[c] | Never | Ever | 0.6 (0.3–1.3) | History of gallbladder disease, age, center, and year of interview |
| Moerman et al,[33] 1994 (Netherlands) | Never | Ever | 1.2 (0.4–3.2) | Age at diagnosis |
| Zatonski et al,[22] 1997[a] | Never | Ever | 1.0 (0.5–2.0) | Age, sex, center, alcohol, smoking, education, and response status |
| **Menopausal status[d]** | | | | |
| Moerman et al,[33] 1994 (Netherlands) | Pre | Natural post | 1.3 (0.3–5.4) | Age at diagnosis/interview |
| Tavani et al,[37] 1996 (Italy) | Pre/peri | Natural post | 0.2 (0.03–0.9) | Age and cholelithiasis |
| Khan et al,[24] 1999 (USA) | Pre | Post | 21.3 (1.1–500) | Age, ethnicity, socioeconomic status, cholelithiasis, hysterectomy, and ever-pregnant |
| Pandey et al,[38] 2003 (India) | Pre | Post | 0.7 (0.5–0.8) | None reported |
| **Hormone replacement therapy use[e]** | | | | |
| Moerman et al,[33] 1994 (Netherlands) | Never | Ever | 0.5 (0.1–1.7) | Age and body mass index |
| Zatonski et al,[22] 1997[a] | Never | Ever | 0.5 (0.2–1.0) | Age, sex, center, alcohol, smoking, education, and response status |
| Gallus et al,[39] 2002 (Italy) | Never | Ever | 3.2 (1.1–9.3) | Age, year of interview, education, smoking, drinking, body mass index, parity, type and age at menopause |

[a] Australia, Canada, Netherlands, Poland.
[b] Summary relative risk for all studies was 0.9 (95% CI, 0.5–1.3) and heterogeneity test between studies was $\chi^2_2 = 1.501$; $P = .472$.
[c] Chile, China, Colombia, Israel, Kenya, Mexico.
[d] Summary relative risk for all studies was 0.9 (95% CI, 0.3–2.6) and heterogeneity test between studies was $\chi^2_3 = 7.566$; $P = .056$.
[e] Summary relative risk for all studies was 0.9 (95% CI, 0.3–3.3) and heterogeneity test between studies was $\chi^2_2 = 8.127$; $P = .0017$.
Data from Randi G, Franceschi S, La Vecchia C. Gallbladder cancer worldwide: Geographical distribution and risk factors. Int J Cancer 2006;118:1591–602.

**Table 4**
**Relative risks for gallbladder cancer by presence of markers or history of selected infections**

| Study | Infecting Organism | Method and Marker | Exposed Cases/Exposed Controls | Unexposed Cases/Unexposed Controls | Participants | RR (95% CI) | Adjustment |
|---|---|---|---|---|---|---|---|
| *Salmonella typhi* and *S paratyphi*[a] | | | | | | | |
| Cohort studies[b] | | | | | | | |
| Caygill et al,[9] 1994 (UK) | Different typhoid and paratyphoid phage types | Chronic carriers (still excreting 2 years after infection) | 5/83 | | | 167 (54.1–389) | Sex, age, and age at infection |
| Yagyu et al,[17] 2004 (Japan) | Typhoid fever | Self-reported | 2/634 | 31/37,974 | Men | 2.1 (0.5–8.7) | Age |
| Case-control studies[c] | | | | | | | |
| Strom et al,[25] 1995 (Bolivia, Mexico) | *S typhi* | Physician-diagnosed typhoid | None reported | None reported | | 12.7 (1.5–598) | Age, sex, and hospital |
| | *S typhi* | Carriers and past exposure (serologic tests) | 7/4 | 8/4 | | 0.9 (0.2–4.3)[d] | |
| Singh et al,[40] 1996 (India) | *S typhi* and paratyphi | Salmonella in bile specimens | 5/2 | 33/65 | | 4.9 (0.9–26.8)[d] | Controls with gallstones |
| Nath et al,[41] 1997 (India) | *S typhi* and paratyphi-A | Salmonella in bile specimens | 4/1 | 24/57 | | 9.2 (1.0–86.4)[d] | Controls with gallstones |
| Shukla et al,[42] 2000 (India) | *S typhi* | Carriers (polysaccharide antigen -Vi-concentration) | 15/2 | 36/38 | | 7.9 (1.7–37.1) | None reported |

| Study | Factor | Detection | | | Ethnicity | RR (95% CI) | Adjustment |
|---|---|---|---|---|---|---|---|
| Dutta et al,[43] 2000 (India) | S typhi | Carriers (polysaccharide antigen -Vi- concentration) | 6/2 | 31/78 | | 14 (1.8–92) | Smoking, age, socioeconomic status |
| Serra et al,[34] 2002 (Chile) | Typhoid fever | Self-reported | 11/9 | 103/105 | | 0.5 (0.2–1.2) | Age, sex, gallstone disease |
| Pandey et al,[38] 2003 (India) | Typhoid fever | Self-reported | 14/13 | 60/88 | | 1.3 (0.9–2.0) | None reported |

*Helicobacter bilis and H pylori*

*Case-control studies[e]*

| Study | Factor | Detection | | | Ethnicity | RR (95% CI) | Adjustment |
|---|---|---|---|---|---|---|---|
| Matsukura et al,[44] 2002 (Japan) | H bilis | PCR: urease A gene and 16S gene | 13/8 | 2/8 | Japanese | 6.5 (1.1–38.6) | Unadjusted/controls with gallstones |
| | H bilis | PCR: urease A gene and 16S gene | 11/10 | 3/16 | Thai | 5.9 (1.3–26.3) | Unadjusted/controls with gallstones |
| Bulajic et al,[45] 2002 (Yugoslavia) | H pylori | PCR: H pylori DNA | 12/3 | 3/8 | | 9.9 (1.4–70.5) | Age and sex |
| Murata et al,[46] 2004 (Japan) | H bilis | PCR: H bilis DNA | 3/2 | 8/14 | | 2.6 (0.6–4.6)[d] | Controls with gallstones |

a Summary relative risk for all studies was 4.8 (95% CI, 1.4–17.3) and heterogeneity test between studies was $\chi^2_9 = 102.129$; $P<.001$, without self-reported information studies was 10.2 (95% CI, 2.0–50.9) and heterogeneity test between studies was $\chi^2_6 = 38.06$; $P<.001$.

b Summary relative risk for cohort studies was 19.3 (95% CI, 0.3–407.7) and heterogeneity test between studies was $\chi^2_1 = 24.417$; $P<.001$.

c Summary relative risk for case-control studies was 2.6 (95% CI, 1.2–6.1) and heterogeneity test between studies was $\chi^2_7 = 22.464$; $P = .002$, without self-reported information studies was 5.2 (95% CI, 2.1–12.7) and heterogeneity test between studies was $\chi^2_3 = 6.846$; $P = .232$.

d Estimated from available data.

e Summary relative risk for all studies was 4.3 (95% CI, 2.1–8.8) and heterogeneity test between studies was $\chi^2_3 = 2.010$; $P = .570$.

*From Randi G, Franceschi S, La Vecchia C. Gallbladder cancer worldwide: Geographical distribution and risk factors. Int J Cancer 2006;118:1591–602; with permission.*

CI, 1.24–5.04) were associated with an increased risk for developing gallbladder cancer. In addition, a younger age at menarche increased the risk for developing gall-bladder cancer almost threefold (OR, 2.63; 95% CI, 1.45–6.03), as did the number of childbirths (OR, 3.69; 95% CI, 1.60–9.60), number of pregnancies (OR, 6.15; 95% CI, 1.70–21.30), age at last childbirth (OR, 2.89; 95% CI, 1.21–7.69), and postmenopausal status (OR, 6.75; 95% CI, 3.10–14.52).

### Bacterial Infections

The best evidence for an association between chronic infection and the development of gallbladder cancer comes from studies on S typhi and S paratyphi (**Table 4**). In a cohort study, Caygill and colleagues[9] provided very strong evidence (RR, 167; 95% CI, 54.1–389) for a relationship between chronic carriers with typhoid and para-typhoid, although these data were only based on five gallbladder cancer cases.

More recently, new organisms, namely Helicobacter bilis and H pylori, have been identified from bile specimens, with data suggesting a relationship with the develop-ment of gallbladder cancer (see **Table 4**). The RRs produced are consistent and range from 5.9 to 9.9 among statistically significant studies. Further research is required on these organisms, and if future studies provide greater evidence of a role in the devel-opment of gallbladder disease or cancer, this may be the impetus for developing treatments.

No evidence suggests that viruses, parasites, or fungi, including yeasts, are associ-ated with the development of gallbladder cancer. However, other infections, including bacteria, have been linked to acute acalculous cholecystitis, but none have been investigated for their potential to induce gallbladder cancer. These bacteria include organisms such as Dengue virus, Epstein-Barr virus, Actinomycosis, Candida species, Dolosigranulum pigrum, Clonorchis sinensis, and Opisthorchis viverrini. Although no current evidence is available regarding these organisms, some might induce chronic inflammation that may lead to cancer. Many of these infections may be endemic to areas that have high incidence of gallbladder cancer and require further research.

### SUMMARY

Current data suggest that the epidemiology of gallbladder cancer is constantly evolving, with much of this change caused by lifestyle, cultural, mixing of different ethnicities, and dietary factors. Constant monitoring of these changes will provide clues to understanding this lethal disease and offer opportunities for screening and early treatment among high-risk groups.

### REFERENCES

1. Stollde M. Rationis Medendi in Noscomio Practico Vindobonensi. In: Rolleston HD, McNee JS, editors. Diseases of the liver, gallbladder and bile ducts. 3rd edition. London: Macmillan; 1929. p. 691.
2. Portincasa P, Moschetta A, Petruzzelli M, et al. Symptoms and diagnosis of gall-bladder stones. Best Pract Res Clin Gastroenterol 2006;20:1017–29.
3. Shaffer EA. Epidemiology of gallbladder stone disease. Best Pract Res Clin Gas-troenterol 2006;20:981–96.
4. No. 160. In: Curado MP, Edwards B, Shin HR, et al, editors, Cancer incidence in five continents, vol. IX. Lyon (France): IARC Scientific Publications; 2007. IARC.
5. Edwards BK, Ward E, Kohler BA, et al. Annual report to the nation on the status of cancer, 1975-2006, featuring colorectal cancer trends and impact of interventions

(risk factors, screening, and treatment) to reduce future rates. Cancer 2010;116: 544–73.

6. Wistuba II, Gazdar AF. Gallbladder cancer: lessons from a rare tumour. Nat Rev Cancer 2004;4:695–706.

7. Zatonski W, La Vecchia C, Levi F, et al. Descriptive epidemiology of gall-bladder cancer in Europe. J Cancer Res Clin Oncol 1993;119:165–71.

8. Hariharan D, Saied A, Kocher HM. Analysis of mortality rates for gallbladder cancer across the world. HPB(Oxford) 2008;10:327–31.

9. Caygill CP, Hill MJ, Braddick M, et al. Cancer mortality in chronic typhoid and paratyphoid carriers. Lancet 1994;343:83–4.

10. Schlenker C, Surawicz CM. Emerging infections of the gastrointestinal tract. Best Pract Res Clin Gastroenterol 2009;23:89–99.

11. Kiran RP, Pokala N, Dudrick SJ. Incidence pattern and survival for gallbladder cancer over three decades: an analysis of 10301 patients. Ann Surg Oncol 2007;14:827–32.

12. Dutta U, Nagi B, Garg PK, et al. Patients with gallstones develop gallbladder cancer at an earlier age. Eur J Cancer Prev 2005;14:381–5.

13. Larsson SC, Wolk A. Obesity and the risk of gallbladder cancer: a meta-analysis. Br J Cancer 2007;96:1457–61.

14. O'Brien K, Cokkinides V, Jemal A, et al. Cancer statistics for Hispanics, 2003. CA Cancer J Clin 2003;53:208–26.

15. Maringhini A, Moreau JA, Melton LJ III, et al. Gallstones, gallbladder cancer, and other gastrointestinal malignancies. An epidemiologic study in Rochester, Minnesota. Ann Intern Med 1987;107:30–5.

16. Chow WH, Johansen C, Gridley G, et al. Gallstones, cholecystectomy and risk of cancers of the liver, biliary tract and pancreas. Br J Cancer 1999;79:640–4.

17. Yagyu K, Lin Y, Obata Y, et al. JACC Study Group. Bowel movement frequency, medical history and the risk of gallbladder cancer death: a cohort study in Japan. Cancer Sci 2004;95:674–8.

18. Lowenfels AB, Lindstrom CG, Conway MJ, et al. Gallstones and risk of gallbladder cancer. J Natl Cancer Inst 1985;75:77–80.

19. Nervi F, Duarte I, Gomez G, et al. Frequency of gallbladder cancer in Chile, a high-risk area. Int J Cancer 1988;41:657–60.

20. WHO. Combined oral contraceptives and gallbladder cancer. The WHO collaborative study of neoplasia and steroid contraceptives. Int J Epidemiol 1989;18: 309–14.

21. Kato K, Akai S, Tominaga S, et al. A case-control study of biliary tract cancer in Niigata Prefecture, Japan. Jpn J Cancer Res 1989;80:932–8.

22. Zatonski WA, Lowenfels AB, Boyle P, et al. Epidemiologic aspects of gallbladder cancer: a case-control study of the SEARCH Program of the International Agency for Research on Cancer. J Natl Cancer Inst 1997;89:1132–8.

23. Okamoto M, Okamoto H, Kitahara F, et al. Ultrasonographic evidence of association of polyps and stones with gallbladder cancer. Am J Gastroenterol 1999;94: 446–50.

24. Khan ZR, Neugut AI, Ahsan H, et al. Risk factors for biliary tract cancers. Am J Gastroenterol 1999;94:149–52.

25. Strom BL, Soloway RD, Rios-Dalenz JL, et al. Risk factors for gallbladder cancer. An international collaborative case-control study. Cancer 1995;76:1747–56.

26. Goldgar DE, Easton DF, Cannon-Albright LA, et al. Systematic population-based assessment of cancer risk in first-degree relatives of cancer probands. J Natl Cancer Inst 1994;86:1600–8.

27. Hemminki K, Li X. Familial liver and gall bladder cancer: a nationwide epidemiological study from Sweden. Gut 2003;52:592–6.
28. Fernandez E, La Vecchia C, D'Avanzo B, et al. Family history and the risk of liver, gallbladder, and pancreatic cancer. Cancer Epidemiol Biomarkers Prev 1994;3: 209–12.
29. Moller H, Mellemgaard A, Lindvig K, et al. Obesity and cancer risk: a Danish record-linkage study. Eur J Cancer 1994;30A:344–50.
30. Calle EE, Rodriguez C, Walker-Thurmond K, et al. Overweight, obesity, and mortality from cancer in a prospectively studied cohort of U.S. adults. N Engl J Med 2003;348:1625–38.
31. Samanic C, Gridley G, Chow WH, et al. Obesity and cancer risk among white and black United States veterans. Cancer Causes Control 2004;15:35–43.
32. Kuriyama S, Tsubono Y, Hozawa A, et al. Obesity and risk of cancer in Japan. Int J Cancer 2005;113:148–57.
33. Moerman CJ, Berns MP, Bueno de Mesquita HB, et al. Reproductive history and cancer of the biliary tract in women. Int J Cancer 1994;57:146–53.
34. Serra I, Yamamoto M, Calvo A, et al. Association of chili pepper consumption, low socioeconomic status and longstanding gallstones with gallbladder cancer in a Chilean population. Int J Cancer 2002;102:407–11.
35. Lambe M, Trichopoulos D, Hsieh CC, et al. Parity and cancers of the gallbladder and the extrahepatic bile ducts. Int J Cancer 1993;54:941–4.
36. De Aretxabala X, Riedeman P, Burgos L, et al. [Gallbladder cancer. Case-control study]. Rev Med Chil 1995;123:581–6 [in Spanish].
37. Tavani A, Negri E, La Vecchia C. Menstrual and reproductive factors and biliary tract cancers. Eur J Cancer Prev 1996;5:241–7.
38. Pandey M, Shukla VK. Lifestyle, parity, menstrual and reproductive factors and risk of gallbladder cancer. Eur J Cancer Prev 2003;12:269–72.
39. Gallus S, Negri E, Chatenoud L, et al. Post-menopausal hormonal therapy and gallbladder cancer risk. Int J Cancer 2002;99:762–3.
40. Singh H, Pandey M, Shukla VK. Salmonella carrier state, chronic bacterial infection and gallbladder carcinogenesis. Eur J Cancer Prev 1996;5:144.
41. Nath G, Singh H, Shukla VK. Chronic typhoid carriage and carcinoma of the gallbladder 211. Eur J Cancer Prev 1997;6:557–9.
42. Shukla VK, Singh H, Pandey M, et al. Carcinoma of the gallbladder—is it a sequel of typhoid? Dig Dis Sci 2000;45:900–3.
43. Dutta U, Garg PK, Kumar R, et al. Typhoid carriers among patients with gallstones are at increased risk for carcinoma of the gallbladder. Am J Gastroenterol 2000; 95:784–7.
44. Matsukura N, Yokomuro S, Yamada S, et al. Association between *Helicobacter bilis* in bile and biliary tract malignancies: *H. bilis* in bile from Japanese and Thai patients with benign and malignant diseases in the biliary tract. Jpn J Cancer Res 2002;93:842–7.
45. Bulajic M, Maisonneuve P, Schneider-Brachert W, et al. Helicobacter pylori and the risk of benign and malignant biliary tract disease. Cancer 2002;95:1946–53.
46. Murata H, Tsuji S, Tsujii M, et al. Helicobacter bilis infection in biliary tract cancer. Aliment Pharmacol Ther 2004;20(Suppl 1):90–4.

# Management of Gallbladder Cancer

Shiva Jayaraman, MD, MESc, William R. Jarnagin, MD*

**KEYWORDS**

- Gallbladder cancer • Epidemiology • Resection
- Gastrointestinal

## EPIDEMIOLOGY AND RISK FACTORS

Gallbladder cancer (GBCA) is the fifth most common gastrointestinal cancer and the most common biliary tract malignancy in the United States, with an incidence of 1.2 per 100,000 persons per year.[1] Because of its tendency to present at an advanced stage, it has historically been considered an incurable disease with a dismal prognosis. In appropriately selected cases, radical surgery is possible and offers some patients a chance at long-term survival. Despite this, in the majority of cases, the outcomes of patients with advanced GBCA remain poor.[2]

There are many known risk factors for GBCA, including cholelithiasis, obesity, multiparity, and typhoid fever.[3–7] In addition, there are geographic variations in the prevalence of the disease, with rates highest in Chile, India, Israel, Poland, and Japan. In the United States, the disease prevails in Native American women from New Mexico.[6] Gallstones are present in the majority of patients; however, the relationship between causation and association is unclear. In some cases of GBCA, a focus of cancer may be found in a gallbladder adenomatous polyp; however, in the majority of cases, small polyps of the gallbladder do not harbor malignancy and are non-neoplastic and may be simply observed.[8–11] Polyps greater than 1 cm, those arising in the setting of primary sclerosing cholangitis, or those discovered in patients older than 50 years of age are more likely to harbor cancers and, therefore, should be treated with cholecystectomy if a patient is an appropriate candidate for surgery.[12]

## CLINICAL PRESENTATION

In general, the symptoms associated with GBCA are nonspecific. As a result, most patients present at an advanced, inoperable stage.[13–15] If patients do have symptoms, they are most commonly abdominal pain or biliary colic.[2,16] It may be seen in the initial assessment as an asymmetric mass detected on a routine ultrasound (US) in the work-up of biliary symptoms (**Fig. 1**). In advanced cases of invasion or compression

Hepatopancreatobiliary Service, Department of Surgery, Memorial Sloan-Kettering Cancer Center, 1275 York Avenue, Room C-891, New York, NY 10065, USA
* Corresponding author.
*E-mail address:* jarnagiw@mskcc.org

Gastroenterol Clin N Am 39 (2010) 331–342
doi:10.1016/j.gtc.2010.02.006
0889-8553/10/$ – see front matter © 2010 Elsevier Inc. All rights reserved.

gastro.theclinics.com

of the porta hepatis, jaundice may ensue and the patients may have systemic signs, such as malaise and weight loss. Jaundice is an ominous finding. In a series from the Memorial Sloan-Kettering Cancer Center from 1995 through 2005, one-third of patients presented with jaundice and only 7% had resectable disease.[14]

## PATHOLOGY AND STAGING

According to the most recent American Joint Committee on Cancer (AJCC) staging algorithm (**Table 1**), GBCAs are staged according to tumor depth of invasion (T), presence of lymph node metastasis (N), and presence of distant metastasis (M).[17] Most GBCA is adenocarcinoma; however, less commonly, other histopathologic variants are seen, such as papillary, mucinous, squamous, and adenosquamous subtypes.

T stage describes how deeply the primary tumor invades through the layers of the gallbladder wall and into adjacent structures. This component is the most important factor in determining appropriate surgical therapy in patients with potentially resectable tumors. The wall of the gallbladder consists of a mucosa, lamina propria, a thin muscular layer, perimuscular connective tissue, and a serosa. The gallbladder wall adjacent to the liver does not have a serosal covering, making the gallbladder and liver more contiguous than the peritoneal viscera. In general, tumors confined to the gallbladder wall are classified as T1 or T2 whereas T3 and T4 tumors have extended beyond the gallbladder (**Fig. 2**).[17]

N staging refers to the presence or absence of metastasis to regional lymph nodes, which are generally confined to the hepatoduodenal ligament, such as hilar, celiac,

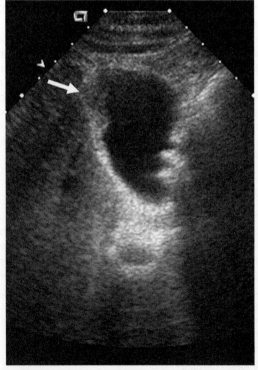

**Fig. 1.** US image depicting asymmetric gallbladder wall thickening (*arrow*) in a patient with GBCA.

**Table 1**
**TNM Groupings for GBCA**

| Category | | T | N | M |
|---|---|---|---|---|
| IS | | Carcinoma in situ | — | — |
| 1 | a | Tumor invades lamina propria | Metastatic lymph nodes | Distant |
| | b | Tumor invades muscle layer | in hepatoduodenal | metastasis |
| | | | ligament | |
| 2 | | Tumor invades perimuscular connective tissue with no extension beyond serosa or into liver | — | — |
| 3 | | Tumor perforates the serosa or directly invades 1 adjacent organ or both or ≤2 cm extension into liver | — | — |
| 4 | | Tumor extends >2 cm into liver or into 2 or more adjacent organs | — | — |

*Data from* American Joint Committee on Cancer. AJCC Cancer Staging Manual. 7th ed. New York: Springer; 2010.

periduodenal, peripancreatic, and superior mesenteric nodes as well as nodes along the pancreatic head. If patients have positive nodes outside these areas, they are considered as having distant metastatic disease. Beyond regional lymph nodes, the most common sites of distant metastasis in GBCA are the peritoneum and the liver.[17] Occasionally, spread to the lung and pleura is seen at presentation, but these sites are uncommon in the absence of apparent metastatic disease in the abdomen.

There is a direct correlation between the incidence of disseminated metastasis or nodal disease and T stage. In other words, tumors that have invaded more deeply into the gallbladder wall are more likely to have spread to regional nodes or distant

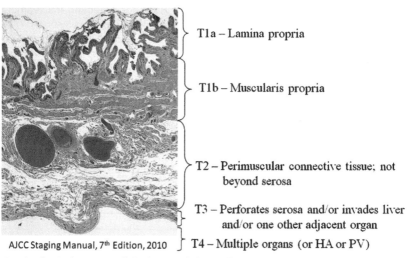

T1a – Lamina propria

T1b – Muscularis propria

T2 – Perimuscular connective tissue; not beyond serosa

T3 – Perforates serosa and/or invades liver and/or one other adjacent organ

AJCC Staging Manual, 7th Edition, 2010

T4 – Multiple organs (or HA or PV)

**Fig. 2.** Histologic depiction of the layers of the gallbladder wall with corresponding T stage for GBCA. HA, hepatic artery; PV, portal vein. (*From* American Joint Committee on Cancer. AJCC Cancer Staging Manual. 7th ed. New York: Springer; 2010; with permission.)

sites. A study from the Memorial Sloan-Kettering Cancer Center demonstrated that distant and nodal metastases increased progressively from 16% to 79% and from 33% to 69%, respectively, in going from T2 to T4 tumors.[13] The current AJCC stage groupings for GBCA reflect the clinical treatment status of the disease, in most cases. GBCA categorized as stages I or II are potentially resectable with curative intent; stage III generally indicates locally unresectable disease as a consequence of vascular invasion or involvement of multiple adjacent organs; and stage IV represents unresectability as a consequence of distant metastases (**Table 2**).

In considering preoperative staging of GBCA, the approach is dependent on a variety of clinical factors related to how a patient presents. Patients generally present in 1 of 3 different ways: GBCA suspected preoperatively; GBCA found intraoperatively at the time of cholecystectomy for presumed benign disease; and, finally, the most common situation, GBCA is diagnosed incidentally on pathologic examination after cholecystectomy.[18] It should be routine to inspect the gallbladder lumen after simple cholecystectomy to ensure there are no suspicious mucosal lesions. This is a safe and fast screening technique while a patient is in the operating room and permits the immediate assessment of suspicious lesions with frozen section.

Staging is primarily achieved through imaging. US is usually the initial radiographic study obtained in the context of the work-up of presumed benign gallbladder diseases. Typically, GBCA has characteristic features on US: a mass replacing or filling the gallbladder or invading the gallbladder bed, an intraluminal growth or polyp, or asymmetric gallbladder wall thickening.[19] In cases of locally advanced disease, US has a sensitivity of 85% and an overall accuracy of 80% in diagnosing GBCA.[14] US can fail to detect GBCA if the cancer is subtle or flat and if there is substantial cholelithiasis.[20] Higher flow on color Doppler US can be indicative of a focus of malignancy and may assist in diagnosis.[21] US also has the ability to determine involvement of the biliary tree and porta hepatis. Similarly, it can accurately assess liver parenchymal invasion.[19]

All patients who have suspected GBCA should undergo staging in the form of cross-sectional imaging with CT or MRI to look for lymph node or distant metastatic disease. These modalities can also help assess depth of invasion into the liver to facilitate operative planning for the extent of potential resection. Ohtani and colleagues[22] reported the positive predictive value of conventional CT scan for detecting involvement in various lymph node stations as 75% to 100% despite lower sensitivity as 17% to 78%. The same group has reported the sensitivity of CT scan to detect of tumor invasion into liver, bile duct, or other adjacent organs, such as pancreas and transverse colon as 50% to 65% and the positive predictive value as 77% to 100%.[23] CT is

| Table 2 | |
|---|---|
| AJCC Staging for GBCA | |
| **Stage** | **TNM Grouping** |
| 0 | TisN0M0 |
| IA | T1N0M0 |
| IB | T2N0M0 |
| IIA | T3N0M0 |
| IIB | T1-3N0M0 |
| III | T4NxM0 |
| IV | TxNxM1 |

Data from American Joint Committee on Cancer. AJCC Cancer Staging Manual. 7th ed. New York: Springer; 2010.

similarly sensitive at detecting invasion into liver or other adjacent organ was with sensitivities ranging from 80% to 100%.[24,25] MRI is less frequently used for staging of GBCA, but sometimes the use of magnetic resonance cholangiography (MRCP) or magnetic resonance angiography provides more information than US or CT. Schwartz and colleagues[26] demonstrated, in a retrospective analysis of 34 patients with GBCA, that combination of conventional MRI and MRCP achieved a sensitivity of 100% for liver invasion and 92% for lymph node involvement.

As in many other intra-abdominal malignancies, fluorodeoxyglucose–positron emission tomography (FDG-PET) scanning is increasingly used. PET scans may have a role in detecting residual disease in the gallbladder fossa post cholecystectomy or in detecting occult metastatic disease.[27,28] It has been shown that additional information from PET alters management in 23% of selected patients with GBCA who were preoperatively staged using US/CT/MRI.[29] Currently, the role of FDG-PET scanning in the work-up of patients with suspected GBCA is not routine. In cases where there is suspicion of metastatic disease that is not completely appreciated on conventional cross-sectional studies, it may be helpful in delineating suspicious masses as malignant or benign.

## SURGICAL MANAGEMENT BASED ON T STAGE

A patient's histologic T stage is the most important determinant of the necessary extent of resection. In the case of patients with incidental GBCAs, it is especially important in aiding in the selection of patients for reoperation and definitive resection. T stage in GBCA is positively correlated with nodal and distant metastasis and the potential for residual liver disease.[13] In general, it is preferable for the first operation for GBCA to be definitive; however, it has been demonstrated that a prior noncurative cholecystectomy may not have an adverse impact on survival after reoperation and definitive R0 resection.[13,16,30] Published series on this topic, however, likely suffer from publication bias, as such analyses only include patients who are submitted to resection and exclude patients with disseminated disease. The logical question that ensues is how many patients with disseminated disease have metastases because the initial operation violated the tumor plane.

There are other reasons why early preemptive identification of patients with GBCA is technically favorable to a reoperative approach. After cholecystectomy, patients naturally form adhesions in the portal hepatis and gallbladder fossa, which can make it difficult to distinguish benign scar tissue and tumor.[31] This in turn may lead to more extensive resections than would otherwise be necessary and could result in unnecessary biliary or liver resections.

In most cases, before proceeding with laparotomy for GBCA, staging laparoscopy is helpful to assess the abdomen for evidence of peritoneal spread or discontiguous liver disease and may spare up to 48% of patients an unnecessary laparotomy.[32] Although laparoscopy is useful in staging, laparoscopic cholecystectomy should be avoided in cases where there is a high preoperative probability of cancer due to the risk of tumor dissemination. In suspicious cases, open assessment should be planned and frozen section should be done to establish a diagnosis of malignancy. If a frozen section is positive for malignancy, hepatic resection may follow. Due caution should be exercised for tumors abutting the liver and preemptive liver resection may be a safer approach in such patients to prevent tumor spillage.

In cases where the diagnosis of GBCA is made at the time of exploration for what had been presumed benign disease, if the treating surgeon is not prepared to perform a hepatic resection, the patient is best served by transfer to a center with experience in performing the appropriate operation.

## T1 TUMORS

T1a tumors are most often discovered after laparoscopic cholecystectomy for presumed benign disease. These lesions are confined to the lamina propria and because the potential for nodal metastasis is small, the cure rate after simple chole-cystectomy is 85% to 100%, if negative margins are attained.[33,34] In the case of T1b tumors, there have been reports of tumor recurrence and death after a simple cholecystectomy. Principe and colleagues[35] have reported only a 50% 1-year survival rate with simple cholecystectomy; therefore, in fit patients, it seems reasonable to proceed with a more radical operation involving portions of segments IVb and V of the liver as well as performing a portal lymphadenectomy. In reoperative cases for these early invasive lesions, patients must be cautioned about the high possibility of not finding residual malignancy in the resected specimen.

## T2 TUMORS

For tumors that extend into the perimuscular connective tissues, simple cholecystec-tomy is inadequate. Therefore, patients with these tumors should be treated with a more extensive resection, which should include partial hepatectomy as well as regional lymphadenectomy. Radical surgery for T2 tumors is supported by studies that show 40% 5-year survival rates after simple cholecystectomy compared with upward of 80% 5-year survival rates after en bloc hepatic resection.[36–38] An extended hepatectomy (right lobe or extended right lobe) may be necessary if there is involve-ment of the hepatic artery or the portal vein. The right portal pedicle is particularly vulnerable due to its proximity to the gallbladder. In the absence of such involvement, segmental resection of segments IVb and V is adequate. Resection and reconstruction of the bile duct should be performed if necessary for proper R0 margins. Thus, assess-ment of the margin status of the cystic duct stump is critical. Regional lymphadenec-tomy should be routine for T2 tumors, because approximately one-third of these cases have lymph node metastases. Although regional nodal involvement is a strong predictor of poor outcome, long-term survival has been reported in patients with N1 disease.[39,40] Lymph nodes within the heptoduodenal ligament are generally included in this resection but not retropancreatic or celiac nodes, as patients with metastases to these nodal basins are unlikely to obtain benefit from resection.

## T3 TUMORS

Like T2 lesions, T3 tumors are not adequately treated by simple cholecystectomy and require hepatic resection with regional lymphadenectomy at minimum. This can include a major hepatectomy if there is extensive extension into the liver or major vascular structures. In many cases, bile duct resection and reconstruction is also required. In cases where direct extension of tumor into adjacent organs (duodenum, stomach, or colon) is suspected, en bloc resection should be performed as it can be difficult to distinguish inflammation from invasion, especially in cases where there has been a prior cholecystectomy. When a complete resection is attained, 5-year survival rates of 30% to 50% can be attained.[13,37,41]

## T4 TUMORS

Unlike in other T stages, T4 tumors are rarely confused for benign gallstone disease and they are nearly always unresectable. Even in cases where extensive resections are performed, they are rarely, if ever, curative. As a result, palliative therapies are often recommended for this stage of disease.

## OTHER SURGICAL ISSUES

Patients with GBCA diagnosed after laparoscopic cholecystectomy for presumed benign disease may be predisposed to early peritoneal spread or port site seeding. This problem may be accentuated by operative spillage of bile or stones.[42,43] In a study of 409 patients who had undergone laparoscopic cholecystectomy for unsuspected GBCA, laparoscopic port site recurrences occurred in 17% of patients at a median of 180 days after surgery.[44] Some surgeons recommend port site removal at reoperation for GBCA; however, there is little evidence showing a benefit of routine port site resection. Port site metastases are a marker for a greater likelihood of subsequent peritoneal disease.[45]

## PROGNOSIS AND OUTCOME

In a broad review of all published cases of GBCA in 1978, a cumulative median survival of 5 to 8 months and 5-year survival rate of only 4% was indentified.[46] Over the past 3 decades, an improvement in the understanding of the characteristics of GCBA and improved surgical techniques has led to less pessimistic attitudes and improved outcomes. Increased surgical experience and safe and standardized techniques of hepatic resection have resulted in a progressive decline in morbidity and mortality associated with these procedures.[37,47] At the Memorial Sloan-Kettering Cancer Center, actuarial 5-year survival of 83% for stage II disease and 63% for stage III have been reported.[37] Similarly, in a long-term retrospective study of aggressive surgical approaches compared with less aggressive approaches, more extensive resections resulted in improved median survival from 9 months to 17 months and 5-year survival rates increased from 7% to 35%.[16]

There are several prognostic factors that can help predict survival after resection. As discussed previously, T stage of the original lesion is an important prognostic factor. Fong and colleagues[13] have shown that in patients who had a noncurative laparotomy, patients with T2 disease had a 59% 5-year survival rate compared with 21% for those with T3 disease. Nodal disease is also associated with poor prognosis with only 2 patients of the 36 with nodal disease surviving beyond 5 years in the same study. Additionally, the number of positive nodes is likely an important prognostic factor as 77% 5-year survival rates have been found in patients without nodal involvement.[48] Conversely, 5-year survival rates of 33% for patients with a single-node metastasis and 0% for patients with 2 or more lymph nodes involved have been reported. As expected, AJCC stage also correlates with outcome.[49] Of the physical findings, the presence of jaundice is an ominous sign in patients with GBCA.[14] The most common finding in jaundiced patients is obstruction of the distal common hepatic duct or proximal common bile duct. This occurs because the gallbladder is situated close to the major extrahepatic biliary ductal and vascular structures, hence the prognostic significance of jaundice. Rates of resectability are exceedingly low in jaundiced patients.[14]

## ADJUVANT THERAPY

Because of the propensity for GBCA to spread to regional lymph nodes at an early stage and the high rate of locoregional recurrence, adjuvant chemotherapy or chemoradiation therapy seems a rational therapeutic option. 5-Fluorouracil (5-FU)–based chemotherapy had been the mainstay of adjuvant regimens and has been used with or without combination of chemoradiation; more recently, gemcitabine, alone or in combination therapy, is favored. There are no strong data, however, to support the efficacy of aduvant therapy. There is only 1 randomized trial examining the efficacy of adjuvant chemotherapy for GBCA.[50] This study reported significant improvement in 5-year overall survival rate (26% vs 14.4%) with postoperative mitomycin C and 5-FU after surgery compared with surgery alone as well as improvement in 5-year disease-free survival rate (20.3% vs 11.6%). This trial is limited by a small sample size and the inclusion of patients with incomplete extirpation of disease. Subgroup analysis in the same study demonstrated that patients who underwent a complete resection had no survival advantage with adjuvant treatment. Most other data for the use of adjuvant or neoadjuvant chemotherapy or chemoradiotherapy in patients with GBCA are derived from phase II trials, in which treated patients were compared with historical controls. Unfortunately, no study has provided conclusive evidence favoring a benefit of adjuvant chemotherapy or chemoradiation treatment for GBCA.[51,52]

## PALLIATIVE CARE

Most patients with GBCA present with advanced, incurable disease and many are not candidates for surgical resection. The median survival of patients with advanced GBCA who are deemed inoperable is only 2 to 4 months,[2,53] thus palliation of symptoms should be the primary goal. The primary objective should be alleviation of symptoms related to the patients' incurable GBCA. These patients typically suffer from jaundice, pain, and gastrointestinal obstruction. Efforts should also be made to prevent serious complications, such as cholangitis. For obstructive jaundice or gastrointestinal obstruction, endoscopic or percutaneous interventions are the preferred approach to palliation to minimize morbidity. In many cases, however, these minimally invasive approaches may not be possible and, therefore, palliative surgery may be necessary. Jaundice due to biliary obstruction can be alleviated with surgical bypass to segment III of the liver. This has been shown an effective strategy in a series of 41 consecutive segment III bypass for patients with advanced GBCA with a 87% success rate with 12% mortality and 51% morbidity rate having been reported.[54] Intestinal bypass should be performed only in patients who have symptomatic obstruction. Endoscopic stenting of the gastrointestinal tract or percutaneous feeding tube insertion should be favored over surgical bypass.

As in the adjuvant setting, palliative chemotherapy and radiation therapy offer little benefit in GBCA. Multiple regimens have been tested, including combinations of 5-FU, leucovorin, mitomycin C, doxorubicin, and methotrexate. Chemotherapy has only shown poor response rates of 10% to 20%.[55] Recent phase II trials, however, using a combination of gemcitabine and oxaliplatin, showed improved response rates ranging 40% to 50%, offering some promise for improved survival as more effective agents emerge.[56–58]

| Table 3 Surgical treatment based on T stage | | |
|---|---|---|
| T Stage | Recommended Operation | Evidence Grade |
| 1a | Simple cholecystectomy | Grade B |
| 1b-2 | Cholecystectomy with en bloc resection of segments IVb and V of liver with regional lymphadenectomy | Grade B |
| 3 | As for T1b-2, but may require right hepatectomy or extended right hepatectomy with bile duct excision and Roux-en-Y biliary reconstruction to obtain R0 margins | Grade B |
| 4 | As for T3, if resectable; most patients likely unresectable so appropriate palliative strategies should be sought | Grade B |

## SUMMARY

Resection is a means of improving survival in patients with GBCA. **Table 3** summarizes the authors' approach to GBCA based on T stage. A more aggressive surgical approach, including resection of the gallbladder, liver, and regional lymph nodes, is advisable for patients with T1b to T4 tumors. T1a lesions are adequately treated with simple cholecystectomy alone. Resection of the bile duct may be necessary to achieve negative margins in more advanced cases. If GBCA is suspected before cholecystectomy, an open approach should be used; however, re-exploration with radical resection in selected patients can be associated with outcomes similar to patients offered aggressive resections from the outset. Aggressive resection is necessary because patients' GBCA stage determines their outcome, not the surgery itself. Therefore, major resections should be offered to appropriately selected patients. Patients with advanced tumors or metastatic disease are not candidates for radical resection and should thus be directed to more suitable palliation.

## REFERENCES

1. Jemal A, Siegel R, Ward E, et al. Cancer statistics, 2008. CA Cancer J Clin 2008; 58(2):71–96.
2. Ito H, Matros E, Brooks DC, et al. Treatment outcomes associated with surgery for gallbladder cancer: a 20-year experience. J Gastrointest Surg 2004;8(2):183–90.
3. Diehl AK. Gallstone size and the risk of gallbladder cancer. JAMA 1983;250(17): 2323–6.
4. Caygill CP, Hill MJ, Braddick M, et al. Cancer mortality in chronic typhoid and paratyphoid carriers. Lancet 1994;343(8889):83–4.
5. Lowenfels AB, Walker AM, Althaus DP, et al. Gallstone growth, size, and risk of gallbladder cancer: an interracial study. Int J Epidemiol 1989;18(1):50–4.
6. Randi G, Franceschi S, La Vecchia C. Gallbladder cancer worldwide: geographical distribution and risk factors. Int J Cancer 2006;118(7):1591–602.
7. Serra I, Calvo A, Baez S, et al. Risk factors for gallbladder cancer. An international collaborative case-control study. Cancer 1996;78(7):1515–7.
8. Chijiiwa K, Tanaka M. Polypoid lesion of the gallbladder: indications of carcinoma and outcome after surgery for malignant polypoid lesion. Int Surg 1994;79(2): 106–9.
9. Ito H, Hann LE, D'Angelica M, et al. Polypoid lesions of the gallbladder: diagnosis and followup. J Am Coll Surg 2009;208(4):570–5.
10. Yang HL, Sun YG, Wang Z. Polypoid lesions of the gallbladder: diagnosis and indications for surgery. Br J Surg 1992;79(3):227–9.
11. Tazuma S, Kajiyama G. Carcinogenesis of malignant lesions of the gall bladder. The impact of chronic inflammation and gallstones. Langenbecks Arch Surg 2001;386(3):224–9.
12. Yeh CN, Jan YY, Chao TC, et al. Laparoscopic cholecystectomy for polypoid lesions of the gallbladder: a clinicopathologic study. Surg Laparosc Endosc Percutan Tech 2001;11(3):176–81.
13. Fong Y, Jarnagin W, Blumgart LH. Gallbladder cancer: comparison of patients presenting initially for definitive operation with those presenting after prior noncurative intervention. Ann Surg 2000;232(4):557–69.
14. Hawkins WG, DeMatteo RP, Jarnagin WR, et al. Jaundice predicts advanced disease and early mortality in patients with gallbladder cancer. Ann Surg Oncol 2004;11(3):310–5.

15. Chan SY, Poon RT, Lo CM, et al. Management of carcinoma of the gallbladder: a single-institution experience in 16 years. J Surg Oncol 2008;97(2):156–64.

16. Dixon E, Vollmer CM Jr, Sahajpal A, et al. An aggressive surgical approach leads to improved survival in patients with gallbladder cancer: a 12-year study at a North American Center. Ann Surg 2005;241(3):385–94.

17. Edge SB, Byrd DR, Compton CC, et al., editors. AJCC cancer staging manual. 7th edition. New York: Springer; 2010.

18. de Aretxabala X, Roa I, Burgos L, et al. Gallbladder cancer: an analysis of a series of 139 patients with invasion restricted to the subserosal layer. J Gastrointest Surg 2006;10(2):186–92.

19. Miller G, Jarnagin WR. Gallbladder carcinoma. Eur J Surg Oncol 2008;34(3): 306–12.

20. Onoyama H, Yamamoto M, Takada M, et al. Diagnostic imaging of early gallbladder cancer: retrospective study of 53 cases. World J Surg 1999;23(7): 708–12.

21. Komatsuda T, Ishida H, Konno K, et al. Gallbladder carcinoma: color Doppler sonography. Abdom Imaging 2000;25(2):194–7.

22. Ohtani T, Shirai Y, Tsukada K, et al. Carcinoma of the gallbladder: CT evaluation of lymphatic spread. Radiology 1993;189(3):875–80.

23. Ohtani T, Shirai Y, Tsukada K, et al. Spread of gallbladder carcinoma: CT evaluation with pathologic correlation. Abdom Imaging 1996;21(3):195–201.

24. Yoshimitsu K, Honda H, Shinozaki K, et al. Helical CT of the local spread of carcinoma of the gallbladder: evaluation according to the TNM system in patients who underwent surgical resection. AJR Am J Roentgenol 2002;179(2):423–8.

25. Kumaran V, Gulati S, Paul B, et al. The role of dual-phase helical CT in assessing resectability of carcinoma of the gallbladder. Eur Radiol 2002;12(8):1993–9.

26. Schwartz LH, Black J, Fong Y, et al. Gallbladder carcinoma: findings at MR imaging with MR cholangiopancreatography. J Comput Assist Tomogr 2002; 26(3):405–10.

27. Petrowsky H, Wildbrett P, Husarik DB, et al. Impact of integrated positron emission tomography and computed tomography on staging and management of gallbladder cancer and cholangiocarcinoma. J Hepatol 2006;45(1):43–50.

28. Rodriguez-Fernandez A, Gomez-Rio M, Llamas-Elvira JM, et al. Positron-emission tomography with fluorine-18-fluoro-2-deoxy-D-glucose for gallbladder cancer diagnosis. Am J Surg 2004;188(2):171–5.

29. Corvera CU, Blumgart LH, Akhurst T, et al. 18F-fluorodeoxyglucose positron emission tomography influences management decisions in patients with biliary cancer. J Am Coll Surg 2008;206(1):57–65.

30. Fong Y, Heffernan N, Blumgart LH. Gallbladder carcinoma discovered during laparoscopic cholecystectomy: aggressive reresection is beneficial. Cancer 1998;83(3):423–7.

31. D'Angelica M, Dalal KM, Dematteo RP, et al. Analysis of the Extent of Resection for Adenocarcinoma of the Gallbladder. Ann Surg Oncol 2009;16(4):806–16.

32. Weber SM, DeMatteo RP, Fong Y, et al. Staging laparoscopy in patients with extrahepatic biliary carcinoma. Analysis of 100 patients. Ann Surg 2002;235(3): 392–9.

33. Yamaguchi K, Tsuneyoshi M. Subclinical gallbladder carcinoma. Am J Surg 1992; 163(4):382–6.

34. Shirai Y, Yoshida K, Tsukada K, et al. Inapparent carcinoma of the gallbladder. An appraisal of a radical second operation after simple cholecystectomy. Ann Surg 1992;215(4):326–31.

35. Principe A, Del Gaudio M, Ercolani G, et al. Radical surgery for gallbladder carcinoma: possibilities of survival. Hepatogastroenterology 2006;53(71):660–4.
36. de Aretxabala XA, Roa IS, Burgos LA, et al. Curative resection in potentially resectable tumours of the gallbladder. Eur J Surg 1997;163(6):419–26.
37. Bartlett DL, Fong Y, Fortner JG, et al. Long-term results after resection for gallbladder cancer. Implications for staging and management. Ann Surg 1996; 224(5):639–46.
38. Oertli D, Herzog U, Tondelli P. Primary carcinoma of the gallbladder: operative experience during a 16 year period. Eur J Surg 1993;159(8):415–20.
39. Shirai Y, Yoshida K, Tsukada K, et al. Radical surgery for gallbladder carcinoma. Long-term results. Ann Surg 1992;216(5):565–8.
40. Onoyama H, Yamamoto M, Tseng A, et al. Extended cholecystectomy for carcinoma of the gallbladder. World J Surg 1995;19(5):758–63.
41. Chijiiwa K, Tanaka M. Carcinoma of the gallbladder: an appraisal of surgical resection. Surgery 1994;115(6):751–6.
42. Winston CB, Chen JW, Fong Y, et al. Recurrent gallbladder carcinoma along laparoscopic cholecystectomy port tracks: CT demonstration. Radiology 1999;212(2):439–44.
43. Fong Y, Brennan MF, Turnbull A, et al. Gallbladder cancer discovered during laparoscopic surgery. Potential for iatrogenic tumor dissemination. Arch Surg 1993;128(9):1054–6.
44. Paolucci V, Schaeff B, Schneider M, et al. Tumor seeding following laparoscopy: international survey. World J Surg 1999;23(10):989–95 [discussion: 996–7].
45. Shoup M, Fong Y. Surgical indications and extent of resection in gallbladder cancer. Surg Oncol Clin N Am 2002;11(4):985–94.
46. Piehler JM, Crichlow RW. Primary carcinoma of the gallbladder. Surg Gynecol Obstet 1978;147(6):929–42.
47. Nakamura S, Sakaguchi S, Suzuki S, et al. Aggressive surgery for carcinoma of the gallbladder. Surgery 1989;106(3):467–73.
48. Endo I, Shimada H, Tanabe M, et al. Prognostic significance of the number of positive lymph nodes in gallbladder cancer. J Gastrointest Surg 2006;10(7): 999–1007.
49. Behari A, Sikora SS, Wagholikar GD, et al. Longterm survival after extended resections in patients with gallbladder cancer. J Am Coll Surg 2003;196(1):82–8.
50. Takada T, Amano H, Yasuda H, et al. Is postoperative adjuvant chemotherapy useful for gallbladder carcinoma? A phase III multicenter prospective randomized controlled trial in patients with resected pancreaticobiliary carcinoma. Cancer 2002;95(8):1685–95.
51. Czito BG, Hurwitz HI, Clough RW, et al. Adjuvant external-beam radiotherapy with concurrent chemotherapy after resection of primary gallbladder carcinoma: a 23-year experience. Int J Radiat Oncol Biol Phys 2005;62(4):1030–4.
52. Kresl JJ, Schild SE, Henning GT, et al. Adjuvant external beam radiation therapy with concurrent chemotherapy in the management of gallbladder carcinoma. Int J Radiat Oncol Biol Phys 2002;52(1):167–75.
53. Shih SP, Schulick RD, Cameron JL, et al. Gallbladder cancer: the role of laparoscopy and radical resection. Ann Surg 2007;245(6):893–901.
54. Kapoor VK, Pradeep R, Haribhakti SP, et al. Intrahepatic segment III cholangiojejunostomy in advanced carcinoma of the gallbladder. Br J Surg 1996;83(12): 1709–11.
55. Hejna M, Pruckmayer M, Raderer M. The role of chemotherapy and radiation in the management of biliary cancer: a review of the literature. Eur J Cancer 1998;34(7):977–86.

56. Andre T, Tournigand C, Rosmorduc O, et al. Gemcitabine combined with oxaliplatin (GEMOX) in advanced biliary tract adenocarcinoma: a GERCOR study. Ann Oncol 2004;15(9):1339–43.
57. Harder J, Riecken B, Kummer O, et al. Outpatient chemotherapy with gemcitabine and oxaliplatin in patients with biliary tract cancer. Br J Cancer 2006; 95(7):848–52.
58. Verderame F, Russo A, Di Leo R, et al. Gemcitabine and oxaliplatin combination chemotherapy in advanced biliary tract cancers. Ann Oncol 2006;17(Suppl 7): vii68–72.

# Acute Acalculous Cholecystitis

Philip S. Barie, MD, MBA[a,b,*], Soumitra R. Eachempati, MD[a,b]

**KEYWORDS**

- Acute acalculous cholecystitis
- Percutaneous cholecystostomy • Ultrasound • CT

Acute cholecystitis may develop at any time in the presence of gallstones, especially once symptoms develop. Acute cholecystitis is especially dangerous during a serious illness or following major surgery, however, whether associated with gallstones or more typically not (acute acalculous cholecystitis [AAC]). Now recognized as a complication of serious medical and surgical illnesses,[1–3] increased numbers of critically ill patients, increased awareness, and improved imaging modalities are resulting in the identification of more cases of AAC.[4] The mortality rate remains at least 30% because the diagnosis of AAC remains challenging to make, affected patients are critically ill, and the disease itself can progress rapidly because of the high prevalence of gangrene (approximately 50%) and perforation (approximately 10%).[5]

## CLINICAL PATTERNS OF AAC

Reports of acute cholecystitis complicating surgery, multiple trauma, or burn injury are numerous. In patients with gallstones, postoperative cholecystitis affects males and females to a similar degree. More than 80% of patients who develop non–trauma-related postoperative AAC, however, are male.[6] The incidence of AAC following open abdominal aortic reconstruction is 0.7% to 0.9%,[7,8] and has also been reported to complicate endovascular aortic reconstruction.[9]

After cardiac surgery, the incidence of acute cholecystitis is 0.12% (42% AAC) in collected reports encompassing 31,710 patients, with an overall mortality rate of 45%.[6] Although rare following cardiac surgery, those undergoing cardiac valve replacement with or without bypass grafting may be at particular risk[10] because of

[a] Division of Critical Care and Trauma, Department of Surgery, Anne and Max A. Cohen Surgical Intensive Care Unit, New York–Presbyterian Hospital, Weill Cornell Medical College, P713A, 525 East 68 Street, New York, NY 0065, USA
[b] Division of Medical Ethics, Department of Public Health, Anne and Max A. Cohen Surgical Intensive Care Unit, New York–Presbyterian Hospital, Weill Cornell Medical College, P713A, 525 East 68 Street, New York, NY 0065, USA
* Corresponding author. Division of Critical Care and Trauma, Department of Surgery, Anne and Max A. Cohen Surgical Intensive Care Unit, New York–Presbyterian Hospital, Weill Cornell Medical College, P713A, 525 East 68 Street, New York, NY 0065.
*E-mail address:* pbarie@med.cornell.edu

Gastroenterol Clin N Am 39 (2010) 343–357
doi:10.1016/j.gtc.2010.02.012
0889-8553/10/$ – see front matter © 2010 Elsevier Inc. All rights reserved.

associated cardiomyopathy. Postoperative cholecystitis, regardless of the antecedent operation, is as likely to develop in the presence of gallstones as in their absence.[11] Patients with trauma[12,13] or burns[14] have a striking predilection to develop AAC, again, mostly among male patients.

The development of AAC is not limited to surgical or injured patients, or even to critical illness. Diabetes mellitus, abdominal vasculitis,[15,16] congestive heart failure, cholesterol embolization of the cystic artery,[17,18] and resuscitation from hemorrhagic shock or cardiac arrest[19] have been associated with AAC. End-stage renal disease is associated with AAC, perhaps because both diabetes mellitus and atherosclerosis are commonplace in patients with end-stage renal disease,[20] who often experience low flow on hemodialysis. Hemorrhagic AAC has been reported in end-stage renal disease, related to either uremic thrombocytopathy or frequent exposure to heparinoids to facilitate blood flow through the circuit.[21] Patients with cancer are also at risk for AAC, including metastasis to the porta hepatis; therapy with interleukin-2 and lymphokine-activated killer cells for metastatic disease[22]; or percutaneous transhepatic catheter drainage of extrahepatic biliary obstruction, wherein the catheter in the common bile duct itself may obstruct the cystic duct.[23] Acute acalculous cholecystitis has been reported with acute myelogenous leukemia.[24] In bone marrow transplant recipients, the incidence of AAC is as high as 4%.[25]

Acalculous cholecystitis may also develop as a secondary infection of the gallbladder during systemic sepsis, for example in disseminated candidiasis,[26,27] leptospirosis,[28] in chronic biliary tract carriers of typhoidal[29] and nontyphoidal *Salmonella*,[30] during active diarrheal illnesses, such as cholera[31] or *Campylobacter* enteritis,[32] and tuberculosis (**Box 1**).[33] Also reported are cases of AAC in malaria,[34] brucellosis,[35] Q fever (*Coxiella burnetii*),[36] and dengue fever.[37] Miscellaneous viral pathogens associated with AAC include hepatitis A[38] and B,[39] and Epstein-Barr virus.[40] Extrahepatic biliary obstruction can lead to AAC from infectious or noninfectious causes. Obstructive infectious causes include ascariasis[41] and echinococcal cysts,[42] whereas noninfectious causes of AAC with extrahepatic biliary obstruction include hemobilia (**Fig. 1**),[43] choledochal cyst,[44] and ampullary stenosis.[45]

Acalculous biliary disease occurs in patients with AIDS, and may take either of two forms: cholestasis,[46] which can be impossible to distinguish from bacterial cholangitis in an acutely jaundiced patient, or AAC.[47] Now increasingly rare because of improved antiretroviral therapy, AIDS-associated AAC has been associated with cytomegalovirus infection[48] or infection with *Cryptosporidium* or microsporidial protozoa.[49]

AAC represents 50% to 70% of all cases of acute cholecystitis in children.[50] Acalculous cholecystitis is recognized in young children and neonates,[51] and older children. Dehydration is a common precipitant, as are acute bacterial infections[52] and viral illnesses, such as hepatitis[38] and upper respiratory tract infections. Portal lymphadenitis with extrinsic cystic duct obstruction may be etiologic in viral infections. Recent reports[51] suggest that the pathogenesis may be similar to that in adults.

## PATHOGENESIS
### Bile Stasis

Bile stasis has been implicated in the pathogenesis of AAC in both experimental and clinical studies. Volume depletion leads to concentration of bile, which can inspissate in the absence of a stimulus for gallbladder emptying (eg, nothing per os). Opioid analgesics increase intralumenal bile duct pressure because of spasm of the sphincter of Oddi. Several early clinical studies suggested that ileus can result in bile stasis, but experimental results are conflicting. Bile stasis may also be induced by mechanical

---

**Box 1**
**Pathogens associated with AAC**

Bacteria

    *Brucella* spp (etiologic agents of brucellosis)

    *Campylobacter jejuni*

    *Coxiella burnetii* (etiologic agent of Q fever)

    *Leptospira* spp (etiologic agents of leptospirosis)

    *Mycobacterium tuberculosis, M bovis*

    *Salmonella* spp

        *S enterica* subsp *enterica* serovar Enteritidis

        *S enterica* subsp *enterica* serovar Typhimurium

        *S typhi* (etiologic agent of typhoid fever)

    *Vibrio cholerae*

Yeasts and molds

    *Candida* spp

Viruses

    Hepatitis A virus

    Hepatitis B virus

    Epstein-Barr virus

    *Flavivirus* (serotypes) (etiologic agents of dengue fever and dengue hemorrhagic fever)

Parasites

    *Ascaris lumbricoides*

    *Echinococcus* spp (etiologic agents of echinococcosis)

        *E granulosus*

        *E multilocularis*

    *Plasmodium* spp (etiologic agents of malaria)

---

ventilation with positive end-expiratory pressure,[53] which also decreases portal perfusion by increasing hepatic venous pressure.

Bile stasis may alter the chemical composition of bile, which may promote gallbladder mucosal injury. Lysophosphatidylcholine has potent effects on gallbladder structure and functional water transport across mucosa.[53] Acute cholecystitis induced in several animal models by lysophosphatidylcholine results in histopathology identical to that of human AAC.[54] Other compounds present in bile (eg, β-glucuronidase) have also been implicated in the pathogenesis of AAC.[55]

### Total parenteral nutrition

Fasting and bile stasis may be aggravated by total parenteral nutrition (TPN) in the pathogenesis of AAC.[56] Parenteral nutrition is associated with gallstone formation and AAC in both adults and children. The incidence of AAC during long-term TPN may be as high as 30%.[57] Formation of gallbladder "sludge" occurs among 50% of patients on long-term TPN at 4 weeks and is ubiquitous at 6 weeks.[58] Neither

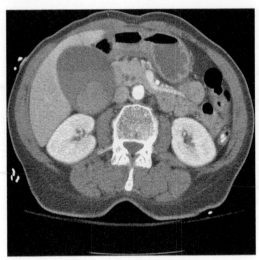

**Fig. 1.** CT of the abdomen revealing a markedly dilated gallbladder containing a globular density compatible with intralumenal blood clot in a patient with severe coronary artery disease, who was receiving aspirin, clopidogrel, and intravenous unfractionated heparin. No gallstones were visualized. At laparoscopic cholecystectomy an acutely inflamed gallbladder was resected. Clot was present in the lumen, but no stones.

stimulation of gallbladder emptying with cholecystokinin nor enteral alimentation, however, can prevent AAC among critically ill patients.[59]

### Gallbladder Ischemia

Gallbladder ischemia is central to the pathogenesis of AAC. An interrelationship between ischemia and stasis has been suggested, leading to hypoperfusion.[60] Perfusion is decreased by hypotension, dehydration, or the administration of vasoactive drugs, whereas intraluminal pressure is increased by bile stasis, thereby decreasing gallbladder perfusion pressure. In this hypothesis, bacterial invasion of ischemic tissue is a secondary phenomenon.[60] Alternatively, reperfusion injury may be the crucial factor. Prolongation of ischemia was associated with increased mucosal phospholipase $A_2$ and superoxide dismutase activities, and increased mucosal lipid peroxide content.[61]

It has been hypothesized that the fundamental lesion leading to AAC is failure of the gallbladder microcirculation with cellular hypoxia.[62] Numerous clinical observations of hypoperfusion leading to AAC support this hypothesis,[6,8,10,16,17] as does the pathologic observation of high rates of gallbladder necrosis and perforation. Gallbladder specimen arteriography reveals marked differences between acute calculous and AAC in humans.[63] Whereas gallstone-related disease is associated with arterial dilatation and extensive venous filling, AAC is associated with multiple arterial occlusions and minimal-to-absent venous filling, reiterating the central role of vascular occlusion and microcirculatory disruption in the pathogenesis of AAC.

### Mediators of Inflammation, Sepsis, and AAC

Vasoactive mediators play a role in the pathogenesis of AAC. Although bacterial infection is likely a secondary phenomenon, the host response to gram-negative bacteremia or splanchnic ischemia-reperfusion injury may be of primary importance. Intravenous injection of *Escherichia coli* lipopolysaccharide, a potent stimulus of inflammation and coagulation that mimics clinical sepsis in several respects, produces AAC in several mammalian species, including opossums[64] and cats.[65] In opossums, lipopolysaccharide decreased the contractile response to cholecystokinin and caused a dose-dependent mucosal injury.[62] The dysmotility was abolished by inhibition of nitric oxide synthase. Human gallbladder mucosal cells stimulated in vitro with lipopolysaccharide secrete eicosanoids and platelet-activating factor.[66] Cholecystitis can also be produced by injection of plant polyphenols that activate coagulation factor XII directly and produce immediate spasm of the cystic artery.[67] AAC has also been produced in cats by infusion of platelet-activating factor into the cystic artery.[68] Platelet-activating factor has been implicated in the pathogenesis of splanchnic hypoperfusion in sepsis and other low-flow states. The inflammation seems to be mediated by proinflammatory eicosanoids, because it is inhibited by nonspecific cyclooxygenase inhibitors.[65]

## DIAGNOSIS

AAC poses major diagnostic challenges.[68] Most afflicted patients are critically ill and unable to communicate their symptoms. Cholecystitis is but one of many potential causes in the differential diagnosis of systemic inflammatory response syndrome or sepsis in such patients. Rapid and accurate diagnosis is essential, because gallbladder ischemia can progress rapidly to gangrene and perforation. Acalculous cholecystitis is sufficiently common that the diagnosis should be considered in every critically ill or injured patient with a clinical picture of sepsis or jaundice and no other obvious source.

Physical examination and laboratory evaluation are unreliable.[69] Fever is generally present but other physical findings cannot be relied on, particularly physical examination of the abdomen.[12] Leukocytosis and jaundice are commonplace, but nonspecific in the setting of critical illness. The differential diagnosis of jaundice in the critically ill patient is complex and context-sensitive, including intrahepatic cholestasis from sepsis or drug toxicity and "fatty liver" induced by TPN, in addition to AAC.[68] Jaundice caused by AAC may be caused most often by sepsis-related cholestasis, or rarely by extrinsic compression of the common duct by the phlegmon (Mirizzi-type syndrome).[70] Other biochemical assays of hepatic enzymes are of little help. The diagnosis of AAC often rests on radiologic studies (**Box 2**).

### Ultrasound

Ultrasound of the gallbladder is the most accurate modality to diagnose AAC in the critically ill patient.[71] Although sonography is accurate for detecting gallstones and measuring bile duct diameter, neither is particularly relevant to the diagnosis of AAC. Thickening of the gallbladder wall is the single most reliable criterion,[72–74] with reported specificity of 90% at 3 mm and 98.5% at 3.5 mm wall thickness, and sensitivity of 100% at 3 mm and 80% at 3.5 mm. Accordingly, gallbladder wall thickness greater than or equal to 3.5 mm is generally accepted to be diagnostic of AAC. Other helpful sonographic findings for AAC include pericholecystic fluid or the presence of intramural gas or a sonolucent intramural layer, or "halo," which represents intramural edema (**Fig. 2**).[71] Distention of the gallbladder of more than 5 cm in transverse diameter has also been reported.[71] False-positive ultrasound examinations have been reported, and may occur in particular when conditions including sludge, nonshadowing stones, cholesterolosis, hypoalbuminemia, or ascites mimic a thickened gallbladder wall.[73]

---

**Box 2**
**Imaging criteria for the diagnosis of AAC**

*Ultrasound*

Either two major criteria, or one major criterion and two minor criteria, satisfy the ultrasound diagnosis of AAC

Major criteria

　Gallbladder wall thickening >3 mm

　Striated gallbladder (ie, gallbladder wall edema)

　Sonographic Murphy sign (inspiratory arrest during deep breath while gallbladder is being insonated; unreliable if patient is obtunded or sedated)

　Pericholecystic fluid (absent either ascites or hypoalbuminemia)

　Mucosal sloughing

　Intramural gas

Minor criteria

　Gallbladder distention (>5 cm in transverse diameter)

　Echogenic bile (sludge)

*Computed tomography*

Either two major criteria, or one major criterion and two minor criteria, satisfy the CT diagnosis of AAC

Major criteria

　Gallbladder wall thickening >3 mm

　Subserosal halo sign (intramural lucency caused by edema)

　Pericholecystic infiltration of fat

　Pericholecystic fluid (absent either ascites or hypoalbuminemia)

　Mucosal sloughing

　Intramural gas

Minor criteria

　Gallbladder distention (>5 cm in transverse diameter)

　High-attenuation bile (sludge)

*Hepatobiliary scintigraphy*

Nonvisualization or questionable visualization of the gallbladder at 1 hour after administration of 5 mCi of a $^{99m}$Tc iminodiacetic acid derivative, in the presence of adequate hepatic uptake of tracer, and excretion into the duodenum

Morphine sulfate, 0.04–0.05 mg/kg intravenously, may be given at 30–40 minutes of nonvisualization to increase specificity at 1 hour

Enhanced accumulation of radiotracer in the gallbladder fossa may be indicative of gallbladder gangrene or perforation

---

## Radionuclide Studies

Although technetium $^{99m}$Tc iminodiacetic acid imaging is approximately 95% accurate to diagnose calculous acute cholecystitis,[75] false-negative hepatobiliary scans are problematic when used for diagnosis of AAC in the setting of critical illness,[75,76]

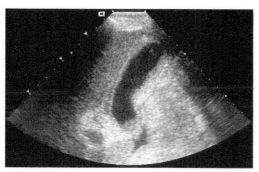

**Fig. 2.** Gallbladder ultrasound of a patient with sepsis and cholestasis. A thick-walled gallbladder is visible with echogenic bile (sludge) within the neck of the gallbladder, but no stones. There is pericholecystic fluid (the echogenic [bright] area) near the neck of the gallbladder. A "halo" sign (intramural edema) is visible just to the left of the gallbladder in the image.

because of false-positive scans associated with fasting, liver disease, or feeding with TPN.[76] The sensitivity of hepatobiliary imaging for AAC is reportedly as low as 68%.[75] Intravenous morphine (0.04–0.05 mg/kg) given after initial nonvisualization of the gallbladder may increase the accuracy of cholescintigraphy among critically ill patients, by enhanced gallbladder filling caused by increased bile secretory pressure.[77,78] Morphine cholescintigraphy has led to a reappraisal of radionuclide imaging for AAC,[71,79] provided the patient can be transported safely to the nuclear medicine suite and can remain there for the 2 hours or more that it may take to complete morphine cholescintigraphy. False-positive studies are reduced dramatically when morphine cholescintigraphy is performed; sensitivity of 67% to 100% and specificity of 69% to 100% have been reported in collected series of morphine cholescintigraphy for the diagnosis of AAC.[71]

## CT

CT seems to be as accurate as ultrasound in the diagnosis of AAC.[80] Diagnostic criteria for AAC by CT are similar to those described for sonography (see **Box 2**; **Figs. 1** and **3**).[81] Only a single retrospective study has compared all three modalities

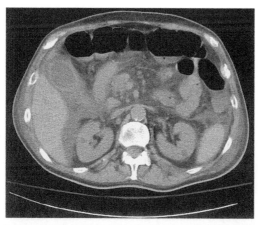

**Fig. 3.** CT of the abdomen showing AAC. Note the thickened, contrast-enhanced wall of the gallbladder, ventral to the right hepatic lobe, and the large amount of surrounding ascites (pericholecystic fluid). No gallstones were visualized.

(ultrasound, hepatobiliary scanning, and CT)[82]; sonography and CT were comparably accurate and superior to hepatobiliary imaging. Low cost and the ability to perform sonography rapidly at the bedside make it the preferred diagnostic modality in possible AAC in the intensive care unit setting. Preference may be given to CT if other thoracic or abdominal diagnoses are under consideration.

### Laparoscopy

Bedside laparoscopy has been used with success for the diagnosis and therapy of AAC,[83–85] but initial enthusiasm has waned because bringing the equipment to the intensive care unit bedside is cumbersome. Laparoscopy can be performed under local anesthesia and intravenous sedation at the bedside, and is possible in patients who have undergone recent abdominal surgery if "gasless" techniques are used. Diagnostic accuracy is high,[84] and both laparoscopic cholecystostomy and cholecystectomy are technically possible to perform.

### THERAPY

The historic treatment for AAC was cholecystectomy,[2] because of the ostensible need to inspect the gallbladder and perform a resection if gangrene or perforation in AAC are present. Pericholecystic fluid collections can be drained during laparoscopy or celiotomy, and other pathology that may mimic acute cholecystitis (eg, perforated ulcer, cholangitis, pancreatitis) may be identified and managed if the diagnosis of AAC is incorrect. Percutaneous cholecystostomy is now established, however, as a lifesaving, minimally invasive alternative.[86,87] Open cholecystostomy can also be accomplished under local anesthesia through a short right subcostal incision, but the ability to visualize elsewhere in the abdomen is limited. Cholecystostomy by either technique does not decompress the common bile duct if cystic duct obstruction is present; therefore, the common duct must be decompressed in addition by some manner (eg, endoscopic retrograde cholangiopancreatography with sphincterotomy, laparoscopic or open common bile duct exploration) if cholangitis is suspected. Patency of the cystic duct can be determined immediately by tube cholangiography (**Fig. 4**), which should always be performed after the patient has recovered to

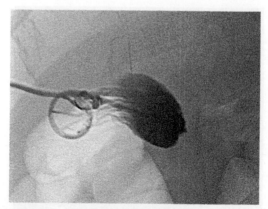

**Fig. 4.** Tube cholangiography following percutaneous cholecystectomy. Contrast fails to enter the common bile duct (incidence approximately 20%), reflecting cystic duct obstruction. In this circumstance, concomitant cholangitis (which is rare) would not be drained without separate instrumentation of the common bile duct.

determine the presence of gallstones that may not have been detected initially. If gallstones are present an elective cholecystectomy is usually recommended, with the drainage tube remaining in place during the interprocedure interval. Interval cholecystectomy is usually not indicated after true AAC[87]; the cholecystostomy tube can be removed after tube cholangiography confirms that gallstones are absent.

Percutaneous cholecystostomy[88–90] controls AAC in 85% to 90% of patients. The gallbladder is usually intubated under sonographic (occasionally laparoscopic) control by an anterior or anterolateral transhepatic approach (through the right hepatic lobe) to minimize leakage of bile, but transperitoneal puncture has been described. Rapid improvement should be expected when percutaneous cholecystostomy is successful. If rapid improvement does not ensue, the tube may be malpositioned or not draining properly, or the diagnosis of AAC may be incorrect, and an open procedure may be required.

Reported causes of failure include gangrenous cholecystitis, catheter dislodgement, bile leakage causing peritonitis, and an erroneous diagnosis.[91,92] Perforated ulcer, pancreatic abscess, pneumonia, and pericarditis have been discovered in the aftermath of percutaneous cholecystostomy when patients failed to improve. Reported major complications occur after 8% to 10% of procedures, including dislodgment of the catheter, acute respiratory distress syndrome, bile peritonitis, hemorrhage, cardiac arrhythmia, and hypotension caused by procedure-related bacteremia.[90] The 30-day mortality of percutaneous and open cholecystostomy are similar, and influenced heavily by the underlying severity of illness.

Empiric percutaneous cholecystostomy has been advocated for patients who have sepsis absent a demonstrable source. In one report of 24 patients receiving vasopressor therapy for septic shock, 14 patients (58%) improved as a result of cholecystostomy.[89] Pneumonia was diagnosed subsequently in 3 of the 10 nonresponders, but an infection was never found in the other seven patients. Such an approach is not recommended routinely, but the importance of considering AAC in the differential diagnosis of occult sepsis is underscored.

Antibiotic therapy does not substitute for drainage of AAC, but is an important adjunct. The most common bacteria isolated from bile in acute cholecystitis are *E coli*, *Klebsiella* spp, and *Enterococcus faecalis*; antibiotic therapy should be directed against these organisms. Critical illness and prior antibiotic therapy alter host flora, however, and resistant or opportunistic pathogens may be encountered. *Pseudomonas*, staphylococci (including methicillin-resistant strains), *Enterobacter* and related species, anaerobic organisms (eg, *Clostridium* spp, *Bacteroides* spp), or fungi may be recovered. Anaerobes are particularly likely to be isolated from bile of patients with diabetes mellitus, in those older than 70 years of age, and from patients whose biliary tracts have been instrumented previously.

## COMPLICATIONS

The prevalence of gallbladder gangrene in AAC exceeds 50%, and leads to additional morbidity, including gallbladder perforation. One variant, emphysematous cholecystitis, is particularly associated with gangrene and perforation. Emphysematous cholecystitis is rare, but shares many traits with AAC; 28% of patients with emphysematous cholecystitis have acalculous disease. More than 70% of cases of emphysematous cholecystitis occur in men, and 20% of patients have diabetes mellitus. Crepitus to palpation of the right upper abdomen or radiographic identification of gas in patients with acute cholecystitis mandates immediate cholecystectomy in view of the fulminant nature of untreated emphysematous cholecystitis (percutaneous cholecystostomy does not achieve source control reliably enough). *Clostridium* spp, rather than aerobic gram-negative bacilli, are isolated most commonly in emphysematous cholecystitis (45% of cases, with *Clostridium welchii* predominating). *E coli* are recovered from approximately one third of affected patients. Antimicrobial therapy specific for *Clostridium* spp (eg, penicillin G) may be added to agents directed against the typical bacteria flora of acute cholecystitis.

Perforation of the gallbladder occurs in 10% or more of cases of AAC,[8] either localized into adjacent duodenum or transverse colon (cholecystoenteric fistula); the subhepatic space, causing abscess formation; or free perforation with generalized peritonitis. Perforation into the liver or biliary tract has been reported rarely in AAC,[93,94] as is perforation into the retroperitoneum with iliopsoas abscess.[95] The usual immediate cause of death with AAC is severe sepsis with multiple organ dysfunction syndrome.[96] Unusual causes of death from gallbladder perforation in AAC include hemorrhage from the liver[97] and pulmonary bile embolism.[98] Serious complications of gallbladder gangrene without perforation include acute pancreatitis,[99] colon perforation,[100] and obstruction of the common hepatic duct.[101] Empyema of the gallbladder may also complicate AAC.[102]

## SUMMARY

AAC should be suspected in every critically ill patient with sepsis in whom the source of infection cannot be found immediately. Suspicion should be especially high if the patient is injured, has undergone recent major surgery, has had a period of hypotension or hypoperfusion for any reason, or becomes jaundiced. The preferred diagnostic modality is ultrasound, which is inexpensive, noninvasive, and can be brought to the bedside of the unstable patient. Once diagnosed, the treatment of choice is percutaneous cholecystostomy, but if the response to drainage is not prompt and favorable, an alternative diagnosis must be considered and abdominal exploration may be required. If percutaneous drainage is successful and the patient truly has no gallstones, then no further treatment may be necessary and the catheter may be removed.

## REFERENCES

1. Gallbladder Survey Committee. Ohio Chapter, American College of Surgeons. 28,621 cholecystectomies in Ohio. Am J Surg 1970;119:714–7.
2. Glenn F, Becker CG. Acute acalculous cholecystitis: an increasing entity. Ann Surg 1982;195:131–6.
3. Johanning JM, Gruenberg JC. The changing face of cholecystectomy. Am Surg 1988;64:643–7.
4. Kalliafas S, Ziegler DW, Flancbaum L, et al. Acute acalculous cholecystitis: incidence, risk factors, diagnosis, and outcome. Am Surg 1998;64:471–5.
5. Barie PS, Fischer E. Acute acalculous cholecystitis. J Am Coll Surg 1995;180:232–44.
6. Barie PS. Acalculous and postoperative cholecystitis. In: Barie PS, Shires GT, editors. Surgical intensive care. Boston: Little, Brown; 1993. p. 837–57.
7. Ouriel K, Green RM, Ricotta JJ, et al. Acute acalculous cholecystitis complicating abdominal aortic aneurysm resection. J Vasc Surg 1984;1:646–8.
8. Hagino RT, Valentine RJ, Clagett GP. Acalculous cholecystitis after aortic reconstruction. J Am Coll Surg 1997;184:245–8.
9. Cadot H, Addis MD, Faries PL, et al. Abdominal aortic aneurysmorraphy and cholelithiasis in the era of endovascular surgery. Am Surg 2002;68:839–43.

10. Leitman IM, Paull DE, Barie PS, et al. Intraabdominal complications of cardiopulmonary bypass surgery. Surg Gynecol Obstet 1987;165:251–4.

11. Gately JF, Thomas EJ. Acute cholecystitis occurring as a complication of other diseases. Arch Surg 1983;118:1137–41.

12. Fabian TC, Hickerson WL, Mangiante EC. Post-traumatic and postoperative acute cholecystitis. Am Surg 1986;52:188–92.

13. Flancbaum L, Majerus TC, Cox EF. Acute post-traumatic acalculous cholecystitis. Am J Surg 1985;150:252–6.

14. McDermott MW, Scudamore CH, Boileau LO, et al. Acalculous cholecystitis: its role as a complication of major burn injury. Can J Surg 1985;28:529–33.

15. Papaioannou CC, Hunder GG, Lie JT. Vasculitis of the gallbladder in a 70 year old man with giant cell arteritis. J Rheumatol 1979;6:71–5.

16. Dessailloud R, Papo T, Vaneecloo S, et al. Acalculous ischemic gallbladder necrosis in the catastrophic antiphospholipid syndrome. Arthritis Rheum 1998; 41:1318–20.

17. Moolenaar W, Lamers CB. Cholesterol crystal embolization to liver, gallbladder, and pancreas. Dig Dis Sci 1996;41:1819–22.

18. Ryu JK, Ryu KH, Kim KH. Clinical features of acute acalculous cholecystitis. J Clin Gastroenterol 2003;36:166–9.

19. Smith JP, Bodai BI. Empyema of the gallbladder-potential consequence of medical intensive care. Crit Care Med 1982;10:451–2.

20. Ini K, Inada H, Satoh M, et al. Hemorrhagic acalculous cholecystitis associated with hemodialysis. Surgery 2002;132:903.

21. Lai YC, Tarng DC. Hemorrhagic acalculous cholecystitis: an unusual location of uremic bleeding. J Chin Med Assoc 2009;72:484–7.

22. Chung-Park M, Kim B, Marmyola G, et al. Acalculous lymphoeosinophilic cholecystitis associated with interleukin-2 and lymphokine-activated killer cell therapy. Arch Pathol Lab Med 1990;114:1073–5.

23. Lillemoe KD, Pitt HA, Kaufman SL, et al. Acute cholecystitis occurring as a complication of percutaneous transhepatic drainage. Surg Gynecol Obstet 1989;168:348–56.

24. Topeli A, Demiroglu H, Dundar S. Acalculous cholecystitis in patients with acute leukaemia. Br J Clin Pract 1996;50:224–5.

25. Wiboltt KS, Jeffrey JB Jr. Acalculous cholecystitis in patients undergoing bone marrow transplantation. Eur J Surg 1997;163:519–24.

26. Hiatt JR, Kobayashi MR, Doty JE, et al. Acalculous *Candida* cholecystitis: a complication of critical surgical illness. Am Surg 1991;57:825–9.

27. Mandak JS, Pollack B, Fishman NO, et al. Acalculous candidal cholecystitis: a previously unrecognized complication after cardiac transplantation. Am J Gastroenterol 1995;90:1333–7.

28. Baelen E, Roustan J. Leptospirosis associated with acute acalculous cholecystitis. Surgical or medical treatment? J Clin Gastroenterol 1997;25:704–6.

29. Khan FY, Elouzi EB, Asif M. Acute acalculous cholecystitis complicating typhoid fever in an adult patient: a case report and review of the literature. Travel Med Infect Dis 2009;7:203–6.

30. McCarron B, Love WC. Acalculous nontyphoidal salmonellal cholecystitis requiring surgical intervention despite ciprofloxacin therapy: report of three cases. Clin Infect Dis 1997;24:707–9.

31. West BC, Silberman R, Otterson WN. Acalculous cholecystitis and septicemia caused by non-01 *Vibrio cholerae*: first reported case and review of biliary infections with *Vibrio cholerae*. Diagn Microbiol Infect Dis 1998;30:187–91.

32. Udayakumar D, Sanaullah N. Campylobacter cholecystitis. Int J Med Sci 2009; 1:374–5.
33. Vallejo EA. Acute tuberculous cholecystitis. Gastroenterology 1950;16:501–4.
34. Khan FY, El-Hiday AH. Acute calculous cholecystitis complicating an imported case of mixed malaria caused by *Plasmodium falciparum* and *Plasmodium vivax*. Int J Infect Dis 2009. [Epub ahead of print].
35. Ashley D, Vade A, Challapali M. Brucellosis with acute acalculous cholecystitis. Pediatr Infect Dis J 2000;19:1112–3.
36. Figtree M, Miyakis Stenos J, et al. Q fever cholecystitis in an unvaccinated butcher diagnosed by gallbladder polymerase chain reaction. Vector Borne Zoonotic Dis 2009. [Epub ahead of print].
37. Bhatty S, Shaikh NA, Fatima M, et al. Acute cholecystitis in dengue fever. J Pak Med Assoc 2009;59:519–21.
38. Souza LJ, Braga LG, Rocha Nde S, et al. Acute acalculous cholecystitis in a teenager with hepatitis A viral infection: a case report. Braz J Infect Dis 2009;13:74–6.
39. Unal H, Korkmaz N, Kirbas I, et al. Acute acalculous cholecystitis associated with acute hepatitis B infection. Int J Infect Dis 2009;13:e310–2.
40. Iaria C, Leonardi MS, Fabiano C, et al. Acalculous cholecystitis during the course of acute Epstein-Barr virus infection and Gilbert's syndrome. Int J Infect Dis 2009;13:e519–20.
41. Kuzu MA, Ozturk Y, Ozbek H, et al. Acalculous cholecystitis: ascariasis as an unusual cause. J Gastroenterol 1996;31:747–9.
42. Mansour K. Acute cholecystitis with echinococcal cyst obstruction of the common bile duct. Postgrad Med J 1963;39:542–3.
43. Sandblom P. Hemorrhage into the biliary tract following trauma: traumatic hemobilia. Surgery 1948;24:571–86, 33.
44. Lin SL, Shank M, Hung YB, et al. Choledochal cyst associated with acute acalculous cholecystitis. J Pediatr Gastroenterol Nutr 2000;31:307–8.
45. Savoye G, Michel P, Hochain P, et al. Fatal acalculous cholecystitis after photodynamic therapy for high-grade dysplasia of the major duodenal papilla. Gastrointest Endosc 2000;51:493–5.
46. Cello JP. AIDS cholangiopathy: spectrum of disease. Am J Med 1989;86: 539–46.
47. French AL, Beaudet LM, Benator DA, et al. Cholecystectomy in patients with AIDS: clinicopathologic correlations in 107 cases. Clin Infect Dis 1995;21:852–8.
48. Keshavjee SH, Magee LA, Mullen BJ. Acalculous cholecystitis associated with cytomegalovirus and sclerosing cholangitis in a patient with acquired immunodeficiency syndrome. Can J Surg 1993;36:321–5.
49. Zar FA, El-Bayouni E, Yungbluth MM. Histologic proof of acalculous cholecystitis due to *Cyclospora cayetanesis*. Clin Infect Dis 2001;33:E140–1.
50. Tsakayannis DE, Kozakewich HP, Lillehei CW. Acalculous cholecystitis in children. J Pediatr Surg 1996;31:127–30.
51. Imamoglu M, Sarrhan H, Sari A, et al. Acute acalculous cholecystitis in children: diagnosis and treatment. J Pediatr Surg 2002;37:36–7.
52. Parithivel VS, Gerst PH, Banerjee S, et al. Acute acalculous cholecystitis in young patients without predisposing factors. Am Surg 1999;65:366–8.
53. Johnson EE, Hedley-White J. Continuous positive-pressure ventilation and choledochoduodenal flow resistance. J Appl Phys 1975;39:937–42.
54. Niderheiser DH. Acute acalculous cholecystitis induced by lysophosphatidyl choline. Am J Pathol 1986;124:559–63.

55. Kouromalis E, Hopwood D, Ross PE, et al. Gallbladder epithelial acid hydrolases in human cholecystitis. J Pathol 1983;139:179–91.
56. Lin KY. Acute acalculous cholecystitis: a limited review of the literature. Mt Sinai J Med 1986;53:305–9.
57. Roslyn JJ, Pitt HA, Mann LL, et al. Gallbladder disease in patients on long-term parenteral nutrition. Gastroenterology 1983;84:148–54.
58. Messing B, Bories C, Kuntslinger F, et al. Does total parenteral nutrition induce gallbladder sludge formation and lithiasis? Gastroenterology 1983;84:1012–9.
59. Merrill RC, Miller-Crotchett P, Lowry P. Gallbladder response to enteral lipids in injured patients. Arch Surg 1989;124:301–2.
60. Orlando R, Gleason E, Drezner AD. Acute acalculous cholecystitis in the critically ill patient. Am J Surg 1983;145:472–6.
61. Taoka H. Experimental study on the pathogenesis of acute acalculous cholecystitis, with special reference to the roles of microcirculatory disturbances, free radicals and membrane-bound phospholipase A2. Gastroenterol Jpn 1991;26: 633–44.
62. Sanda RB. Acute acalculous cholecystitis after trauma: the role of microcirculatory hypoxia and cellular hypoxia. South Med J 2008;101:1087–8.
63. Hakala T, Nuuiten PJ, Ruokonen ET, et al. Microangiopathy in acute acalculous cholecystitis. Br J Surg 1997;84:1249–52.
64. Cullen JJ, Maes EB, Aggarwal S, et al. Effect of endotoxin on opossum gallbladder motility: a model of acalculous cholecystitis. Ann Surg 2000;232:202–7.
65. Kaminski DL, Feinstein WK, Deshpande YG. The production of experimental cholecystitis by endotoxin. Prostaglandins 1994;47:233–45.
66. Kaminski DL, Amir G, Deshpande YG, et al. Studies on the etiology of acute acalculous cholecystitis: the effect of lipopolysaccharide on human gallbladder mucosal cells. Prostaglandins 1994;47:319–30.
67. Ratnoff OD, Crum JD. Activation of Hageman factor by solutions of ellagic acid. J Lab Clin Med 1964;63:359–77.
68. Kaminski DL, Andrus CH, German D, et al. The role of prostanoids in the production of acute acalculous cholecystitis by platelet-activating factor. Ann Surg 1990;212:455–61.
69. Trowbridge RL, Rutkowski NK, Shojania KG. Does this patient have acute cholecystitis? JAMA 2003;289:80–6.
70. Ahwalat SK. Acute acalculous cholecystitis simulating Mirizzi syndrome: a very rare condition. South Med J 2009;102:188–9.
71. Huffman JL, Schwenker S. Acute acalculous cholecystitis: a review. Clin Gastroenterol Hepatol 2010;8:15–22.
72. Deitch EA, Engel JM. Acute acalculous cholecystitis: ultrasonic diagnosis. Am J Surg 1981;142:290–2.
73. Deitch EA, Engel JM. Ultrasound in elective biliary tract surgery. Am J Surg 1980;140:277–83.
74. Deitch EA, Engel JM. Ultrasonic detection of acute cholecystitis with pericholecystic abscess. Am Surg 1981;47:211–4.
75. Ziessmann HA. Nuclear medicine hepatobiliary imaging. Clin Gastroenterol Hepatol 2009. [Epub ahead of print].
76. Ohrt HJ, Posalaky IP, Shafer RB. Normal gallbladder cholescintigraphy in acute cholecystitis. Clin Nucl Med 1983;8:97–100.
77. Shuman WP, Roger JV, Rudd TG, et al. Low sensitivity of sonography and cholescintigraphy in acalculous cholecystitis. AJR Am J Roentgenol 1984;142: 531–4.

78. Flancbaum L, Choban PS, Sinha R, et al. Morphine cholescintigraphy in the evaluation of hospitalized patients with suspected acute cholecystitis. Ann Surg 1994;220:25–31.
79. Krishnamurthy S, Krishnamurthy GT. Cholecystokinin and morphine pharmacological intervention during 99mTc-HIDA cholescintigraphy: a rational approach. Semin Nucl Med 1996;26:16–24.
80. Mirvis SE, Whitley NN, Miller JW. CT diagnosis of acalculous cholecystitis. J Comput Assist Tomogr 1987;11:83–7.
81. Cornwell EE III, Rodriguez A, Mirvis SE, et al. Acute acalculous cholecystitis in critically injured patients: preoperative diagnostic imaging. Ann Surg 1989;210: 52–5.
82. Mirvis SE, Vainright JR, Nelson AW, et al. The diagnosis of acute acalculous cholecystitis: a comparison of sonography, scintigraphy, and CT. AJR Am J Roentgenol 1986;147:1171–5.
83. Yang HK, Hodgson WJ. Laparoscopic cholecystostomy for acute acalculous cholecystitis. Surg Endosc 1996;10:673–5.
84. Almeida J, Sleeman D, Sosa JL, et al. Acalculous cholecystitis: the use of diagnostic laparoscopy. J Laparoendosc Surg 1995;5:227–31.
85. Brandt CP, Preibe PP, Jacobs DG. Value of laparoscopy in trauma ICU patients with suspected acute cholecystitis. Surg Endosc 1994;8:361–4.
86. Granlund A, Karlson BM, Elvin A, et al. Ultrasound-guided percutaneous cholecystostomy in high-risk surgical patients. Langenbecks Arch Surg 2001;386: 212–7.
87. Davis CA, Landercasper J, Gundersen LH, et al. Effective use of percutaneous cholecystostomy in high-risk surgical patients: techniques, tube management, and results. Arch Surg 1999;134:727–31.
88. Akhan O, Akinci D, Oznen MV. Percutaneous cholecystostomy. Eur J Radiol 2002;43:229–36.
89. Lee MJ, Saini S, Brink JA, et al. Treatment of critically ill patients with sepsis of unknown cause: value of percutaneous cholecystostomy. AJR Am J Roentgenol 1991;156:1163–6.
90. van Sonnenberg E, D'Agostino HB, Goodacre BW, et al. Percutaneous gallbladder puncture and cholecystostomy: results, complications, and caveats for safety. Radiology 1992;183:167–70.
91. Lo LD, Vogelzang RL, Braun MA, et al. Percutaneous cholecystostomy for the diagnosis and treatment of acute calculous and acalculous cholecystitis. J Vasc Interv Radiol 1995;6:629–34.
92. McLoughlin RF, Patterson EJ, Mathieson JR, et al. Radiologically guided percutaneous cholecystostomy for acute cholecystitis: long-term outcome in 50 patients. Can Assoc Radiol J 1994;45:455–9.
93. Shah SH, Webber JD. Spontaneous cystic duct perforation associated with acalculous cholecystitis. Am Surg 2002;68:895–6.
94. Fujii H, Kubo S, Tokuhara T, et al. Acute acalculous cholecystitis complicated by penetration into the liver after coronary artery bypass grafting. Jpn J Thorac Cardiovasc Surg 1999;47:518–21.
95. Ishiwatari H, Jisai H, Kanisawa Y, et al. [A case of secondary iliopsoas abscess induced by acalculous cholecystitis]. Nippon Shokakibyo Gakkai Zasshi 2002; 99:985–9 [in Japanese].
96. Barie PS, Hydo LJ, Pieracci FM, et al. Multiple organ dysfunction syndrome in critical surgical illness. Surg Infect (Larchmt) 2009;10:369–77.

97. Elde J, Norbye B, Hartvett F. Fatal hemorrhage following atraumatic liver rupture secondary to postoperative perforation of the gallbladder. Acta Chir Scand 1975;141:316–8.

98. Proia AD, Fetter BF, Woodard BH, et al. Fatal pulmonary bile embolism following acute acalculous cholecystitis. Arch Surg 1986;121:1206–8.

99. Wagner DS, Flynn MA. Hemorrhagic acalculous cholecystitis causing acute pancreatitis after trauma. J Trauma 1985;25:253–6.

100. Brady E, Welch JP. Acute hemorrhagic cholecystitis causing hemobilia and colonic necrosis. Dis Colon Rectum 1985;28:185–7.

101. Ippolito RJ. Acute acalculous cholecystitis associated with common hepatic duct obstruction: a variant of Mirizzi's syndrome. Conn Med 1993;57:451–5.

102. Fry DE, Cox RA, Harbrecht PJ. Empyema of the gallbladder: a complication in the natural history of acute cholecystitis. Am J Surg 1981;141:366–9.

# Diagnosis and Management of Gallbladder Polyps

William C. Gallahan, MD, Jason D. Conway, MD, MPH*

**KEYWORDS**
- Gallbladder polyp • Gallbladder neoplasm
- Endoscopic ultrasound

The increasing use and constantly improving resolution of abdominal imaging modalities in clinical practice often lead to "abnormal" findings that are of unclear significance. Polypoid lesions of the gallbladder are a prime example of this, as they are frequently diagnosed on routine transabdominal ultrasounds. Any projection of mucosa into the lumen of the gallbladder is defined as a polypoid lesion of the gallbladder, regardless of the neoplastic potential. Many gallbladder polyps are often diagnosed incidentally following cholecystectomy for gallstones or biliary colic. The estimated prevalence of gallbladder polyps varies by the demographics of the studied population, but it is generally considered to be around 5%.[1,2] The vast majority of gallbladder polyps are benign, and gallbladder cancer is a very rare disease. The estimated new cases of gallbladder and other biliary cancers only represented 0.66% of the estimated new cancer cases in the United States in 2009, accounting for only 0.60% of estimated new cancer deaths.[3] This article discusses the clinical presentation, diagnosis, and natural history of gallbladder polyps, as well as risk factors for malignant polyps and indications for cholecystectomy.

## CLASSIFICATION

A classification of benign tumors and pseudotumors of the gallbladder was first proposed in 1970.[4] Benign tumors include adenomas, lipomas, hemangiomas, and leiomyomas. Benign pseuodotumors include adenomyomas, cholesterol polyps, inflammatory polyps, and heterotopic mucosa from the stomach, pancreas, or liver. The current accepted classification divides these polyps into neoplastic (adenomas, carcinoma in situ) and non-neoplastic, with the non-neoplastic polyps accounting for about 95% of these lesions.[5]

There are no financial disclosures to report.
Section on Gastroenterology, Wake Forest University School of Medicine, Medical Center Boulevard, Winston-Salem, NC 27157, USA
* Corresponding author.
*E-mail address:* jconway@wfubmc.edu

Gastroenterol Clin N Am 39 (2010) 359–367
doi:10.1016/j.gtc.2010.02.001
0889-8553/10/$ – see front matter © 2010 Elsevier Inc. All rights reserved.

The most common of the non-neoplastic polyps is the cholesterol polyp. These result when the lamina propria is infiltrated with lipid-laden foamy macrophages. Cholesterol polyps account for about 60% of all gallbladder polyps and are generally less than10 mm. Often, multiple cholesterol polyps are present.[5] Adenomyomatosis of the gallbladder is a benign, hyperplastic lesion caused by excessive proliferation of surface epithelium, which can then invaginate into the muscularis. Adenomyomatosis accounts for about 25% of gallbladder polyps and usually localizes to the gallbladder fundus appearing as a solitary polyp ranging in size from 10 to 20 mm. Adenomyomatosis is not considered neoplastic.[5] Inflammatory polyps account for about 10% of gallbladder polyps and result from granulation and fibrous tissue secondary to chronic inflammation. They are typically less than 10 mm in size and are not neoplastic.[5]

Adenomas account for about 4% of gallbladder polyps and are considered neoplastic. They range in size from 5 to 20 mm, are generally solitary, and are often associated with gallstones.[5] Whether or not gallbladder adenomas progress to adenocarcinomas is not clear. Several studies do support this potential progression. Kozuka and colleagues[6] analyzed 1605 cholecystectomy specimens and found histological, traceable transitions from the 11 benign adenomas, 7 adenomas with malignancy changes, and 79 invasive carcinomas. Other case reports support this adenoma-to-cancer progression.[7] However, this progression is not felt to be the predominant pathway of carcinogenesis in the gallbladder, and K-ras mutations have not been detected in gallbladder carcinomas associated with an adenoma.[8]

Finally, rare miscellaneous neoplastic polyps of varying sizes account for the remaining 1% of gallbladder polyps and include leiomyomas, lipomas, neurofibromas, and carcinoids.[5]

## CLINICAL PRESENTATION

Gallbladder polyps are generally thought not to cause any symptoms, though most of the prevalence studies did not assess symptoms.[9] Polyps are sometimes identified on transabdominal ultrasounds done for right upper quadrant pain. In the absence of other findings, the gallbladder polyp may be considered a source of biliary colic.[10] Terzi and colleagues[11] reported that, in a series of 74 patients undergoing cholecystectomy for gallbladder polyps, 91% had symptoms, most commonly right upper quadrant pain, nausea, dyspepsia, and jaundice. However, about 60% of the patients also had gallstones, so it is unclear whether the polyps were primarily driving the symptoms. There was no difference in presenting symptoms between patients with benign versus malignant polyps. In another large retrospective analysis of 417 patients found to have gallbladder polyps on abdominal ultrasound, 64% of these polyps were diagnosed during a work-up of unrelated illness. Twenty-three percent had abdominal symptoms, and 13% had elevated liver function tests.[12]

Cholesterol polyps may detach and behave clinically as a gallstone, causing biliary colic, obstruction, or even pancreatitis.[5] There are also reports of gallbladder polyps causing acalculous cholecystitis[13] and, even, massive hemobilia.[14]

### Risk Factors

In contrast to the well-known risk factors for gallstones, attempts to identify risk factors for developing gallbladder polyps have not shown any consistent relationship between formation of polyps and age, gender, obesity, or medical conditions such as diabetes.[9] There is some literature to suggest an inverse relationship between gallbladder polyps and stones. Jorgensen and Jensen[1] studied 3608 asymptomatic patients and found gallbladders with both polyps and stones in only 3 patients. The investigators hypothesized that polyps either mechanically disrupt the formation of stones or that polyps are harder to diagnose radiographically when stones are present. Patients with congenital polyposis syndromes such as Peutz-Jeghers and Gardner syndrome can also develop gallbladder polyps.[15,16] A recent large retrospective analysis of risk factors for gallbladder polyps in the Chinese population identified chronic hepatitis B as a risk factor.[17] Proposed patient risk factors for malignant gallbladder polyps include age greater than 60, presence of gallstones, and primary sclerosing cholangitis. Polyp risk characteristics include a size greater than 6 mm, solitary, and sessile.

## DIAGNOSIS

Most gallbladder polyps are diagnosed during a routine abdominal ultrasound. They appear as fixed, hyperechoic material protruding in to the lumen of the gallbladder, with or without an acoustic shadow (**Fig. 1**).[9] However, the accuracy of abdominal ultrasound for diagnosing these lesions has been questioned. Abdominal ultrasound is often limited by the body habitus of the patient, and technical limitations can lead to intraobserver variability in interpretation. Yang and colleagues[18] found that abdominal ultrasound was quite sensitive (90%) and specific (94%) in diagnosing gallbladder polyps, particularly when there are no gallstones present. However, Akyurek and colleagues[19] found that abdominal ultrasound was only 20% sensitive in diagnosing polyps less than 1 cm and 80% sensitive in diagnosing polyps greater than 1 cm. The investigators concluded that abdominal ultrasound was inaccurate in 82% of cases of these polyps. Also, in another large retrospective study of 417 patients with gallbladder polyps found on abdominal ultrasound, one-third of those patients did not have polyps found at cholecystectomy.[12] Chattopadhyay and colleagues[20] analyzed a retrospective case series of 23 patients who were diagnosed preoperatively with a gallbladder polyp by abdominal ultrasound. When using 10 mm size as the cut-off criteria, the investigators noted 100% sensitivity, 87% specificity, and positive predictive value of 50% in the diagnosis of malignancy in gallbladder polyps. Abdominal ultrasound is generally considered the first of line study for making this diagnosis, it is by no means a definitive indicator of the presence of a gallbladder polyp or its malignant potential.

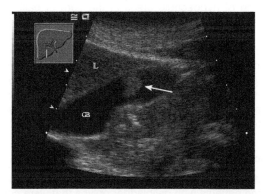

**Fig. 1.** Ultrasound image: sagittal grayscale sonogram of the gall bladder. A solid soft issue mass within the gall bladder is noted (*white arrow*). This mass appears adherent to the nondependent wall of the gall bladder without posterior shadowing. This mass was not mobile during real-time dynamic imaging with the patient in different positions. The sonographic features are consistent with a polyp. GB, gall bladder; L, liver. (*Courtesy of* Hisham Tchelepi, MD.)

### Role of Endoscopic Ultrasound

Endoscopic ultrasound (EUS) has gained widespread use for the diagnosis of gastro-intestinal malignancies, submucosal lesions of the gastrointestinal tract, and abnormalities seen on cross-sectional imaging. Its role in evaluating the biliary tree has been well defined, and this includes a possible role in the management of gallbladder polyps.[21] Because the gallbladder lies directly on the gastric antrum and duodenal bulb, the EUS probe can be placed immediately adjacent to the gallbladder. This small distance between the probe and the gallbladder allows for scanning at high frequencies, thereby creating very high-resolution images. Sugiyama and colleagues[22] examined a case series of 194 patients who underwent both abdominal ultrasound and EUS for evaluation of gallbladder polyps less than or equal to 20 mm. Fifty-eight of these patients went to surgery, and the EUS preoperative diagnosis was cholesterol polyp in 34 patients, adenomyomatosis in 7 patients, and neoplastic lesions in 17 patients. The accuracy of EUS in correctly distinguishing the polyp was 97%, superior to the 76% accuracy of abdominal ultrasound. Another study attempted to define EUS criteria that could help determine the risk of underlying neoplasia in gallbladder polyps between 5 and 15 mm in diameter. Polyps were more likely to be neoplastic if there was loss of definition of the muscularis propria; if they were solitary, sessile, and lobulated; and if their echo pattern was isoechoic to the liver with heterogeneous echotexture. These criteria were used to create an EUS score ranging from 0 to 20 points. When a cut-off score of 6 or greater was used, the sensitivity, specificity, and accuracy of diagnosing a neoplastic polyp was 81%, 86%, and 83.7%, respectively.[23]

Whether EUS alone can be used to determine a treatment strategy for gallbladder polyps is not clear. Cheon and colleagues[24] reviewed a case series of 365 patients who underwent EUS for evaluation of gallbladder polyps less than 20 mm in diameter. Of these, 94 patients underwent cholecystectomy. Neoplastic lesions were found in 19 patients (17 adenomas and 2 adenocarcinomas), and, of these patients, 10 had polyps 5 to 10 mm in diameter. EUS was 88.9% sensitive in diagnosing neoplastic disease in polyps greater than 1.0 cm. However, EUS was only 44.4% sensitive in diagnosing malignant disease in polyps less than 1.0 cm, leaving the investigators to conclude that EUS alone is not sufficient in determining the course of treatment in polyps less than 1.0 cm. On the other hand, Cho and colleagues[25] found that the finding of hypoechoic areas in the core of gallbladder polyps less than 20 mm in size was 90% sensitive and 89% specific in predicting neoplastic polyps. Akatsu and colleagues,[26] in cases series of 29 patients with gallbladder polyps 10 to 20 mm, determined that aggregation of hyperechoic spots and multiple microcysts are predictors of cholesterol polyps and adenomyomatosis, respectively, which are non-neoplastic polyps. EUS may be more accurate than transabdominal ultrasound in determining whether gallbladder polyps are neoplastic, though there is not enough evidence to suggest that EUS is the one definitive diagnostic modality for making this determination.

### Other Imaging Modalities

Other imaging modalities have also been studied. Koh and colleagues[27] presented a case series of three patients with gallbladder polyps that were correctly diagnosed preoperatively as benign or malignant with the use of positron emission tomography scanning with 18F-labelled deoxyglucose. Jang and colleagues[28] prospectively followed 144 patients found to have 1 cm gallbladder polyps who eventually underwent cholecystectomy. Preoperatively, each patient underwent evaluation with high-resolution transabdominal ultrasound, EUS, and CT scan. High-resolution ultrasound is a new technology using a broad bandwidth MHz linear array probe. The diagnostic sensitivity for malignancy of the high-resolution ultrasound was comparable to that of EUS (90% vs 86%, respectively), and both were better than CT scan (72%). The investigators concluded that high-resolution transabdominal ultrasound may therefore be another important imaging modality for gallbladder polyps.

## MANAGEMENT

When a gallbladder polyp is identified on abdominal ultrasound, the two major questions are (1) is this causing any symptoms and (2) does this need to be removed? As discussed above, most polyps are generally thought to be asymptomatic. Therefore, the main role for the clinician in managing these polyps is recommending when to proceed with surgery and when to take a watchful waiting approach, recognizing that gallbladder cancer, while quite rare, carries a poor prognosis (**Fig. 2**).

### Risk Factors for Malignancy

Numerous studies have attempted to define characteristics which increase the likelihood that a given gallbladder polyp may be malignant. Polyp size has long been noted to be an important factor. Koga and colleagues[29] reviewed 411 patients who underwent cholecystectomy and found 40 gallbladder polyps, 8 of which were adenocarcinomas. Ninety-four percent of the benign polyps were less than 1.0 cm, whereas 88% of the malignant polyps were larger than 1.0 cm. Therefore, 1.0 cm was their recommended size cut-off for considering malignancy. Terzi and colleagues[11] found a similar size cut-off in their review of 100 patients undergoing cholecystectomy for gallbladder polyps, and they noted patient age greater than 60 and the coexistence of gallstones as risk factors for malignancy. Gallstones are known to be a major risk factor for developing gallbladder carcinoma, likely because they can lead to long-term chronic inflammation within the gallbladder.[8]

Yang and colleagues[18] used an age cut-off of 50 and found that benign lesions were found in 99% of patients under age 50. Shinkai and colleagues[30] analyzed 134 patients who either underwent cholecystectomy for gallbladder polyps or had gallbladder polyps noted on abdominal ultrasound. They found that neoplastic polyps tended to

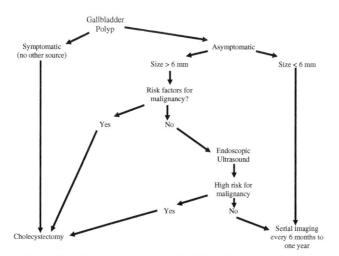

**Fig. 2.** Proposed algorithm for management of gallbladder polyps.

be solitary, whereas cholesterol polyps were typically multiple. If less than three polyps were noted, then the incidence of neoplasm was 37%, even in polyps 5 to 10 mm in diameter. Kwon and colleagues[31] reviewed 291 patients with confirmed gallbladder polyps on cholecystectomy and found that age over 60, sessile morphology, and size of 10 mm were all clear risk factors of malignant gallbladder polyps.

Besides age and cholelithiasis, another patient risk factor for malignancy in a gallbladder polyp is the diagnosis of primary sclerosing cholangitis (PSC). Leung and colleagues[32] report a cases series of four patients with PSC and gallbladder cancer who presented with gallbladder polyps ranging from 7 to 14 mm. The investigators concluded that any gallbladder polyp, regardless of size, in a patient with PSC should be considered for cholecystectomy.

Solitary sessile polyps greater than 10 mm in patients over age 50 should be considered for cholecystectomy, particularly in patients with cholelithiasis and PSC.

### Natural History of Gallbladder Polyps

Recent studies have attempted to more clearly define the natural history of gallbladder polyps. Ito and colleagues[12] retrospectively analyzed 417 patients with gallbladder polyps detected on abdominal ultrasound. No invasive neoplasms were found, and no neoplastic lesions were found in patients with polyps less than 6 mm on abdominal ultrasound. In patients who were monitored with serial abdominal ultrasounds, 86% of the polyps did not change in size, while 6% grew in size. The significance of growth of gallbladder polyps has also been studied. Shin and colleagues[33] retrospectively reviewed 145 patients who, following at least two abdominal ultrasounds at least 6 months apart, eventually underwent cholecystectomy. Age greater than 60 and polyp size greater than 10 mm were associated with neoplastic polyps, but the rate of polyp growth was not significantly associated with neoplastic polyps. Thus, the investigators concluded that gallbladder polyps less than 10 mm do not need to be removed simply because they grow. Colecchia and colleagues[34] prospectively followed 56 patients with small gallbladder polyps (ie, <10 mm) over 5 years with annual abdominal ultrasounds. No patients developed any clinical symptoms, and no changes in polyp morphology were observed, suggesting that the natural history of small gallbladder polyps is benign.

A recent study, however, yields conflicting results. Park and colleagues[35] analyzed 1558 patients diagnosed with gallbladder polyps and followed them over an average of 37 months. Thirty-three cases of neoplastic polyps were found, and polyp size greater than or equal to 10 mm and the presence of gallstones were the most significant risk factors for malignancy. However, 46% of the neoplastic polyps were less than 10 mm at the time of diagnosis, leading the investigators to conclude that even small polyps warrant close follow-up. A recent retrospective study from the Mayo Clinic also challenged the notion of the 1 cm cut-off for malignancy. One hundred and thirty patients with preoperative ultrasound and subsequent cholecystectomy were reviewed. It was found that 7.4% of polyps less than 1 cm were neoplastic, and a polyp size greater than or equal to 6 mm was a statistically significant risk factor for malignancy. The negative predictive value of abdominal ultrasound to predict malignancy was 100% when the 6 mm cut-off was used.[36]

## INDICATIONS FOR SURGERY AND RECOMMENDED FOLLOW-UP

Any gallbladder polyp that is felt to be symptomatic should be removed from a patient otherwise fit for surgery. In asymptomatic patients, the data presented above argues against the previous standard size cut-off of 1 cm to consider surgical resection. In patients at risk for malignancy, a polyp of 6 mm or greater should likely be resected. Patients without risk factors are good candidates for EUS for further evaluation. Those polyps that are considered high risk by EUS criteria should be considered for resection. The surgery of choice is laparoscopic cholecystectomy, except in cases where there is a high suspicion for malignancy. Kubota and colleagues[37] concluded that a gallbladder polyp greater than 1.8 cm has a high likelihood of being an advanced cancer and should be removed with open cholecystectomy, partial liver resection, and possible lymph node dissection. Lee and colleagues[38] also support open exploration when the suspicion of malignancy is high.

Gallbladder polyps that are not resected should be followed with serial ultrasound examinations. Clear guidelines on a screening interval are not available, and individual patient characteristics need to be considered. However, recent studies support a screening interval of every 6 to 12 months, to be continued for as long as 10 years.[9,34,35]

## SUMMARY

The primary goal in the management of gallbladder polyps is to prevent the development of gallbladder carcinoma, which is a rare illness. Often patients with gallbladder polyps undergo cholecystectomy because of symptoms. However, asymptomatic gallbladder polyps can be a dilemma for the clinician. Polyp size has long been known to be the simplest predictor for malignant potential. However, recent studies suggest that the cut-off size should be 6 mm as opposed to the traditional 10 mm recommendation. Age and presence of gallstones are other important patient factors to consider. EUS may play an important role in stratifying polyps into high or low risk for malignancy. The natural history of small gallbladder polyps suggests that polyps less than 6 mm in size can be confidently monitored with serial imaging.

## REFERENCES

1. Jorgensen T, Jensen KH. Polyps in the gallbladder. A prevalence study. Scand J Gastroenterol 1990;25:281–6.
2. Okamoto M, Okamoto H, Kitahara F, et al. Ultrasonographic evidence of association of polyps and stones with gallbladder cancer. Am J Gastroenterol 1999;94: 446–50.
3. Jemal A, Siegel R, Ward E, et al. Cancer statistics, 2009. CA Cancer J Clin 2009; 59:225–49.
4. Christensen AH, Ishak KG. Benign tumors and pseudotumors of the gallbladder. Report of 180 cases. Arch Pathol 1970;90:423–32.
5. Persley KM. Acalculous cholecystitis, cholesterolosis, adenomyomatosis, and polyps of the gallbladder. In: Feldman M, Friedman LS, Brandt LJ, editors. Sleisenger & Fordtran's gastrointestinal and liver disease. 8th edition. Philadelphia (PA): Saunders; 2006. p. 1450–6.
6. Kozuka S, Tsubone N, Yasui A, et al. Relation of adenoma to carcinoma in the gallbladder. Cancer 1982;50:2226–34.
7. Harbison J, Reynolds JV, Sheahan K, et al. Evidence for the polyp-cancer sequence in gallbladder cancer. Ir Med J 1997;90:98.
8. Goldin RD, Roa JC. Gallbladder cancer: a morphological and molecular update. Histopathology 2009;55:218–29.
9. Myers RP, Shaffer EA, Beck PL. Gallbladder polyps: epidemiology, natural history and management. Can J Gastroenterol 2002;16:187–94.
10. Persley KM. Gallbladder polyps. Curr Treat Options Gastroenterol 2005;8:105–8.

11. Terzi C, Sokmen S, Seckin S, et al. Polypoid lesions of the gallbladder: report of 100 cases with special reference to operative indications. Surgery 2000;127: 622–7.

12. Ito H, Hann LE, D'Angelica M, et al. Polypoid lesions of the gallbladder: diagnosis and followup. J Am Coll Surg 2009;208:570–5.

13. Jones DB, Soper NJ, Brewer JD, et al. Chronic acalculous cholecystitis: laparoscopic treatment. Surg Laparosc Endosc 1996;6:114–22.

14. Cappell MS, Marks M, Kirschenbaum H. Massive hemobilia and acalculous cholecystitis due to benign gallbladder polyp. Dig Dis Sci 1993;38:1156–61.

15. Wada K, Tanaka M, Yamaguchi K. Carcinoma and polyps of the gallbladder associated with Peutz-Jeghers syndrome. Dig Dis Sci 1987;32:943–6.

16. Komorowski RA, Tresp MG, Wilson SD. Pancreaticobiliary involvement in familial polyposis coli/Gardner's syndrome. Dis Colon Rectum 1986;29:55–8.

17. Lin WR, Lin DY, Tai DI, et al. Prevalence of and risk factors for gallbladder polyps detected by ultrasonography among healthy Chinese: analysis of 34 669 cases. J Gastroenterol Hepatol 2008;23:965–9.

18. Yang HL, Sun YG, Wang Z. Polypoid lesions of the gallbladder: diagnosis and indications for surgery. Br J Surg 1992;79:227–9.

19. Akyurek N, Salman B, Irkorucu O, et al. Ultrasonography in the diagnosis of true gallbladder polyps: the contradiction in the literature. HPB (Oxford) 2005;7:155–8.

20. Chattopadhyay D, Lochan R, Balupuri S, et al. Outcome of gall bladder polypoidal lesions detected by transabdominal ultrasound scanning: a nine year experience. World J Gastroenterol 2005;11:2171–3.

21. Mishra G, Conway JD. Endoscopic ultrasound in the evaluation of radiologic abnormalities of the liver and biliary tree. Curr Gastroenterol Rep 2009;11:150–4.

22. Sugiyama M, Atomi Y, Yamato T. Endoscopic ultrasonography for differential diagnosis of polypoid gall bladder lesions: analysis in surgical and follow up series. Gut 2000;46:250–4.

23. Choi WB, Lee SK, Kim MH, et al. A new strategy to predict the neoplastic polyps of the gallbladder based on a scoring system using EUS. Gastrointest Endosc 2000;52:372–9.

24. Cheon YK, Cho WY, Lee TH, et al. Endoscopic ultrasonography does not differentiate neoplastic from non-neoplastic small gallbladder polyps. World J Gastroenterol 2009;15:2361–6.

25. Cho JH, Park JY, Kim YJ, et al. Hypoechoic foci on EUS are simple and strong predictive factors for neoplastic gallbladder polyps. Gastrointest Endosc 2009; 69:1244–50.

26. Akatsu T, Aiura K, Shimazu M, et al. Can endoscopic ultrasonography differentiate nonneoplastic from neoplastic gallbladder polyps? Dig Dis Sci 2006;51: 416–21.

27. Koh T, Taniguchi H, Kunishima S, et al. Possibility of differential diagnosis of small polypoid lesions in the gallbladder using FDG-PET. Clin Positron Imaging 2000;3: 213–8.

28. Jang JY, Kim SW, Lee SE, et al. Differential diagnostic and staging accuracies of high resolution ultrasonography, endoscopic ultrasonography, and multidetector computed tomography for gallbladder polypoid lesions and gallbladder cancer. Ann Surg 2009;250:943–9.

29. Koga A, Watanabe K, Fukuyama T, et al. Diagnosis and operative indications for polypoid lesions of the gallbladder. Arch Surg 1988;123:26–9.

30. Shinkai H, Kimura W, Muto T. Surgical indications for small polypoid lesions of the gallbladder. Am J Surg 1998;175:114–7.

31. Kwon W, Jang JY, Lee SE, et al. Clinicopathologic features of polypoid lesions of the gallbladder and risk factors of gallbladder cancer. J Korean Med Sci 2009;24: 481–7.
32. Leung UC, Wong PY, Roberts RH, et al. Gall bladder polyps in sclerosing cholangitis: does the 1-cm rule apply? ANZ J Surg 2007;77:355–7.
33. Shin SR, Lee JK, Lee KH, et al. Can the growth rate of a gallbladder polyp predict a neoplastic polyp? J Clin Gastroenterol 2009;43(9):865–8.
34. Colecchia A, Larocca A, Scaioli E, et al. Natural history of small gallbladder polyps is benign: evidence from a clinical and pathogenetic study. Am J Gastroenterol 2009;104:624–9.
35. Park JY, Hong SP, Kim YJ, et al. Long-term follow up of gallbladder polyps. J Gastroenterol Hepatol 2009;24:219–22.
36. Zielinski MD, Atwell TD, Davis PW, et al. Comparison of surgically resected polypoid lesions of the gallbladder to their pre-operative ultrasound characteristics. J Gastrointest Surg 2009;13:19–25.
37. Kubota K, Bandai Y, Noie T, et al. How should polypoid lesions of the gallbladder be treated in the era of laparoscopic cholecystectomy? Surgery 1995;117:481–7.
38. Lee KF, Wong J, Li JC, et al. Polypoid lesions of the gallbladder. Am J Surg 2004; 188:186–90.

# Functional Gallbladder Disorder: Gallbladder Dyskinesia

Stephanie L. Hansel, MD, MS[a], John K. DiBaise, MD[b],*

**KEYWORDS**

- Functional biliary pain • Gallbladder • Cholecystectomy
- Cholescintigraphy

The occurrence of abdominal pain thought is to resemble gallbladder pain but in the absence of gallstones confronts the clinician with regularity and results in significant health care costs.[1] The estimated prevalence of this disorder is about 8% in men and 21% in women according to population-based studies involving persons with biliary-like pain and normal gallbladder ultrasounds.[2–4] The pathogenesis of this condition, referred to by various names including gallbladder dyskinesia, chronic acalculous gallbladder dysfunction, acalculous biliary disease, chronic acalculous cholecystitis, and biliary dyskinesia, is poorly understood. The term functional gallbladder disorder is currently the accepted Rome consensus nomenclature for this condition and will be used throughout this article. The aim of this article is to clarify the identification and management of patients with suspected functional gallbladder disorder.

## CLINICAL PRESENTATION

A critical question that has plagued clinicians for many years is what exactly constitutes biliary-like abdominal pain? Biliary-like abdominal pain originally was described as a pain in the right upper quadrant that was colicky in nature and associated with fatty food intake and various nonspecific gastrointestinal (GI) symptoms.[5] In contrast, the definition recently endorsed by the Rome committee on functional biliary and pancreatic disorders describes biliary-like pain as episodic, severe, steady pain located in the epigastrium or right upper quadrant that lasts at least 30 minutes and is severe enough to interrupt daily activities or require consultation with a physician (**Box 1**).[6,7] The pain may be accompanied by nausea and vomiting, radiate to the back or infrascapular region, or awaken the patient from sleep. In general, an irregular

[a] Division of Gastroenterology and Hepatology, Mayo Clinic, 200 First Street Southwest, Rochester, MN 55905, USA
[b] Division of Gastroenterology and Hepatology, Mayo Clinic, 13400 East Shea Boulevard, Scottsdale, AZ 85259, USA
* Corresponding author.
*E-mail address:* dibaise.john@mayo.edu

Gastroenterol Clin N Am 39 (2010) 369–379
doi:10.1016/j.gtc.2010.02.002
0889-8553/10/$ – see front matter © 2010 Elsevier Inc. All rights reserved.

gastro.theclinics.com

---

**Box 1**
**Rome III criteria for the diagnosis of functional gallbladder disorder**

Episodes of pain in the right upper quadrant or epigastrium and all of the following:

Gallbladder is present

Normal liver enzymes, conjugated bilirubin, amylase and lipase

Pain lasts 30 minutes or longer

Recurrent episodes occur at different intervals (not daily)

Pain builds up to a steady level

Pain is severe enough to interrupt the patient's current activities or lead to a visit to a clinician/emergency room

Pain is not relieved by bowel movements, postural change, or antacids

Other structural diseases that may explain the symptoms have been excluded

---

periodicity between episodes is characteristic, and the relationship to eating is unreliable. Importantly, pain lasting more than 6 hours is unlikely to be related to the gallbladder when gallstones are not present, and serologic liver and pancreas tests are normal unless due to a complication of gallstone disease (eg, acute cholecystitis, pancreatitis). Despite this clarification of the clinical criteria, there continues to be confusion and significant overlap with other functional GI disorders requiring further validation of these criteria.

## PATHOGENESIS

Presumably, the pain associated with functional gallbladder disorder may occur due to increased gallbladder pressure caused by either structural or functional outflow obstruction. Similar to other functional GI disorders, the pathophysiology of functional gallbladder disorder remains poorly understood and may, in fact, represent a constellation of mechanisms. Multiple theories of pathogenesis have been proposed including cholesterolosis, microlithiasis, biliary sludge, chronic cholecystitis, gallbladder dysmotility, narrowed cystic duct, cystic duct spasm, sphincter of Oddi dysfunction, and visceral hypersensitivity.[2,8–10] Two studies, one by Velanovich[11] and one by Brugge,[12] reported a significant association between crystal formation in the bile or in the walls of the gallbladder in patients with functional biliary pain who had undergone cholecystectomy, suggesting that bile saturation or gallbladder dysmotility may lead to crystal growth and eventually gallstones or chronic inflammation. Presumably, pain may occur at any point during the process. Abnormal gallbladder histology, however, has not been a universal finding in patients who experience symptom relief following cholecystectomy for presumed functional biliary pain, with studies reporting changes of chronic cholecystitis ranging from 44% to 100%.[13–15] Furthermore, it remains unclear whether the histologic changes in the gallbladder are a cause or an effect of poor gallbladder contractility.

Impaired gallbladder emptying resulting from hypokinesia of the gallbladder or dyskinesia due to partial obstruction distal to the gallbladder, either structural or functional, also might be responsible for functional gallbladder disorder.[16] Interestingly, given the not uncommon occurrence of abnormalities in gastric emptying and colon transit in these patients, it has been suggested that functional gallbladder disorder may reflect a panenteric motility disorder.[17] The role of dysfunction at the level of the sphincter of Oddi in patients with presumed functional gallbladder disorder remains unclear.[18–20] To clarify this relationship, Ruffolo and colleagues[19] conducted a prospective study of patients with biliary-type pain and normal-appearing gallbladder. Patients were tested extensively with quantitative cholescintigraphy, sphincter of Oddi manometry, and endoscopic retrograde cholangiopancreatography (ERCP). Approximately 50% of patients were found to have a normal gallbladder ejection fraction (GBEF), and within this group, 57% were found to have sphincter of Oddi dysfunction. Of the patients with low GBEF, 50% also were found to have sphincter of Oddi dysfunction. These findings are supported by results from another study that also failed to find a correlation between sphincter of Oddi pressure and GBEF.[21] Thus, it appears abnormalities in GBEF and sphincter of Oddi pressure occur independent of one another.

## NATURAL HISTORY

The natural history of functional gallbladder disorder is poorly understood. Information can be gleaned from a recent study by Krishnamurthy and colleagues[22] They found that a low GBEF based on cholecystokinin-cholescintigraphy (CCK-CS) remains low on repeat testing months to years later. The severity of GBEF reduction increased with time. In those with a normal GBEF, about 30% became abnormally low after a mean duration of about 53 months between studies. How these changes correlate with symptoms over time remains poorly defined.

Additional information on the natural history of this disorder can be learned from an assessment of the outcome of the nonsurgical arms of studies conducted on patients with suspected functional gallbladder disorder. Yap and colleagues[23] randomized 21 patients with abnormal GBEF to cholecystectomy versus no surgery and followed the patients for up to 54 months. Of the 10 patients in the no surgery group, all continued to report symptoms of functional gallbladder disorder. A more recent study reported similar findings, with 50% of patients with abnormal GBEF reporting resolution in symptoms up to 4 years after cholecystectomy, compared with only 16% of those with abnormal GBEF who elected not to pursue cholecystectomy ($P$ = .039).[24] In contrast, a retrospective study by Ozden and DiBaise[25] found that 50% of patients with an abnormal GBEF who did not undergo cholecystectomy reported clinical remission of symptoms after up to 3 years of follow-up, similar to the 64% of patients with a normal GBEF who reported resolution of their symptoms. Another retrospective study gathered information from 58 patients treated at two community hospitals, 42 of whom had an abnormal GBEF.[26] Of those 42 patients, 12 of 15 who did not undergo cholecystectomy reported lessening or resolution of symptoms. Finally, a study by Gonclaves and colleagues[27] reported 75% of patients with suspected functional gallbladder disorder who did not have cholecystectomy had persistent symptoms, and only 25% had resolution of symptoms without any treatment. Clearly, these results need to be interpreted with caution given the retrospective nature of most of these studies, the variable length of follow-up and criteria of symptom outcome, and the small number of patients evaluated.

## DIAGNOSTIC TESTS

In the setting of biliary-like abdominal pain and a normal gallbladder on transcutaneous ultrasound, the diagnosis of functional gallbladder disorder requires a careful evaluation to exclude other causes of the symptoms, and, at a minimum, serologic testing of liver and pancreatic enzymes and upper endoscopy.[6] Several tests have been developed in an attempt to more objectively implicate the gallbladder as the source of the symptoms. The technique of analyzing aspirated bile from the biliary system or duodenum to assess for microlithiasis has not been widely accepted due to technical issues with the procedure and poor specificity.[28,29] The use of CCK-provocation of abdominal pain when deciding whether to proceed with cholecystectomy is discouraged. Smythe and colleagues[30] evaluated 58 patients with functional biliary pain who underwent CCK provocation test and gallbladder volumetry before cholecystectomy and did not find a significant difference in symptom outcome following cholecystectomy between CCK provocation positive and negative patients. Furthermore, CCK administration, particularly when infused over a few minutes, is known to stimulate not only the gallbladder but also the duodenum and colon. Because small stones (<5 mm) may be missed with traditional transabdominal ultrasonography, three studies[31–33] have prospectively evaluated patients with biliary-type pain and a normal transabdominal ultrasound using endoscopic ultrasound of the gallbladder, finding a significant number of patients with cholecystolithiasis. In one of these studies, 76% of the patients offered cholecystectomy were pain-free at their 1-year follow-up.[33] Despite these encouraging reports, this technique is not yet widely available, and further studies are necessary to determine its clinical utility, cost-effectiveness, and overall place in the evaluation of these patients.

Functional assessment of gallbladder emptying before and after gallbladder stimulation using either a fatty meal or CCK is currently the most common test used to evaluate patients with suspected functional gallbladder disorder. Oral cholecystography, both with and without CCK stimulation,[34] has demonstrated variable results regarding symptom outcome and is considered insufficiently reliable as a measure of gallbladder function. Presently, CCK-CS with measurement of the GBEF is the most commonly used test to aid in the diagnosis of functional gallbladder disorder.[35,36] Although controversial, the use of CCK-CS has been supported by the Rome committee, which has recommended that, in the presence of biliary-like pain, an absence of gallstones on abdominal ultrasound, and normal liver and pancreatic enzymes, CCK-CS should be the next diagnostic step (**Fig. 1**).[7]

## CAVEATS RELATING TO THE USE OF CHOLECYSTOKININ–CHOLESCINTIGRAPHY

CCK-CS involves the intravenous administration of $^{99m}$technetium-labeled hepatoiminodiacetic acid, which is taken up by the liver and excreted into the biliary system, where it accumulates in the gallbladder. A GBEF then can be measured reliably after stimulating gallbladder emptying, most commonly with CCK. A low GBEF has been suggested to be indicative of gallbladder dysfunction and supportive of a diagnosis of functional gallbladder disorder; however, its use is not without controversy.[37] This is reflected in clinical practice by the not uncommon scenario of patients with suspected functional biliary pain and a reduced GBEF reporting no or incomplete relief of symptoms or recurrence of symptoms following cholecystectomy.

It is important to recognize that the finding of a low GBEF is not specific for functional gallbladder disorder and may occur in asymptomatic, healthy individuals, in patients with various medical conditions including diabetes, celiac disease, or irritable bowel syndrome,[37] and as a result of a number of medications such as opioid analgesics, calcium channel blockers, oral contraceptive agents, histamine-2 receptor antagonists, and benzodiazepines.[38] It also must be recognized that the gallbladder may not be responsible for a decreased GBEF as, occasionally, outflow obstruction from abnormalities of the cystic duct or sphincter of Oddi may be responsible.[39] Therefore, this test should be considered only when there is a high index of suspicion

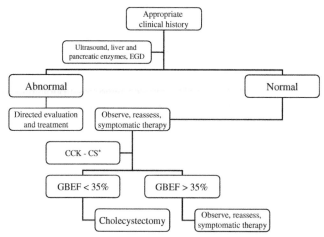

**Fig. 1.** Suggested algorithm for the diagnosis and treatment of suspected functional biliary pain in patients with a gallbladder. *using slow CCK infusion for at least 30 minutes. CCK-CS, cholecystokinin cholescintigraphy; GBEF, gallbladder ejection fraction. (*Reproduced from* DiBaise JK. Evaluation and management of functional biliary pain in patients with an intact gallbladder. Expert Rev Gastroenterol Hepatol 2009;3(3):305–13; with permission.)

of a gallbladder origin of the symptoms and other diagnoses have been eliminated. Furthermore, when considering whether to perform CCK-CS, it is preferable for it to be performed as an outpatient procedure on a patient who is not having pain at the time given the potential of confounding effects of acute illness in the hospitalized patient who may be receiving multiple medications.[37]

The clinician should be familiar with how the test is performed and interpreted at his or her institution. At present, there is no consensus on the dose, rate, and duration of CCK infusion used in CCK-CS. Many CCK-CS studies are conducted using a rapid infusion of CCK over 2 to 3 minutes, a methodology that has been shown to yield highly variable results.[37] In contrast, the slow infusion of CCK over 30 to 60 minutes results in an overall increase in mean GBEF compared with its rapid infusion and less inter- and intrasubject variability.[40–42] Regarding CCK-CS interpretation, there remains no consensus on the definition of an abnormal GBEF, although most clinicians consider a value of less than 35% as abnormal.[20,38] A multicenter trial is in progress that is attempting to determine the best methodology and establish normal values in a large healthy population.[43]

## TREATMENT

The Rome committee also has proposed criteria to confirm successful treatment in long-term follow-up studies.[6] The criteria are threefold and include an abnormal GBEF less than 40% after prolonged CCK infusion; an absence of gallbladder sludge, stones, or microlithiasis; and an absence of recurrent pain for at least 12 months.

Currently, the evidence for medical therapy in functional gallbladder disorder is lacking. Evaluation of psychological conditions and treatment for visceral hyperalgesia have been proposed but not well studied[20] as has the case for prokinetic agents, bile acid composition modifiers, and anti-inflammatory agents. Even though evidence-based recommendations cannot be made, the use of neuromodulators, similar to their use in other functional GI disorders, seems reasonable to consider in those with suspected functional gallbladder disorder.[44]

## EVIDENCE SUPPORTING CHOLECYSTECTOMY FOR PATIENTS WITH FUNCTIONAL GALLBLADDER DISORDER

Many retrospective, generally low-quality, studies have been published that support the performance of cholecystectomy in patients with suspected functional gallbladder disorder, particularly in patients with a GBEF less than 35%.[20] To date, Yap and colleagues[23] have published the only randomized controlled study of cholecystectomy in functional gallbladder disorder. They studied 21 patients with suspected functional biliary pain and a GBEF less than 40% based on a 45-minute infusion of CCK. Eleven patients were randomized to cholecystectomy and 10 to no surgery. Over a 3-year period, 10 patients became asymptomatic after cholecystectomy, and one reported improved symptoms after surgery. In contrast, most patients in the no surgery group reported their symptoms to be unchanged; two of these requested cholecystectomy. Based on these findings, the authors concluded that CCK-CS is useful in identifying a group of patients with acalculous gallbladder disease and biliary-like pain who respond to cholecystectomy. Although encouraging, these results are limited by the small size of the study, lack of concealed allocation to treatment group, and a lack of a sham-control group.

More recently, Paajanen and colleagues[24] completed a prospective, uncontrolled study of patients with presumed functional gallbladder disorder who were categorized into one of three groups based on the results of their CCK-CS. The first group consisted of 32 patients with a GBEF less than 35% who underwent laparoscopic cholecystectomy. The second group included 52 patients with a GBEF less than 35% but who did not undergo surgery. The third group consisted of 38 patients with a normal GBEF. All patients were followed for a mean follow-up of 4 years (range, 1 to 7 years). They found that over 90% of patients in the laparoscopic cholecystectomy group reported their pain had resolved or was substantially improved. In contrast, in the low GBEF and no surgery group, only 16% of patients reported their pain had resolved, and 50% reported no change in symptoms. In the group with a normal GBEF and no surgery, 33% reported their pain had resolved, and 26% reported no change in symptoms. The authors concluded that laparoscopic cholecystectomy is an effective treatment in patients with high clinical suspicion of functional gallbladder disorder and GBEF less than 35%.

Carr and colleagues[45] reported similar findings. They identified 93 patients with suspected functional gallbladder disorder and GBEF less than 35%. Patients were separated into two groups based on symptoms, classical or atypical, and followed for up to 1 year. Sixty of the 61 patients in the classic group underwent cholecystectomy; 58 reported their symptoms resolved. In the atypical group, 23 patients eventually underwent cholecystectomy; 13 reported resolution of their symptoms. The authors concluded that classic biliary symptoms were more predictive of success after cholecystectomy than the GBEF. They also suggested that patients with atypical symptoms such as bloating and upper abdominal fullness should be observed rather than offered surgery.

## EVIDENCE AGAINST CHOLECYSTECTOMY FOR PATIENTS WITH FUNCTIONAL GALLBLADDER DISORDER

Despite excellent symptom improvement after cholecystectomy for gallstone disease, the clinical improvement in patients with presumed functional biliary pain is not as good. Fenster and colleagues[46] prospectively evaluated the effects of cholecystectomy on the presenting symptoms in 225 patients undergoing laparoscopic cholecystectomy. Fifteen percent of the patients were believed to have functional gallbladder disorder, while 48% described atypical pain, and 82% experienced bothersome nonpain symptoms. A key finding was a cure rate for what was described as classic biliary pain of 82% in those with gallstones compared with 52% in those without gallstones. As expected, nonpain symptoms were infrequently completely relieved, in only 46% with gallstones and 38% without gallstones ($P>.05$), emphasizing that these symptoms should not necessarily be attributed to functional gallbladder disease, particularly in the absence of biliary-like abdominal pain. This study demonstrates that while cholecystectomy may relieve classical pain in most patients with cholelithiasis, pain relief in presumed functional gallbladder disorder, even when described as classic biliary pain by the physician, is generally poor.

A recent review on the management of acalculous biliary-type abdominal pain pointed out that the response range for cholecystectomy in patients with biliary-type pain and abnormal GBEF is quite variable between studies, ranging from 38% to greater than 90%.[20] In addition to this wide variation in results, they pointed out that many of the studies are not methodically sound and cautioned of the possibility of publication bias. Therefore, any conclusions drawn from these studies must be interpreted cautiously.

A Cochrane review[47] of the evidence for cholecystectomy in suspected functional gallbladder disorder analyzed randomized clinical trials comparing cholecystectomy versus no cholecystectomy in patients with gallbladder dyskinesia. Only one study was found that met this criteria, but it too was deemed to be at high risk for bias.[23] It was concluded there is a lack of sufficient data to assess the role of cholecystectomy in gallbladder dyskinesia, and randomized clinical trials are necessary.

## DOES GBEF PREDICT OUTCOME IN FUNCTIONAL GALLBLADDER DISORDER?

A systematic review and meta-analysis by Delgado-Aros and colleagues[48] of studies dating back to 1966 found only nine articles eligible for inclusion in their study to determine whether patients with suspected functional biliary pain with decreased GBEF have better symptomatic outcome after cholecystectomy than those with normal GBEF. They found that 94% of patients with reduced GBEF had a positive outcome compared with 85% among those with normal GBEF. The odds ratio for positive outcome was 1.37 (95% confidence interval [CI] 0.56 to 3.34; $P = .56$). Thus, based on their pooled analysis, they found no difference in outcomes after cholecystectomy between patients with abnormal GBEF and normal GBEF. In addition, they demonstrated evidence of publication bias, commented on the poor quality of the studies included, and recommended further study be conducted to definitively answer this question.

Similarly, a systematic review assessed the utility of CCK-CS with calculation of the GBEF in predicting symptomatic outcome following cholecystectomy in patients with suspected functional gallbladder disorder and came to the same conclusion.[49] Even though 19 of 23 studies reviewed reported the calculation of GBEF was useful, these authors pointed out there were significant methodological limitations with all of the studies making this conclusion. Therefore, the question as to whether GBEF is useful in predicting symptom outcome remains to be answered.

---

**Box 2**
**Areas requiring further study in functional gallbladder disorder**

Clinical utility of the diagnostic criteria as defined by the Rome committee

Pathogenesis and natural history

Role of endoscopic ultrasound in the diagnosis

Optimization of CCK-CS technique and interpretation

Clinical utility of CCK-CS with calculation of the GBEF

Role of medical therapy

Large, multicenter, randomized, controlled study comparing cholecystectomy to no surgery

---

## SUMMARY

It is readily apparent that there is a lack of high-quality data to aid in good decision making regarding the role of CCK-CS in the diagnosis and cholecystectomy in the treatment of functional gallbladder disorder. Nevertheless, this does not necessarily negate their utility when used in the patient with a high clinical suspicion of functional gallbladder disorder—suspicion that may be enhanced by using the Rome diagnostic criteria. Several areas have been identified that require further study to have a better understanding of the optimal diagnosis and management of functional gallbladder disorder (**Box 2**). For now, it is recommended that patients with suspected functional gallbladder disorder be carefully evaluated to exclude other causes for their symptoms. As proposed by the Rome committee,[6] initial work-up should include transabdominal ultrasound, liver and pancreatic laboratory studies, and an upper endoscopy (grade B). If these studies are normal, the patient should be observed, provided symptomatic therapy, and reassessed in a few months time. If symptoms warrant further work-up, then CCK-CS with slow infusion over at least 30 minutes is recommended by the Rome group (grade B). If the GBEF is less than 35%, cholecystectomy should be considered; however, if the GBEF is greater than 35%, continued observation and follow-up are advised (grade B). Despite concerns raised about the clinical utility of CCK-CS, with proper patient selection and use of optimal testing technique, on the basis of currently available evidence, this seems to be a reasonable approach. On the other hand, given its limitations and the suggestion of similar results following cholecystectomy in those with reduced and normal GBEF, foregoing CCK-CS testing in a patient with a high index of clinical suspicion after adequate follow-up and exclusion of other disease entities and counseling the patient on postoperative expectations is not entirely unreasonable in the authors' opinion.

## REFERENCES

1. Ko SW, Lee SP. Gallbladder disease. Clin Perspect Gastroenterol 2000;3:87–96.
2. Rome group for epidemiology and prevention of cholelithiasis (GREPCO). Prevalence of gallstone disease in an Italian adult female population. Am J Epidemiol 1984;119(5):796–805.
3. Barbara L, Sama C, Labate AM, et al. A population study on the prevalence of gallstone disease: the Sirmione study. Hepatology 1987;7(5):913–7.
4. Rome group for the epidemiology and prevention of cholelithiasis (GREPCO). The epidemiology of gallstone disease in Rome, Italy. Part 1. Prevalence data in men. Hepatology 1988;8(4):904–6.

5. DenBesten L, Roslyn JJ. Gallstones and cholecystitis. In: Moody FG, Carey LC, Jones RS, et al, editors. Surgical therapy of digestive disease. Chicago: Year Book Medical Publishers; 1986. p. 277–95.

6. Behar J, Corazziari E, Guelrud M, et al. Functional gallbladder and sphincter of Oddi disorders. Gastroenterology 2006;130(5):1498–509.

7. Drossman DA, Dumitrascu DL. Rome III: new standard for functional gastrointestinal disorders. J Gastrointest Liver Dis 2006;15(3):307–12.

8. Schwesinger WH, Diehl AK. Changing indications for laparoscopic cholecystectomy: stones without symptoms and symptoms without stones. Surg Clin North Am 1996;76(3):493–504.

9. Ponsky TA, DeSagun R, Brody F. Surgical therapy for biliary dyskinesia: a meta-analysis and review of the literature. J Laparoendosc Adv Surg Tech A 2005; 15(5):439–42.

10. Desautels SG, Slivka A, Huston WR, et al. Postcholecystectomy pain syndrome: pathophysiology of abdominal pain in sphincter of Oddi type III. Gastroenterology 1999;116(4):900–5.

11. Velanovich V. Biliary dyskinesia and biliary crystals: a prospective study. Am Surg 1997;63(1):69–74.

12. Brugge WR, Brand DL, Atkins HL, et al. Gallbladder dyskinesia in chronic acalculous cholecystitis. Dig Dis Sci 1986;31(5):461–7.

13. Shaffer E. Acalculous biliary pain: new concepts for an old entity. Dig Liver Dis 2003;35(Suppl 3):S20–5.

14. Barron LG, Rubio PA. Importance of accurate preoperative diagnosis and role of advanced laparoscopic cholecystectomy in relieving chronic acalculous cholecystitis. J Laparoendosc Surg 1995;5(6):357–61.

15. Patel NA, Lamb JJ, Hogle NJ, et al. Therapeutic efficacy of laparoscopic cholecystectomy in the treatment of biliary dyskinesia. Am J Surg 2004; 187(2):209–12.

16. Amaral J, Xiao ZL, Chen Q, et al. Gallbladder muscle dysfunction in patients with chronic acalculous disease. Gastroenterology 2001;120(2):506–11.

17. Penning C, Gielkens HA, Delemarre JB, et al. Gallbladder emptying in severe idiopathic constipation. Gut 1999;45(2):264–8.

18. Soto DJ, Arregui ME. Kinevac stimulated ultrasound correlated with biliary manometry and clinical outcome in patients with chronic acalculous cholecystitis [abstract]. Gastroenterology 2001;120:471.

19. Ruffolo TA, Sherman S, Lehman GA, et al. Gallbladder ejection fraction and its relationship to sphincter of Oddi dysfunction. Dig Dis Sci 1994;39(2):289–92.

20. Rastogi A, Slivka A, Moser AJ, et al. Controversies concerning pathophysiology and management of acalculous biliary-type abdominal pain. Dig Dis Sci 2005; 50(8):1391–401.

21. Kalloo AN, Sostre S, Meyerrose GE, et al. Gallbladder ejection fraction. Nondiagnostic for sphincter of Oddi dysfunction in patients with intact gallbladders. Clin Nucl Med 1994;19(8):713–9.

22. Krishnamurthy GT, Krishnamurthy S, Brown PH. Constancy and variability of gallbladder ejection fraction: impact on diagnosis and therapy. J Nucl Med 2004;45(11):1872–7.

23. Yap L, Wycherly AG, Morphett AD, et al. Acalculous biliary pain: cholecystectomy alleviates symptoms in patients with abnormal cholescintigraphy. Gastroenterology 1991;101(3):786–93.

24. Paajanen H, Miilunpohja S, Joukainen S, et al. Role of quantitative cholescintigraphy for planning laparoscopic cholecystectomy in patients with gallbladder

dyskinesia and chronic abdominal pain. Surg Laparosc Endosc Percutan Tech 2009;19(1):16–9.

25. Ozden N, DiBaise JK. Gallbladder ejection fraction and symptom outcome in patients with acalculous biliary-like pain. Dig Dis Sci 2003;48(5):890–7.

26. Mishkind MT, Pruitt RF, Bambini DA, et al. Effectiveness of cholecystokinin-stimulated cholescintigraphy in the diagnosis and treatment of acalculous gallbladder disease. Am Surg 1997;63(9):769–74.

27. Gonclaves RM, Harris JA, Rivera DE. Biliary dyskinesia: natural history and surgical results. Am Surg 1998;64(6):493–7.

28. Moskovitz M, Min TC, Bavaler JS. The microscopic examination of bile in patients with biliary pain and negative imaging tests. Am J Gastroenterol 1986;81(5):329–33.

29. Susann PW, Sheppard F, Baloga AJ. Detection of occult gallbladder disease by duodenal drainage collected endoscopically. A clinical and pathologic correlation. Am Surg 1985;51(3):162–5.

30. Smythe A, Majeed AW, Fitzhenry M, et al. A requiem for the cholecystokinin provocation test? Gut 1998;43(4):571–4.

31. Dahan P, Andant C, Lévy P, et al. Prospective evaluation of endoscopic ultrasonography and microscopic examination of duodenal bile in the diagnosis of cholecystolithiasis in 45 patients with normal conventional ultrasonography. Gut 1996;38(2):277–81.

32. Dill JE, Hill S, Callis J, et al. Combined endoscopic ultrasound and stimulated biliary drainage in cholecystitis and microlithiasis-diagnosis and outcomes. Endoscopy 1995;27(6):424–7.

33. Thorboll J, Vilmann P, Hassan H. Endoscopic ultrasonography in detection of cholelithiasis in patients with biliary pain and negative transabdominal ultrasonograpy. Scand J Gastroenterol 2004;39(3):267–9.

34. Griffen WO, Bivins BA, Rogers EL, et al. Cholecystokinin cholecystography in the diagnosis of gallbladder disease. Ann Surg 1980;191(5):636–40.

35. Weissmann HS, Frank MS, Rosenblatt R, et al. Role of 99mTc-IDA cholescintigraphy in evaluating biliary tract disorders. Gastrointest Radiol 1980;5(3):215–23.

36. Krishnamurthy GT, Bobba VR, Kingston E. Radionuclide ejection fraction: a technique for quantitative analysis of motor function of the human gallbladder. Gastroenterology 1981;80(3):482–90.

37. Ziessman HA. Cholecystokinin cholescintigraphy: victim of its own success? J Nucl Med 1999;40(12):2038–42.

38. Ziessman HA. Cholecystokinin cholescintigraphy: clinical indications and proper methodology. Radiol Clin North Am 2001;39(5):997–1006.

39. Wald A. Functional biliary-type pain: update and controversies. J Clin Gastroenterol 2005;39(5 Suppl 3):S217–22.

40. Ziessman HA. Functional hepatobiliary disease: chronic acalculous gallbladder and chronic acalculous biliary disease. Semin Nucl Med 2006;36(2):119–32.

41. Sarva RP, Shreiner DP, Van Thiel D, et al. Gallbladder function: methods for measuring filling and emptying. J Nucl Med 1985;26(2):140–4.

42. Hopman WP, Jansen JB, Rosenbusch G, et al. Gallbladder contraction induced by cholecystokinin: bolus injection or infusion? Br Med J (Clin Res Ed) 1986;292(6517):375–6.

43. Dose response of intravenous sincalide (CCK-8) for gallbladder emptying. Clinical trials Web site Available at: http://clinicaltrials.gov/ct2/show/NCT00685477?term=sincalide&rank=1. Accessed November 23, 2009.

44. Grover M, Drossman DA. Psychopharmacologic and behavioral treatments for functional gastrointestinal disorders. Gastrointest Endosc Clin N Am 2009; 19(1):151–70.
45. Carr JA, Walls J, Bryon LJ, et al. The treatment of gallbladder dyskinesia based upon symptoms: results of a 2-year, prospective, nonrandomized, concurrent cohort study. Surg Laparosc Endosc Percutan Tech 2009;19(3):222–6.
46. Fenster LF, Lonborg R, Thirlby RC, et al. What symptoms does cholecystectomy cure? Insights from an outcome measurement project and review of literature. Am J Surg 1995;169(5):533–8.
47. Gurusamy KS, Junnarkar S, Farouk M, et al. Cholecystectomy for suspected gallbladder dyskinesia. Cochrane Database Syst Rev 2009;(1):CD007086.
48. Delgado-Aros S, Cremonini R, Bredenoord AJ, et al. Systematic review and meta-analysis: does gallbladder ejection fraction on cholecystokinin cholescintigraphy predict outcome after cholecystectomy in suspected functional biliary pain? Aliment Pharmacol Ther 2003;18(2):167–74.
49. DiBaise JK, Oleynikov D. Does gallbladder ejection fraction predict outcome after cholecystectomy for suspected chronic acalculous gallbladder dysfunction? A systematic review. Am J Gastroenterol 2003;98(12):2605–22.

# Index

*Note:* Page numbers of article titles are in **boldface** type.

Gastroenterol Clin N Am 39 (2010) 381–391
doi:10.1016/S0889-8553(10)00036-1
0889-8553/10/$ – see front matter © 2010 Elsevier Inc. All rights reserved.

**gastro.theclinics.com**

# *Moving?*

## *Make sure your subscription moves with you!*

To notify us of your new address, find your **Clinics Account Number** (located on your mailing label above your name), and contact customer service at:

**E-mail: elspcs@elsevier.com**

**800-654-2452 (subscribers in the U.S. & Canada)**
**314-453-7041 (subscribers outside of the U.S. & Canada)**

**Fax number: 314-523-5170**

**Elsevier Periodicals Customer Service**
11830 Westline Industrial Drive
St. Louis, MO 63146

*To ensure uninterrupted delivery of your subscription, please notify us at least 4 weeks in advance of move.

ELSEVIER

Printed and bound by CPI Group (UK) Ltd, Croydon, CR0 4YY

03/10/2024

01040457-0007